*In the Shadow of Diagnosis*

∴

# In the Shadow
# of Diagnosis

∵

PSYCHIATRIC POWER AND QUEER LIFE

Regina Kunzel

THE UNIVERSITY OF CHICAGO PRESS

CHICAGO AND LONDON

The University of Chicago Press, Chicago 60637
The University of Chicago Press, Ltd., London
© 2024 by The University of Chicago
Published 2024

33  32  31  30  29  28  27  26  25  24      2  3  4  5

ISBN-13: 978-0-226-83019-3 (cloth)
ISBN-13: 978-0-226-83185-5 (paper)
ISBN-13: 978-0-226-83184-8 (e-book)
DOI: https://doi.org/10.7208/chicago/9780226831848.001.0001

Library of Congress Cataloging-in-Publication Data

Names: Kunzel, Regina G., 1959– author.
Title: In the shadow of diagnosis : psychiatric power and queer life /
    Regina Kunzel.
Description: Chicago : The University of Chicago Press, 2024. |
    Includes bibliographical references and index.
Identifiers: LCCN 2023028646 | ISBN 9780226830193 (cloth) |
    ISBN 9780226831855 (paperback) | ISBN 9780226831848 (e-book)
Subjects: LCSH: Homosexuality—Diagnosis—United States—History—
    20th century. | Homosexuality—Diagnosis—United States—Case studies. |
    Psychiatry—United States—History—20th century. | Psychoanalysis
    and homosexuality—United States—History—20th century. | Mental
    illness—Classification.
Classification: LCC RC558.K86 2024 | DDC 616.890086/64—dc23/
    eng/20230710
LC record available at https://lccn.loc.gov/2023028646

# Contents

*Introduction 1*

CHAPTER ONE
The Violent Optimism of American Psychiatry · 18

CHAPTER TWO
Fixing Queerness · 38

CHAPTER THREE
Psychiatric Power and Queer Life · 70

CHAPTER FOUR
Psychiatric Encounters · 94

CHAPTER FIVE
The Queer Politics of Health · 117

EPILOGUE
The Queer Afterlives of Psychiatric Power · 150

*Acknowledgments 161*
*List of Archives 165*
*Notes 169*
*Index 225*

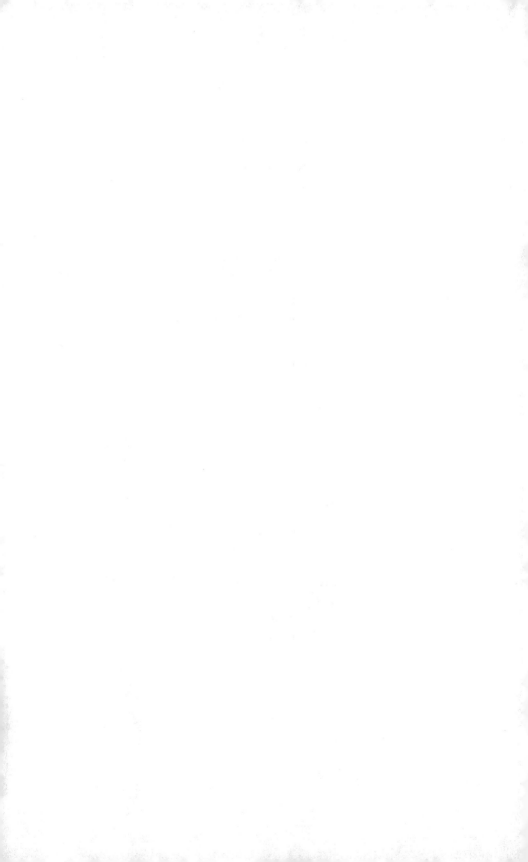

A few years ago, I came across something in a box of my belongings at my parents' house that I had forgotten about: a letter that I had written to them in 1978. I was nineteen years old, and I had recently come out to them. They were distraught, and among the evidence that I marshaled in my defense was the decision of the American Psychiatric Association (APA) just five years earlier, in 1973, to declassify homosexuality as a mental disorder. I don't remember how that information had come to me, but I remember hanging on to it like a life raft. My parents, as I recall, were not impressed, nor were they dissuaded from their belief in the value of a medical approach to what they took to be a dire psychological condition (and they were far from alone in that belief in 1978, the APA's decision notwithstanding). They consulted first with my pediatrician, who recommended that they meet with a psychiatrist. When that psychiatrist assured them that I could be treated with psychotherapy, they insisted that I see a therapist affiliated with my university.

Eventually my parents came around, as did countless other parents of that time, and we found our way. Meanwhile, over the next decade or so, in addition to learning how to be queer, I was also learning how to be a historian. After writing my first book, I began to think about a potential project in the then-developing field of gay history. Returning to my own encounter with psychiatry years earlier, one that left its mark even though it was only brief and glancing, I began to plot out a project on the history of psychiatric thinking about homosexuality. I still have my notes from that early work, based mostly on my reading of the writing of the mid-twentieth-century American psychoanalysts Edmund Bergler, Irving Bieber, and Charles Socarides, all of whom promoted an understanding of homosexuality as pathological.[1] They were leaders in the move on the part of psychiatrists, beginning in 1940 and continuing into the 1970s, to promote an understanding of homosexuality as a mental disorder, one they claimed to be able to diagnose, treat, and "cure." A novel proposition, that claim countered and competed with older understandings of homosexuality as organic in its etiology and older ones still that marked it as an acquired vice, willful crime, moral failing, or sin. Casting aside what they viewed as the needless reticence and therapeutic pessimism of psychiatrists and psychoanalysts before them (and of Sigmund Freud in particular), a new generation of psychiatrists boasted of their successes in sexual conversion.

It is hard to overstate psychiatry's dominance over the understanding and regulation of homosexuality in those decades. More than an aggregate of practitioners, clinics, and institutions, psychiatry represented a new epistemology and a new operation of power. Psychiatrists promoted a sense of psychic interiority and selfhood, introduced a new understanding of normality and deviance, and established new modes of regulation.[2] Early lesbian activist Barbara Gittings found it "difficult to explain to anyone who didn't live through that time how much homosexuality was under the thumb of psychiatry."[3] Historian Jonathan Ned Katz denounced psychiatric treatment as "one of the more lethal forms of homosexual oppression" and devoted a chapter of his foundational 1976 work, *Gay American History*, to documenting psychiatrists' use of insulin and electroconvulsive shock, lobotomy, aversive conditioning, and psychotherapy in their efforts to "cure" homosexuality.[4] As one of the most powerful regimes of judgment and authority in the twentieth-century United States, psychiatric diagnosis also sanctioned and underwrote larger structures of discrimination and criminalization and cast a stigmatizing pall over gay men, lesbians, and gender-nonconforming people for decades.

Along with the primary psychiatric texts on the topic, I began reading in the historical literature. I discovered that Ronald Bayer had written a book on the challenge that gay activists posed to the APA and to the reigning psychiatric conception of homosexuality as a mental disorder.[5] I read psychologist Kenneth Lewes's insider analysis and forceful takedown of post-Freudian psychoanalytic ideas about homosexuality.[6] Martin Duberman had written candidly and movingly about his own painful encounters with psychoanalysts in the 1950s and 1960s in his memoir *Cures*.[7] I couldn't imagine what I might be able to add to the story, and I couldn't find a way into the questions that most interested me from the available sources, mostly the published works of psychiatrists: How and why did American psychiatrists at mid-century believe they could "cure" homosexuality and normalize gender identification? Why were homosexuality and gender variance so important to them? How did psychiatrists' ideas about etiology and cure translate into practice? Most elusive but most intriguing to me, How were those ideas and judgments received by their intended audiences and what was their effect? What did it mean, in short, that queer people were understood as sick people in need of treatment at the moment when queerness was becoming consolidated as an identity and assuming its modern form?

As I was pondering this history of psychiatry and medicalization, historians of queer life were turning their attention elsewhere. In his pioneering history of the early gay rights movement, John D'Emilio observed that "the medical model is one area that has received relatively extensive treatment in the history of homosexuality."[8] As early as 1983, then, before there was anything like a field of the history of sexuality or LGBT history, D'Emilio suggested that the story of sickness and medicalization had already been told too many times. Seeming to follow the cue of gay liberationists' early 1970s protest slogan, "off the couches and into the streets," urging gay men and lesbians to reject psychiatrists' characterization of them as sick and instead to enter the political fray, historians turned from early explorations of the medicalization of homosexuality to histories of sociality, citizenship, community, culture, politics, and the state.[9] Some positioned that turn as a social history corrective to Michel Foucault's emphasis on the role of doctors and sexologists in the construction of the new category of homosexuality in the nineteenth century. In his pathbreaking book, *Gay New York*, for example, George Chauncey directed readers away from "the official maps of the culture" drawn by doctors and other authorities and drew attention instead to "the maps etched in the city streets by daily habit, the paths that guided men's practices" and created the vibrant gay male geography of early twentieth-century New York City.[10] Martin Duberman identified a historiographical turn in the late 1980s away from "a history of repression and more toward an analysis of how gay people have viewed *themselves* through time."[11] More recently, historians have moved to consider different regulatory structures that exerted power over queer life. In her important exploration of the evolution of the federal regulation of homosexuality and how the "straight state" made the homosexual an "anti-citizen," Margot Canaday reminds us that homosexuality was "a legal category as much as a medical or psychiatric one."[12] Historians of trans life and experience, too, encourage a turn away from histories of medicalization, documenting trans histories that both precede and exceed the clinic. As Jules Gill-Peterson and others have shown, the medical archive of transsexuality overrepresents white, class-privileged trans life, restricting our view of a broad and diverse array of gender imaginaries, meanings, and identifications.[13]

After a few months of reading in that dispiriting psychiatric literature, I abandoned my fledgling project and moved on. Fast-forward a couple of decades to 2008, my first year on the faculty at the University of Minnesota. One day I got a call from Jean-Nickolaus Tretter, the founder of the

Jean-Nickolaus Tretter Collection in Gay, Lesbian, Bisexual, and Transgender Studies, housed in the University of Minnesota's Archives and Special Collections. Jean was an avid and intrepid collector, and he wanted to show me a sample from a collection he was trying to acquire for the library. He arrived at my office, pulled a thick bunch of papers out of his satchel, and told me it was a file of someone who had been institutionalized at Saint Elizabeths Hospital, the federal institution for the mentally ill in Washington, DC, for being gay. It was one of over one hundred such files, he said, discovered by a contractor hired by the General Services Administration who had been assigned the task of salvaging historically significant material from the ruins of Saint Elizabeths prior to its makeover into the Department of Homeland Security.

Interested as I had long been in queer histories and histories of carceral spaces, my curiosity about these records was piqued, to say the least. When I was invited to work with the collection, I had just finished work on my book *Criminal Intimacy*, about the shifting fascinations and anxieties circulating around same-sex sexuality in prisons and the queer cultures that took shape behind bars, and I recognized Saint Elizabeths as part of what Foucault called the "carceral archipelago"—the sprawling set of institutions beyond the formal prison that distribute carceral practices and thinking so widely.[14] The collection also revived my interest in psychiatry's investment in "treating" homosexuality and gender nonconformity. Given the sensitivity of the documents and anticipating the library's concerns about acquiring them, Jean asked me to help him make the case for their historical significance. It took some work, first on Jean's and my part and then on the part of archivists, librarians, and university lawyers, but we were ultimately successful, and nineteen boxes of materials, many of them disintegrating with age and mold and filed in no easily discernible order, were delivered from Washington, DC, to the Tretter Collection in Minneapolis.[15]

As I began to work with the collection, I was able to identify it as consisting of case files of people in treatment with Dr. Benjamin Karpman, a psychoanalytically oriented psychiatrist at Saint Elizabeths. A Russian-born Jew, Karpman had immigrated to the United States at the turn of the twentieth century, attending college at the University of North Dakota and then, by remarkable coincidence, training in psychology and medicine at the University of Minnesota. He was hired at Saint Elizabeths in 1922 by William Alanson White, the hospital's director, who was among the first American psychiatrists to embrace psychoanalysis and to imagine that it might be practiced in state institutions as well as private hospitals and clinics. Like many of his most ambitious and intellectually curious contemporaries, Karpman took up the psychoanalytic project with gusto. He spent the next thirty-five years treating patients at Saint Elizabeths and in his private clinical practice until his retirement in 1957.

While the people represented in the collection are mostly (though, importantly, not all) white and male, they reflect some of the diversity of the Saint Elizabeths patient population in those years. Founded in 1855 as the Government Hospital for the Insane and the only federal facility for the mentally ill, Saint Elizabeths served an array of people under federal jurisdiction: active-duty members and veterans of the U.S. armed services, Native Americans residing on reservations, people incarcerated in federal penitentiaries, and residents of Washington, DC, especially those too poor to afford private care.[16] At its peak in the late 1940s and early 1950s, the hospital was nearly a city unto itself, housing over eight thousand patients. People came to Saint Elizabeths from a range of class backgrounds; many struggled to make ends meet in jobs as common laborers or domestic workers.[17] Among Karpman's patients were teachers and itinerant laborers, homemakers and servicemen, civil service workers and waiters. Some of the people whose files are included in the collection were in out-patient psychoanalysis with Karpman and others were in court-ordered treatment. Some were institutionalized by family members, while others were committed by the court, some under the Washington, DC, sexual psychopath law, passed in 1948, which authorized the indefinite institutionalization of those diagnosed as sexual psychopaths. Some were transferred to Saint Elizabeths from federal prisons. All had either sought or were compelled to undertake psychiatric treatment for gender or sexual difference of some kind—homosexuality, fear of homosexuality, nonnormative gender expression and identification, or sex with minors. Read alongside psychiatric texts, oral histories, memoirs, and activist accounts, these case files and the people represented in them illuminate the impact of psychiatric thinking and treatment on queer and gender-nonconforming people and the experience of psychiatric scrutiny from the position of those whose same-sex sexual desires and cross-gender identifications marked them as mentally ill.

Historians have often looked to case files—medical, legal, social welfare, and disciplinary—for evidence of the histories of marginalized people. At the same time, historians recognize that the materials that typically comprise a case file—medical evaluations, clinical observations, family histories, disciplinary records—inevitably reflect the investments and agendas of their authors rather than their subjects.[18] The case history assumed a central place in psychiatric thinking and practice, functioning as a clinical record of the personal and medical histories of patients, a tool for diagnosing their disorders, and a methodological anchor securing new forms of disciplinary authority.[19] The voices of the subjects of case files, then, come to us in muted, mediated, and distorted form, shaped by what Lauren Berlant identifies as "the idiom of judgment" that characterized the genre and marked by the disciplinary machinery and dynamics of power that brought them to the attention of the case-building authority.[20] As Foucault famously observed about the "infamous" subjects illuminated by prison records,

> What snatched them from the darkness in which they could, perhaps should, have remained was the encounter with power; without that collision, it's very unlikely that any word would be there to recall their fleeting trajectory. The power that watched these lives, that pursued them . . . and marked them with its claw was what gave rise to the few words about them that remain for us.[21]

This is true of the cases in Karpman's files: the jazz musician who worried that he was "queer" and was hospitalized by his wife. The college student who heard voices telling him he was a "sexual pervert" and was committed by his parents. The high school teacher forced into treatment by the court after having sex with his students. The aspiring Black politician institutionalized after being arrested for having sex in a public restroom. The married woman who descended into alcoholism after falling in love with her best friend. The navy sailor who felt "entombed" in a male body. The conditions of their entry into the historical record and the traces they left there are bound up with expressions of power: the power of the law; the power exercised by parents, spouses, and family; the power of community norms and exclusions; the power of a binary gender regime.

Because the sources that comprise the archive of queer history are often authored by people who judge, police, diagnose, condemn, and punish nonnormative sexuality and gender, historians have learned to read against their grain, scrutinizing sources for dominant meanings; attending to their gaps, silences, and contradictions; and reading for the possibility of insurgent meanings and voices. Jennifer Terry calls this analytic method a form of "vengeful countersurveillance" that queer historians might use to locate how marginalized subjects "have spoken back against the terms of a pathologizing discourse which has relied upon us parasitically to establish its own authority."[22]

Reading against the grain is a method to which the Saint Elizabeths files make themselves abundantly available. In part, that is thanks to a generative idiosyncrasy of this particular archive. Psychoanalysis, known as the "talking cure," is structured around a private encounter between analyst and analysand that typically leaves no historical trace. But early in his career, Karpman developed the unusual and perhaps unique practice of requiring his patients to write.[23] He asked them to write autobiographies, to record and analyze their dreams, to respond to detailed questionnaires, to keep diaries. He boasted that his method involved "little to no couch work"; one man under Karpman's care described it less charitably as "therapy by correspondence."[24] And so the files include not only Karpman's memoranda and reports, but also his patients' life narratives, journals, free associative writing, and reviews and critiques of psychiatric texts. Some wrote autobiographies that ran hundreds of pages long. Some, with Karpman's encouragement, recorded details of every sexual encounter they could recall, an assignment that produced astonishing documents of queer sexual life. And so, admittedly, one can often simply *read*, rather than read against the grain: the people represented in this collection authored their own narratives of self, although they did so, importantly, under some degree of coercion, sometimes within the narrative conventions of psychoanalysis, and always in circumstances marked by radically unequal relations of power.[25]

The Karpman collection became the inspiration and springboard for this book and for its broader consideration of the meaning and consequences of the encounter of queer and gender-nonconforming people with psychiatric power and authority. In widening the analytic lens (and its source base), *In the Shadow of Diagnosis* explores the complex and multiple ways in which people experienced psychiatric scrutiny, diagnosis, and treatment. It examines their intimate engagements with psychiatry and the ways in which they assimilated, accommodated, challenged, rejected, and rearticulated the judgment that they were sick. It moves from there to consider how that encounter continued to reverberate in queer psychic and political life after the declassification of homosexuality from the register of psychiatric conditions collected in the APA's *Diagnostic and Statistical Manual of Mental Disorders (DSM)* in 1973. The book explores the imbrication of psychiatric and state power within which modern queer and trans identities were forged and the politics that queer and gender-variant people crafted in response. The book, then, examines the accrual of a form of power that was implicated in nearly every discriminatory structure arrayed against queer and gender-nonconforming people. It also considers the complex and subject-making effects of that power, examining how it was variously received, negotiated, internalized, and subverted—what Cameron Awkward-Rich describes, in his astute examination of the field of trans studies, as "the political, epistemic, and psychic effects of being subject to diagnosis."[26]

The history of psychiatry's impact on queer and gender-nonconforming people has been told as a relatively straightforward allegory, one with villains, heroes, a linear time line, and a gratifying and triumphant narrative arc. It begins with an account of psychiatrists' abusive and oppressive treatment of gay men and lesbians. That oppression is met by the resistance of gay and lesbian activists, who ultimately prevail in their assault on psychiatric authority and are rewarded with the declassification of homosexuality as a mental disorder. Retracing the outlines of that story, I aim to shift its register—from an oppression-to-liberation or pathology-to-politics telos to one more attentive to complexity, more open to surprise and contradiction, and more alert to unexpected consequences.

I do so by foregrounding the dynamic of *encounter*—in some cases the literal encounter of queer and gender-variant people with psychiatrists and psychiatric treatment and in others an encounter with psychiatric ideas and authority that was an inevitable part of living in a culture saturated with psychiatric power. Physicians use *encounter* to describe the point at which transactions between the patient and the medical professional take place and the basis for decisions about diagnosis and treatment. In considering the encounter with psychiatry, I draw from observations made by historians who use the concept of encounter to examine the meanings and consequences of other kinds of meetings in different historical contexts that are also structured by radical asymmetry. Sometimes attended by violence and conquest, such meetings can also be sites in which new forms of knowledge and subjectivity are forged and new strategies of resistance conceived. Theorizing the encounter in the context of colonial relations between the United States and Latin America, historian Gilbert Joseph writes that such interactions "are usually fraught with inequality and conflict, if not coercion, but *also* with interactive, improvisational possibilities."[27] The encounter "is not a meeting between already constituted subjects who know each other," theorist Sara Ahmed writes; rather, it plays an active part in constituting and reconstituting its participants.[28] Those observations prompt questions about the encounter of queer and gender-variant people with psychiatry that take us beyond a simple story of oppression and resistance. What did those encounters mean to people and how did they navigate them? What understandings and forms of knowledge were produced in encounters shaped by dramatically unequal relations of power that often took place under coercion? What transformative effects might such encounters have had on psychiatrists? How did queer and gender-nonconforming people come to understand themselves through and against those encounters, what imprint did they leave, and what kind of politics did people forge in response?

∵

My exploration of these questions is abetted by my access to a collection of rich and remarkable sources. It is made possible, too, with the help of new analytic lenses and insights from scholars in disability studies, critical health studies, and queer and trans studies—fields that emerged after the first generation of scholarship in gay history and that have the potential to help us rethink histories of medicalization and the encounter with psychiatry.

Queer history and disability history may seem oddly paired; when they are brought into conversation, it is often by way of analogy. Lesbian and gay history often appears in disability histories and analyses as a model and object lesson in the successful transformation of a medicalized and pathologized status to a political one. In *Claiming Disability*, for example, Simi Linton calls for critiques of medical models of disability "similar to those that have been done on the self-loathing homosexual figures in [the 1968 Off-Broadway play and 1970 film] *Boys in the Band*."[29] Anthropologist Emily Martin likewise stages an analogy between the political reconceptualization of homosexuality—from a medicalized condition to an unfairly stigmatized minority status—and the destigmatizing reconceptualization that she proposes for mania and depression.[30] In her survey of disability history, historian Kim Nielson writes that "like gay and lesbian activists, people with disabilities insisted that their bodies did not render them defective. Indeed, their bodies could even be sources of political, sexual, and artistic strength."[31]

It is easy to understand the appeal of these analogies. At the same time, it is useful to recall the vexed politics of analogical reasoning and the perils as well as the promises of analogizing histories and experiences of social difference in particular. Scholars critical of analogical arguments have focused most closely and critically on "like race" claims that compare the struggles of various groups to those of African Americans.[32] In their staging of likeness across forms of difference, such analogies can work to elide important distinctions and experiential specificity. Analogies can also effectively erase the existence of subjects who occupy both the positions being compared. Analogies can elide incongruences; they can also, paradoxically, *create* them: something posited as *like* something else, by definition, is not that thing. And so analogies can function to deny the rich intersections across axes of difference and marginalization and obscure the ways in which forms of difference work together, constituting and compounding each other.[33]

Exploring the encounter between queer and gender-variant people and psychiatry invites a consideration of the intersections and coconstitutions between sexual and gender difference and disability. The psychiatric discourse on homosexuality at mid-century drew heavily on the idioms and tropes of disability: the homosexual as emotional cripple, homosexuality as a form of mental illness, the promise and prospect of "cure." Rather than simply rhetorical or metaphorical, that language attests to the material, discursive, and ideological histories that link disability and queerness. For many in the mid-twentieth century, homosexuality was not *like* disability. For some, it was indistinguishable from an experience of disability as well, literally disabling as it was to one's emotional, relational, economic, and social life.

Disability studies scholars Robert McRuer and Anna Mollow describe queer studies as being "on the cusp" of engaging with disability while maintaining an "uneasy distance."[34] What might we learn if we considered queer history as part of disability history rather than akin to it (and vice versa)? In this book, I join an ongoing conversation among scholars interested in the generative possibilities of bringing queer, trans, and disability into conversation. Disability studies' long-standing interest in normativity and stigma invites us to reflect on the power exercised by a pathologizing diagnosis as well as its impact. Assessing the significance of psychiatric thinking and practice for modern queer life requires us to attend to what literary critic and queer theorist Heather Love calls the "history of injury" that lies at the underexamined heart of queer history.[35] Reckoning with that history requires that we see queer and trans subjects not simply as heroic actors in defiance of the culture's norms, but, to borrow from Kadji Amin, as complex persons "too often assigned the psychically flat role of righting the ills of an unjust social order and denied the right to be damaged, psychically complex, or merely otherwise occupied."[36] As this book shows, there was no universal response on the part of queer people to psychiatrists' insistence that they suffered from a mental disorder. George Chauncey challenges the assumption that gay men internalized the shaming attitudes of the broader postwar U.S. culture, arguing that "the truly remarkable thing about 1950s queers was their refusal to play the role assigned them by the hostility of their own time."[37] But while some gay men and lesbians resisted the mid-twentieth-century orthodoxy that they were sick, it should not surprise us that many others located the source of their oppression within themselves rather than the social and political order.

Disability studies scholars also offer critiques of medical discourses of "cure" that expose and name the violence that is often done in its name. "At the center of cure lies eradication," writes Eli Clare, "and the many kinds of violence that accompany it."[38] Mid-century American psychiatrists often described their curative goals with queer patients in progressive terms, as a compassionate response to their misery and a more modern and humane stance than that undertaken by religious or legal authorities. Disability studies critiques help bring into view the goal of eradication—the effort to eliminate the existence of queerness and gender nonconformity—that lay at the heart of the curative projects of mid-century American psychiatry.

Beyond stigma and violence, disability studies scholars encourage us to see disability as a form of difference that allows for an altered perspective, a site from which new knowledge might be produced, a source of insight and even revelation, and a "tool of diagnosis" that can identify disabling policies, practices, architectures, and values and cultivate new modes of resistance to regimes of normativity.[39] Psychiatry was not simply an obstacle to flourishing for queer and gender nonnormative people—or not uniformly, or only, or uncomplicatedly so. It also presented new institutional locations, new vocabularies, and new critical lenses for people to make sense of themselves and the world around them, even when they took up those new forms of knowledge to resist psychiatric ideas and treatment.

The story of the removal of homosexuality from the *DSM* in 1973 has been understandably celebrated as a civil rights victory for gay people. The history of that decision and the political strategies that led to it, though, also look different when viewed through the lenses provided by disability studies. "We Are the Experts on Homosexuality," a petition to the American Psychiatric Association that appeared in a lesbian newspaper in 1971, echoed the disability activist principle of "nothing about us without us" in its insistence on wresting authority and self-definition from medical experts.[40] The removal of homosexuality from the *DSM* was "one of the founding moments of contemporary gay liberation," McRuer observes, but also "a distancing from disability."[41] Increasingly, in the appraisal of activists, arguments for gay and lesbian civil rights seemed to hang on making persuasive claims about the health and happiness of gay men and lesbians. That mandate required activists to disassociate what they presented as the healthy gay majority from histories of shame and stigma and a minority rightly identified as "sick." Among the critical insights of disability studies scholars, however, is the understanding that health is not simply a self-evident and universal good. Health also functions as a normalizing ideology that mobilizes a set of prescriptions and hierarchies of worth.[42] Critical lenses developed by disability studies scholars and others allow us to see the norms and values that attach to health; they also illuminate the distancing moves and exclusions that so often accompanied gay claims to health and prompt us to ask at whose expense such claims were made.

Gay activists worked to disaggregate those they posed as the healthy majority from the sick; they also worked to sever ties between gayness and gender nonnormativity. In doing so, they challenged psychiatrists who understood same-sex desire and cross-gender identification to be constitutionally linked. The new diagnosis of "Gender Identity Disorder" was included in the third revised version of the *DSM* in 1980, the first edition of the manual to omit homosexuality from its pages. Exploring the encounter with psychiatry tells us more about how queerness and transness were historically bound together; it also tells us how they came to be disentangled and distinguished from one another, and with what consequences.

∵

The assertion of psychiatric authority over queer and gender-variant people and the encounters that followed were consequential, I propose, in ways that historians have yet to consider. The chapters that follow explore the complexity of those encounters and advance a set of claims about their significance.

The first of those claims is that psychiatrists' assertion to expertise regarding gender and sexual difference was essential to the expansion of psychiatric power and authority during the decades that historians have characterized as psychiatry's "golden age."[43] In the decades before the mid-twentieth century, most psychiatrists held custodial jobs in asylums and state institutions overseeing chronically mentally ill and elderly dementia patients and battled public skepticism about their professional status as medical doctors. By the 1940s, 1950s, and 1960s, psychiatrists had innovated careers that were fully integrated into American medicine and American public life. Crucial to their enhanced power and prestige in this period was their claim to an enlarged purview—from the treatment of serious mental disorders to addressing the problems of everyday life.[44] Psychiatrists' substantial authority in the wartime and postwar United States derived, in large part, from their successful bid to expertise regarding what psychiatrist Harry Stack Sullivan called "problems in living." "In consequence," historian Elizabeth Lunbeck writes, "psychiatrists now had access to a stratum of society, composed of the sane but not entirely normal, that had eluded their predecessors' institutional net."[45]

Criminality, juvenile delinquency, women's discontent, men's emasculation, troubled marriages—psychiatrists built their authority at mid-century by staking a claim to expertise regarding these issues of "maladjustment" and more. Key among the "problems in living" that psychiatrists claimed to be able to treat and ease were those presented by same-sex desire and gender nonconformity. What distinguished homosexuality from the myriad other issues that psychiatrists claimed to be able to treat was that sexual and gender nonconformity were of heightened state interest and concern in this period, competing with communism (and often linked with it) as a threat to national security.[46] Psychiatrists used their claim to expertise regarding homosexuality to broker some of their most important and strategic collaborations with various arms of the state.[47] At the beginning of the Second World War, psychiatrists allied with the federal government to establish guidelines for the psychological screening of military inductees to weed out those deemed "unfit" for service, homosexuals among them. Psychiatrists also made themselves useful to the state, enhancing their own influence and expanding their power in the process, first by helping legitimize a national wave of sexual psychopath laws that vastly expanded the criminalization of nonnormative sex and especially consensual sex between men, and then by agreeing to treat people who were carcerally committed as sexual psychopaths.[48] On a much wider scale, psychiatrists became intimately involved in the criminal legal system, called on to serve as experts of sexual and gender difference, staffing psychiatric clinics attached to the courts, and building clinical practices by accepting patients ordered by judges to undertake psychiatric treatment.[49] American psychiatrists would come to form a symbiotic relationship with the U.S. state at mid-century, a relationship premised on their role as arbiters of gender and sexual normativity. That means that a story that is typically told within the confines of the history of medicine or the history of the oppression of gay men and lesbians is also a story about American state and carceral power. In this history, therapeutic and carceral spaces, practices, and logics blend and blur.[50]

And so, I propose, psychiatric power, at its apex in the mid-twentieth century, *depended* on psychiatrists' claims to expertise regarding homosexuality and gender variance. Psychiatrists' new confidence in their ability to convert the sexual orientation of people from homosexual to heterosexual and normalize gender identification was central to their project of enlarging their professional jurisdiction. As Benjamin Karpman contended, "There is at present no problem in psychiatry more important than that of homosexuality" because "its roots and branches ramify themselves beyond psychiatry proper and into virtually every field of human behavior" and "press upon us from every side for some solution."[51] Psychiatry's power in this period extended far beyond the hospital and the clinic and into the courtroom and the broader culture.

If it is impossible to conceive of the triumph of psychiatric power at mid-century without considering its claim to expertise regarding homosexuality and gender variance, likewise it is impossible to conceive of modern queer life sealed off from the influence of psychiatric thinking or stripped entirely clean of its assumptions.[52] The encounter with psychiatric thinking and treatment was a formative condition of queer life in the mid-twentieth-century United States, I propose, with consequences for queer experience and subjectivity. Historians have argued that earlier medical conceptualizations of sexual difference had only a limited impact on ordinary people's understanding of themselves, in large part because the circulation of medical texts, especially those having to do with sex and sexuality, was so tightly restricted. But while it would have been possible for ordinary people to remain ignorant of sexological and medical theories of homosexuality in the late nineteenth and early twentieth centuries, it would have been hard to avoid the psychiatric and psychoanalytic conceptualizations that circulated so widely in the popular culture just a few decades later. That is not to say that queerness did not exist beyond the frame of psychiatric influence and authority at mid-century or that psychiatry's capture of queerness was anywhere near complete. Nor is it to agree with some readings of Foucault that the birthplace of modern homosexuality was the clinic. But for queer people at mid-century, psychiatry had to be reckoned with, if only, for some, to disavow it.

The encounter with psychiatric thinking and practice also mattered to a wider and more diverse group of people than we have been led to expect. Given the dominance of psychoanalysis in American psychiatry in this period and its reputation as an elite and expensive practice with European origins and an arcane lexis, we might assume that psychiatric scrutiny and treatment were limited to upper-class white men in coastal cities. But psychoanalysis was practiced in many state institutions as well as private hospitals and clinics and, especially because of psychiatry's involvement in the criminal legal system, psychiatrists' reach extended far beyond the clinic and the narrow demographic we usually associate with it. Institutionalization and psychotherapy were often imposed by the court, and low-income people and people of color were then, as now, caught up disproportionately in the carceral net. In fact, I find that the most violent and invasive forms of psychiatric "treatment" in this period (and those that loom largest in popular accounts of this history and in lesbian and gay collective memory)—electroconvulsive shock, lobotomy, and aversive behavior modification—were often performed with punitive or behavior-managing aims rather than putatively curative intentions and in carceral rather than clinical contexts. That means that they may well have been suffered disproportionately by queer and gender-nonconforming people of color.

Psychiatric approaches to homosexuality also had an impact far beyond their diagnostic targets, affecting people who did not understand themselves as gay or lesbian or as gender nonconforming. The pathologizing diagnoses that were granted such authority in this period created hierarchies of health and privilege; they also disciplined straight/cis people's sexuality and expressions of masculinity and femininity and fostered anxieties around border crossing or blurring.

Finally, the encounter with psychiatry mattered to the shape that gay politics would take. Beginning in the 1950s and accelerating in the 1960s and early 1970s, gay activists struggled to unburden homosexuality of its association with mental illness. Given the consequences attached to being labeled mentally disordered, it was perhaps inevitable that gay activists would insist on the normalcy of homosexuality and embrace a politics of health. Activists would come to believe that this project required distancing homosexuality from mentally ill, gender-nonconforming, and other minoritized subjects, setting in motion a politics of disassociation and exclusion.

∴

I conclude here with a few words on concepts, terminology, and ethical considerations raised by this work. My use of *psychiatry* as an umbrella term to refer to a range of orientations and modalities may rankle some historians of medicine and psychiatry, who might rightly counter that there is no singular practice of psychiatry but instead a heterogeneous set of practitioners with different and often competing conceptions of mental disorder, and with diverse understandings of homosexuality and gender variance more specifically. Psychoanalysts often distinguished themselves from their more medically oriented colleagues. Benjamin Karpman, for instance, disparaged the psychiatrist, who made "rounds to cover five or six hundred patients, prescribe a pill or a powder here, restraint there, and that is all there is to it," in contrast to the psychoanalyst, who "does not deal with quantity but quality."[53] As learning theory and behavior modification gained popularity in the 1960s, psychologists began to challenge psychiatrists' understandings of the etiology of mental disorders and their methods of treatment. While I discuss some of those lines of division when they are important to this story, I am less interested in the details of the debates among clinician-theorists of the so-called psy-sciences than I am in encounters with psy-authority more generally. While psychiatrists, psychoanalysts, and psychologists debated the origins of sexual and gender difference and argued over how to treat them most effectively, those distinctions would have been less meaningful to people on the receiving end of psychiatric power.

Language changes over time, dramatically so when it comes to gender and sexual difference, making terminology an inevitably vexed decision in historical writing. Because language exerts a determinative power, reflecting but also shaping the way people think about themselves and are thought about by others, the choice of terms is a consequential decision as well. The terminology of modern sexuality took shape over the course of the decades covered in this book, and my general practice is to recognize and use the terms used by the people I write about. By the 1940s, some same-sex-desiring men were using *gay*, a term first taken up as coded insiders' argot used to distinguish its adopters from gender-variant fairies.[54] By the 1960s, politically minded gay men and lesbians embraced it as a bold and affirmative alternative to the medical term *homosexual*. I retain the use of *homosexual* in its historical context. *Queer* circulated vernacularly in the decades I write about in this book, whether lobbed as a slur, applied in casual and often contemptuous description, or taken up in bold self-identification.[55] I use it more expansively here, and admittedly sometimes anachronistically, beyond subjects who might identify or be identified as queer, to depict an array of desires and identifications that existed aslant to or in active defiance of sexual and gender norms and as a critical lens with which to investigate challenges to normative modes of gender and sexuality and the unsettling of modern sexual identity itself. As the historian Laura Doan observes, "What 'queer' teaches us is that no matter how many new words we invent, none will ever adequately capture the contradictions and confusions of individuals as sexual beings; simply put, according to [Eve Kosofsky] Sedgwick's first axiom, 'people are different from each other.'"[56] Taking Sedgwick's observation as a guiding principle, I do my best to attend to the range of identifications among my subjects and their widely varying engagements with psychiatry.

*Transgender* is of newer vintage, having been first used in 1965 by psychiatrist John Oliven to describe an "urge for gender 'sex' change" and then a few years later by cross-dressing advocate and activist Virginia Prince in her magazine *Transvestia* to distinguish cross-dressers from transsexuals.[57] *Transgender* was taken up more broadly beginning in the 1990s as an expansive umbrella term to collect a range of expressions of gender nonconformity. While *trans* is not a term that people in earlier decades would have used, I sometimes invoke it here to conjure that collectivity.[58] The risk, of course, is that my use of contemporary terms projects contemporary meanings onto the lived experiences of people a half-century ago and more, whose desires, identifications, and embodiments took shape in worlds differently structured than our own. *Transsexual* and *transvestite*, "the two primary signifiers of trans life for the majority of the twentieth century," appear more often in the records, both as diagnostic categories and as terms of self-identification.[59] Historians Emmet Harsin Drager and Lucas Platero characterize those terms and subject positions as forged "in conversation with medicine," a valuable formulation that captures my interest in the subject-making effects of the encounter with psychiatric thinking and psychiatric power.[60] The question of what pronouns to use for gender-nonconforming people presents another quandary. Psychiatrists typically, and pointedly, used the pronouns aligned with the sex assigned at birth to refer to their gender-variant patients, regardless of the person's own practice or preference and sometimes in active defiance of it, and often after that person's social or medical transition. Because that practice reveals much about psychiatrists' belief that cross-gender identification was a symptom of mental illness as well as about their relationship to their patients, I retain that usage when I quote from published sources, even as I note its disrespect and sometimes violent disregard. I use pronouns that people used for themselves in the cases in which that is clear. When I am not certain about what pronouns gender-nonconforming people used, I use the pronouns *they* and *them*.

The question of respect raises the more challenging question of ethics. Historians sometimes feel that our study of the past absolves us from having to wrestle with ethical questions in our work, especially when that work involves people who are no longer alive.[61] But because my exploration of these questions involved my examination of medical records and personal writing about the most intimate details of people's lives, the question of my ethical relationship to my subjects was unavoidable and often worrying. As a step toward respecting their privacy, I have masked patients' identities with the use of pseudonyms and have not included any other personally identifying information, such as an address, a birthplace, or a birthdate. Those practices satisfy lawyers, archival policies, and institutional review boards, but to tell this history, I must live with the discomfiting fact that I am training an analytical gaze on people whose personal lives were already overburdened by scrutiny.[62] As small compensation, and guided and enabled by these subjects' own remarkable writing, I have tried to write them into a history that they would recognize and perhaps appreciate in its effort to weigh the meaning and complexity of life in the shadow of diagnosis.

## CHAPTER ONE

# The Violent Optimism
# of American Psychiatry

"Homosexuality is widespread and involves all classes of society," psychiatrist George W. Henry observed in 1937. "An intelligent attitude toward this problem" required that it be "studied and understood." Psychiatrists, he concluded, "are best qualified to make this study."[1] Henry's own ambitious study of homosexuality, *Sex Variants: A Study of Homosexual Patterns*, would be published in two weighty volumes just a few years later, proving this claim to be both immodest and self-interested.[2] It was also relatively novel. Rather than a problem of vice or criminality to be rooted out by the police and adjudicated by the courts or a religious or moral issue to be judged by the church, homosexuality was a problem of mental health, Henry insisted, and thus the proper province of psychiatry and psychiatrists.

Henry was far from alone among psychiatrists in making this claim or unusual in his hubris. Beginning in the 1940s, and with increasing confidence in the decades that followed, psychiatrists declared their expertise regarding homosexuality and, even more boldly, an ability to "cure" it. They represented that stance as one of a new therapeutic "optimism," a keyword that marked their distance from their predecessors, whom they characterized as pessimistic or nihilistic, and that communicated their newfound confidence in an ability to convert homosexuals into heterosexuals. Appearing mantralike in nearly every work by psychiatrists on homosexuality in this period, "optimism" appealed to an enduring stereotype of American life and culture and was one of the hallmarks of American exceptionalism, observed as early as 1840 by the French political philosopher Alexis de Tocqueville, who noted in Americans "a lively faith in the perfectibility of man."[3] A century later, the optimistic therapeutic stance of mid-twentieth-century American psychiatrists aligned with a broader postwar American confidence, chiming with a national mood buoyed by the U.S. defeat of the Axis powers along with economic growth and prosperity (however unevenly distributed) and a new superpower status.

American optimism in the postwar period was tempered, though, by deep anxiety about national security, a security believed to be threatened by communism at home and abroad as well as by the perceived subversive influence of homosexuality and other forms of sexual and gender difference, which might "soften" American resolve and undermine Americans' ability to fight communism.[4] At a time when homosexuality was understood to constitute a threat linked ominously to communism and perhaps surpassing it in menace, psychiatrists' promise to promote healthy heterosexuality and eradicate homosexuality bought them considerable influence and authority. Psychiatrists who were confident in their ability to "cure" homosexuality framed their own expertise as responsive to the needs and concerns of the Cold War American state. Psychiatric hostility toward homosexuality and psychiatrists' participation in the "intimate governance" of American wartime and postwar statecraft underwrote the evolution of psychiatric power.[5]

The consolidation of psychiatric power in the 1940s, 1950s, and 1960s, then, depended in large part on psychiatry's claims to expertise regarding homosexuality. The rise of psychiatric power and psychiatric homophobia happened in tandem, coconstitutively, with each depending on the other. Psychiatrists' optimistic therapeutic stance masked the violent project that underlay it: the promise to eradicate homosexuality and gender nonconformity. Eve Kosofsky Sedgwick rightly detects in postwar American psychiatry "the wish that gay people *not exist,*" an enactment of "a culture's desire that gay people *not be.*"[6] By claiming the ability to grant that wish, psychiatrists were rewarded with enhanced power and prestige in what historians would characterize as psychiatry's "golden age."[7]

## Earlier Etiologies

By the time American psychiatrists turned their attention to homosexuality in the 1940s, it had been the object of scientific and medical study across the Atlantic for nearly a century. Beginning in the 1860s, European and British physicians, psychiatrists, forensic scientists, and neurologists debated the etiology of same-sex sexual desire and the nonnormative gender expression with which it was assumed to be causally related. Rather than seeking to treat or "cure" sexual and gender nonconformity, the group of scientists and physicians that would become known as sexologists endeavored to catalog and classify its various forms, producing elaborate compendia of sexual aberrations and identifying and naming new sexual and gender types: the homosexual, the sadist, the fetishist, the masochist, the exhibitionist, the transvestite, and the pedophile key among them.[8]

At the heart of sexologists' taxonomical project was the effort to discern the cause of sexual and gender difference. Most located the origin of same-sex sexual desire in the human constitution.[9] By *constitution*, sexologists referred to a broad collection of physical conditions and drives, collapsing what would later be distinguished as the somatic and the psychic. They were admittedly uncertain, though, about the specific locus of the anomaly that resulted in same-sex attraction. German lawyer and writer Karl Heinrich Ulrichs understood people who desired others of the same sex to constitute a "third sex," formed by what he described poetically as a "migration of the soul": a woman's soul in a man's body explained a man's desire for men and vice versa.[10] Others favored more organic explanations. The German physician Magnus Hirschfeld proposed a theory of congenital sexual "intermediacy," occurring naturally and akin to (and sometimes inclusive of) what is now understood as intersex embodiment.[11] Austrian psychiatrist Richard von Krafft-Ebing admitted that the "anatomical and functional foundation" of an "abnormal psycho-sexual constitution" was "absolutely unknown," but he was intrigued by the theory of one of his patients who alerted him to "the actual bi-sexuality shown by the foetus anatomically up a certain age." "It is conceivable," Krafft-Ebing wrote, "that, under the influence of a factor inimical to the normal development of the brain (hereditary taint, etc.), these rudimentary organs likewise exercise an influence" in inverting the sexual drive.[12] Embedded in all these ideas was the assumption of a fundamental human bisexuality, either physical, psychic, or some combination of the two, that explained what sexologists called "contrary sexual feeling," or inversion.[13]

The notion of universal human bisexuality was central to the theories of an Austrian neurologist in this period, Sigmund Freud. Historians debate the extent to which Freud's early ideas were aligned with or broke from the theories of sexologists working around the same time and with whom he was in conversation.[14] Freud distanced himself from the theories of hereditary degeneration that Krafft-Ebing and others had advanced to explain the inheritance of homosexuality. But he frequently referenced the work of sexologists including Ellis, Iwan Bloch, and Hirschfeld, and he credited Hirschfeld and others for the theory of constitutional bisexuality, a concept that Freud embraced and used to assert the existence of homoerotic desire in everyone. Freud held to the belief in a biological component or "bedrock," existing prior to the psychosexual forces that he believed shaped a person from infancy, which naturally predisposed some to homosexuality.[15] "In human beings," Freud wrote, "pure masculinity or femininity is not to be found in either a psychological or a biological sense. Every individual to the contrary displays a mixture of the character-traits belonging to his own and to the opposite sex; and he shows a combination of activity and passivity whether or not these last character traits tally with his biological ones."[16] Here Freud offered a way to conceive of the predisposition of some people toward homosexuality; he also detached masculinity and femininity from a necessary and inevitable alignment with biological sex.

At the same time, Freud came to posit a dynamic model of psychosexual development in which individuals progressed through a series of stages, homosexuality key among them, culminating ideally in mature heterosexuality. Breaking from earlier somatic theories, Freud stressed the importance of family dynamics and other environmental factors in psychic development. In retrospect, and especially when one's view is shaped by the legacy of mid-twentieth-century American psychoanalytic thinking, which would both draw from and disavow Freud, the pathologization of homosexuality can seem to be hardwired into the psychoanalytic paradigm of normative psychosexual development. But Freud vacillated on the subject over the course of his career, offering a number of explanations, sometimes contradictory, for same-sex attraction. Homosexuality to Freud was both a normal feature of human development and a sign of arrest or regression, a stop at a stage shy of mature heterosexuality. At various points and in different publications he characterized homosexual desire as narcissistic, fetishistic, arrested, regressive, paranoid, and sometimes associated with creative genius. As a clinician, Freud did not believe that homosexuality was a neurosis or perversion, that it was a unitary phenomenon or constitutive of a special category of person, or that it should, or could, be "treated." Indeed, he conjectured provocatively, it was as difficult to "convert a fully developed homosexual into a heterosexual" as it was "to do the reverse" (adding that "for good practical reasons the latter is never attempted").[17] "It is not for psycho-analysis to solve the problem of homosexuality," Freud concluded in his 1920 case study of an eighteen-year-old woman who had fallen in love with an older woman. Instead, Freud wrote, psychoanalysis must "remain content with disclosing the psychical mechanisms that resulted in determination of the object-choice, and with tracing the paths leading from them to the instinctive basis of the disposition. There its work ends," he concluded, "and it leaves the rest to biological investigation."[18] In his most famous and widely circulated statement on the subject, a letter he wrote in 1935 to an American woman concerned about her son's sexuality, Freud wrote that while homosexuality was "assuredly no advantage," neither was it something "to be ashamed of, no vice, no degradation, [and] it cannot be classified as an illness."[19] Freud understood *heterosexuality* as an object choice that required explanation as well, one that necessitated the sublimation or repression of a natural homosexuality.[20]

The word that Freud's American psychoanalytic successors used to describe the perspective of Freud and his contemporaries toward homosexuality was *pessimism*. There is little evidence, however, that Freud or others of this first generation of sexologists and psychoanalysts understood their own stance as pessimistic, a term that seems to have been more often deployed in retrospect by the generation of self-declared "optimists" that succeeded them. Havelock Ellis's pronouncement in 1896 that he had "little sympathy with those who are prepared to 'cure' the invert at any price," for instance, was less an expression of pessimism than of compassion and support. Ellis was particularly critical of German psychiatrist Albert von Schrenck-Notzing, who purported to cure homosexuals through hypnosis and visiting prostitutes, emboldened by "large doses of alcohol."[21] Ellis suspected that these methods "seldom succeed in eradicating the original inverted instinct."[22] Rather than attempt to cure homosexuals, Ellis proposed that psychiatrists might, by "psychic methods . . . refine and spiritualize the inverted impulse, so that the invert's natural perversion may not become a cause of acquired perversity in others." Reviewing cases of people whose inversion was "really organic and deep-rooted," Ellis supported an early version of homosexual respectability: "If we can enable an invert to be healthy, self-restrained, and self-respecting," he wrote, "we have often done better than to convert him into the mere feeble simulacrum of a normal man." As a model for this kind of transformation, Ellis referenced the "'manly love' celebrated by Walt Whitman" as a "wholesome and robust ideal."[23] "It is better that a man should be enabled to make the best of his own strong natural instincts, with all their disadvantages," Ellis proposed, "than that he should be unsexed and perverted, crushed into a position which he has no natural aptitude to occupy."[24]

Magnus Hirschfeld went even further in his recommendation to therapists to first "calm the patient" in distress about homosexuality. He then instructed them to tell the patient that they possessed "an inborn, undeserved condition which has become a misfortune not because of the nature of homosexuality but for the unjust judgment which it encounters," and further, "that the misfortune of being homosexual is often exaggerated" and that they are members of "a great group of human beings." Thus apprised of their place in a larger community, "homosexuals may look at their position altogether differently than as isolated eccentrics stamped with the mark of monstrosity."[25] It often helped, Hirschfeld added, to introduce patients to "other homosexuals of good character . . . , for to meet someone who has already reached the harbor of self-knowledge is of great value to the lonely homosexual."[26] Hirschfeld took it on himself to build queer community as part of his therapeutic practice, hosting salons and parties in his Institute of

Sexual Science in Berlin, and committed himself to what he called "adjust-ment therapy or a method of adaptation." Hirschfeld concluded in 1920 that a review of the research would show that "homosexuality cannot be cured by any of the known methods of science, neither by means of operative or medicinal methods, nor by psychotherapy."[27]

While the early psychiatric consensus leaned strongly against the possi-bility of "curing" homosexuality, some psychiatrists and the first generation of psychoanalysts in the late nineteenth and early twentieth centuries did attempt it. Krafft-Ebing experimented with hypnosis, but he admitted that his results were mixed and that "homo-sexual feelings" may "become per-manent, leading to enduring and exclusive contrary sexual instinct."[28] Aus-trian psychoanalyst Wilhelm Stekel, first an analysand of Freud's and later one of his earliest followers (and also one of the first to fall out of favor after challenging Freud's authority and deviating from psychoanalytic ortho-doxy), shared the belief of his mentor that "all persons are bisexual" and that "the disposition toward homosexuality exists in everyone."[29] But he broke from the notion that homosexuality was a "congenital condition," proclaim-ing it instead a "psychic disease . . . curable by psychic treatment."[30] Stekel believed that he could "reestablish the heterosexual instincts" through a form of short-term therapy that he called "active analysis." Most cases, Stekel reported, required a relatively short analytic course of two to three months' duration. Distancing himself from "Magnus Hirschfeld and his school," Stekel argued that Hirschfeld's sympathetic approach effectively *produced* homosexuals: sexologists like Hirschfeld "hatch homosexuals," Stekel wrote, "by removing from these people all sense of responsibility" and cultivating in them a sense that their "condition can neither be changed nor cured."[31]

For the most part, these early debates about the ontological status, etiol-ogy, and proper treatment of homosexuality took place among doctors and scientists in Germany, Austria, and Great Britain. Among the first Ameri-cans to contribute, Chicago physician James G. Kiernan presaged the more judgmental and punitive approaches that would take shape in the United States a few decades later. In an article published in 1894, one of the first in the American context to use the word *homosexual*, Kiernan described a case of a twenty-two-year-old woman with "neurotic ancestry" on her father's side, whose friendship with another girl had become "a perverted love." While the invert could not be regarded as a "lunatic," Kiernan wrote, the condition was "closely akin to that of the hysteric or sexual neurasthenic," and thus should be considered treatable by psychotherapy. Kiernan agreed with his European colleagues that homosexuality had roots in both the hu-man constitution and psychological development. But he concluded that "there is entirely too much sympathy wasted on these patients," who will not "'will' to be cured while they are the subjects of sympathy." Kiernan condemned a tendency that he detected among homosexuals to consider themselves "interesting invalids to whom sympathy is due," a notion that he believed cultivated a "hypochondriac gloating in sexual pervert notions" and impeded their "proper management."[32]

## Mid-Century Optimists

From the late nineteenth century through the early twentieth, conversations and debates about sexual and gender difference were held in the salons, clinics, and psychoanalytic societies of Europe and Great Britain. Beginning in the 1930s, with the rise of Nazism and fascism, psychoanalysts, many of them Jewish, were among the tens of thousands who fled wartime Europe and settled in the United States. The historian Eli Zaretsky counts nearly two hundred refugee psychoanalysts, some leaders in the field, who arrived in the United States from Germany, Austria, and Central Europe during the Second World War.[33] By 1939, one historian writes, "substantial parts of entire local European psychoanalytic communities [had] transferred from Central Europe to America."[34]

European psychoanalysts joined and invigorated a small American psychoanalytic community that had been growing since Freud's electrifying visit to the United States in 1909. The New York Psychoanalytic Society was founded in 1910. In 1911, Ernest Jones, a Welsh psychoanalyst and Freud's official biographer, established the American Psychoanalytic Association.[35] The Washington Psychoanalytic Society was organized by psychiatrists at Saint Elizabeths Hospital in 1914—evidence of the close tie between psychoanalysis and psychiatric medicine in the United States. European wartime émigrés joined an eclectic American psychoanalytic community, one that was generally less philosophical and more empirical and instrumentalist in orientation than its European counterpart. While European psychoanalysts had registered a "genuine rejection of the prevailing notions in psychiatry and medical psychology," American practitioners were more practical in orientation and eager to tether psychoanalysis to the medical discipline of psychiatry.[36] Also unlike European psychoanalysts, American psychoanalysts were required to have a medical degree to conduct clinical practices or join psychoanalytic societies. Psychoanalysts enjoyed tremendous prestige in the American psychiatric profession in these decades; by the 1930s, psychiatrists had "incorporated psychoanalytic ideation in their thinking," and psychoanalysts dominated the discipline's leadership positions through the early 1970s.[37]

Psychoanalysts confronted a European sexological tradition that diagnosed homosexuality as a hereditary condition, sited its locus in the human constitution, and for the most part, argued for sympathy and tolerance rather than cure. Despite the efforts of some early adherents of psychoanalysis to treat "inversion," the skepticism of Freud and others about conceiving of homosexuality as a curable disorder prevailed for nearly four decades. However, American analysts were more enthusiastic about the curative potential of psychoanalytic treatment generally, and about the possibility of curing homosexuality in particular, than were their European predecessors.

In 1940, New York psychiatrist Sandor Rado set the theoretical machinery in motion for a radical change. Born in Hungary in 1890, Rado was drawn to psychoanalysis early in his career and became a student and disciple of Freud's. Earning a reputation as an astute theoretician, he became secretary of the German Psychoanalytic Society in Berlin, and in 1924 Freud appointed him managing editor of the two international journals of psychoanalysis, *Internationale Zeitschrift für Psychoanalyse* and *Imago*. In 1931, Rado moved to the United States to serve as education director of the New York Psychoanalytic Society, and later he founded the first American training school for psychoanalysis at Columbia University. Rado served as director of that program from its founding in 1944 until his retirement in 1955.

Empowered by his European psychoanalytic credentials and his direct ties to Freud, Rado charted a boldly heterodox course, just a year after Freud's death in 1939, by rejecting the Freudian concept of constitutional bisexuality.[38] Freud had made a scientific error, Rado asserted, in assuming that a sexually mixed biological development resulted in the presence of both masculine and feminine characteristics in the psyche. Countering arguments based in the new science of endocrinology and drawing on theories of evolution, Rado argued that heterosexual object choice was biologically ordained, dictated by the reproductive drive and the survival of the species. "The desire to fulfill the male-female pattern is a sexual characteristic shared by all members of our civilization," he wrote.[39] Homosexuality, Rado proposed, resulted from "hidden but incapacitating fears" of the opposite sex produced by trauma in infancy and early childhood.[40]

Rado's argument deployed the kind of functionalist reasoning, grounded in a biological drive to reproduction, that Freud had argued strongly against. Still, Rado's views gained enormous influence in U.S. psychoanalytic circles, creating the intellectual foundation for a new stance toward homosexuality that psychiatrists characterized as "optimistic." Psychoanalysts who trained with Rado at Columbia, including Irving Bieber, Lionel Ovesey, and Charles Socarides, would go on to elaborate theories and establish clinical practices that combined a dogmatic hostility toward homosexuality with therapeutic optimism about the possibility of conversion and cure.

Among the most influential of the new generation of psychoanalysts, Edmund Bergler had abandoned his private practice and position as associate director of the Psychoanalytic Society in Vienna and fled Austria in advance of the Nazi annexation in 1937. He settled in New York City, where he established a clinical practice and pursued a prolific writing career, publishing twenty-seven books and over three hundred articles during his lifetime. Bergler first focused his attentions on analyzing frigidity in women, impotence in men, and unhappy marriages and divorce, but he then turned to the topic of homosexuality. He began lecturing in psychoanalytic circles on the prospects for curing homosexuality in the 1940s; in 1956, he took those ideas to a broad public with the publication of his best-selling book, *Homosexuality: Disease or Way of Life?* The book's title seemed to stage a debate, but for Bergler, the conclusion was foregone: "*there are no healthy homosexuals*," he emphasized. Rather, homosexuality was an "*illness* as painful, as unpleasant and as disabling as any other serious affliction." That illness, Bergler theorized, was rooted in a fundamental masochism, a "wish to suffer" that made homosexuals, in Bergler's estimation, irrational, narcissistic, depressive, megalomaniacal, infantile, and "essentially disagreeable people."[41]

Bergler's characterization of homosexuality was harshly pathologizing; at the same time, he offered a promise, that "*today, psychiatric-psychoanalytic treatment can cure homosexuality*."[42] Countering what he characterized as the "therapeutic pessimism of the past" and distancing himself from his predecessors who could only offer to help reconcile homosexuals to their fate, Bergler contended that homosexuality now "has an excellent prognosis in psychiatric-psychoanalytic treatment."[43] Initially recommending an analysis of one to two years' duration with a minimum of three appointments each week, Bergler accommodated himself to his American audience by proposing successively shorter analyses in later publications, the shortest being eight months.[44] He boasted a near-perfect cure rate of 99 percent.

Bergler identified a pre-Oedipal attachment to the mother and a displaced projection of the maternal breast to the penis as among the primary causes of male homosexuality. Irving Bieber, another New York City–based psychoanalyst, elaborated on the theory that a pathological family formation caused homosexuality in what became the most influential work on the subject, *Homosexuality: A Psychoanalytic Study of Male Homosexuals*, published in 1962. Bieber was less bombastic in tone than Bergler and less overtly judgmental toward the gay men that were both his patients and re-search subjects; he also garnered attention and authority through the sheer volume of evidence he collected. While the unit of analysis in published psychoanalytic research was often a single case study of an individual per-son presented in narrative form, Bieber based his work on a quantitative analysis of 106 case studies of homosexual men contributed by 77 New York psychiatrists and a 450-item questionnaire, analyzed over the course of nine years. In a bid for the recognition of his study as empirical, large-scale, sci-entific research, Bieber noted that it was "the first time that voluminous and detailed data obtained in individual psychoanalyses have been collected for such a large number of homosexuals and subjected to clinical and statistical analysis," adding that the data were put on "IBM cards for processing."[45]

From an analysis of this data set, Bieber and his team concluded that a pathological family constellation caused homosexuality in men. "Close-binding," overprotective, and sometimes seductive mothers babied and emasculated their sons, inhibited boyish aggressiveness, and interfered with their heterosexual development. In those claims, psychiatrists joined a larger misogynistic chorus decrying "momism," a term coined by writer Philip Wylie to assert the allegedly emasculating effect of America's ideal-ization of motherhood.[46] Absent, hostile, or abusive fathers shouldered less blame in accounts by Bieber and other psychoanalysts (and in the broader American postwar culture), but they often figured in these explanations as well as the third prong in a dysfunctional family triangle.

"What about Lesbians?," the title of one of Bergler's chapters in *Homo-sexuality: Disease or Way of Life?*, unwittingly betrayed the extent to which lesbianism was an afterthought and an addendum for him and for most of his psychoanalytically oriented colleagues in this period. As studies about gay men proliferated in the 1950s and 1960s, featured on bestseller lists as well as in medical journals, psychiatric studies devoted to lesbians were al-most nonexistent. That the subjects of most psychoanalytic writing were white and male was rarely remarked on. When psychoanalysts did include women in their studies, they explained the etiology of lesbianism with awk-ward reference to the same pathological family narrative that they used to explain homosexuality in men. Homosexuality in women was understood to be produced by an overbearing, controlling mother and a distant and detached father, with emphasis on a dysfunctional relationship with the mother, resulting in the same pathological triangular relationship that purportedly produced homosexuality in boys.[47] The "typical mother" of a lesbian, psychiatrist Cornelia Wilbur wrote in 1965, was an "overbearing individual who is dominant in the family and excessively controlling of the girl who is destined to become a homosexual"; the "typical father" was a "submerged" individual, often "quiet, withdrawn, and unassertive," who "may even absent himself, using the pressure of work as a rationalization."[48]

At the same time that American psychiatrists and psychoanalysts were theorizing the origins of homosexuality, they also pondered the etiology of what they termed "transvestism," or the desire to cross-dress, and later of "transsexuality," which they understood to be a more wholesale (and less eroticized) cross-gender identification. Counter to the theories of endocrinologists, including most prominently Harry Benjamin, who searched for organic causes of cross-gender identification and promoted hormone treatment and surgery as the appropriate medical intervention, most psychiatrists in the 1940s, 1950s, and 1960s understood transgender identification as the result of pathological psychogenic processes and people's desire to cross-dress or identify as a gender contrary to the one assigned at birth as a "harking back to their neurotic past, to their infantile fears and pleasures."[49] In 1949, physician and editor of *Sexology* magazine David O. Cauldwell coined the term "psychopathia transexualis" to describe the "unusual mental condition" that created a desire for gender transition.[50] Many psychoanalysts understood gender nonconformity as a subset of homosexuality, likewise caused by an overattachment to the mother, which created "too strong a feminizing symbiosis in infancy."[51] For psychiatrist Benjamin Karpman, a "homosexual component" was "always present" in people diagnosed with transvestism (and also, he believed, "present in a great deal in most neuroses").[52] Some turned to Freud's theory of fetishism—the boy's symbolic substitution for the traumatic discovery of his mother's "lack" of a penis and subsequent fear of castration—to explain people's attachment to clothes of the "opposite" sex. Psychologist Danica Deutsch described transgender women as engaged in a form of "masculine protest," a revolt against the father's role in the family and the responsibilities of men.[53]

Psychoanalysts understood homosexuality and gender nonconformity as mental disorders, but they differed over whether they were best understood as neuroses or instead represented more severe forms of mental illness better characterized as psychoses. New York psychologist Albert Ellis insisted that most homosexuals, cross-dressers, and "transsexualists" were "not merely neurotic, but are actually borderline or outright psychotics," suffering from delusion and detached from reality.[54] Psychoanalysts painted a deeply pathologizing portrait of homosexuality and gender nonconformity, sometimes to the point of self-contradiction and incoherence. Homosexuals were simultaneously lacking in self-esteem and convinced of their own superiority. Self-pitying and loveless, they were also driven by emotion and often violently and irrationally jealous. Historian Dagmar Herzog captures the contradictions of psychoanalytic theories of male homosexuality promoted by psychoanalysts as "a way of attempting to avoid castration by the father—or as a way to unite with the father. It signaled an overidentification with a seductive or domineering mother—or it was a sign of a profound fear of the female genitals. It functioned as a hapless way to repair one's sense of inadequacy as a male—or it was a powerful sexual compulsion that required better control."[55]

Running through the psychoanalytic debates and claims about etiology was the language of disease. Psychiatrists sometimes invoked disease as metaphor or by way of comparison. Combating what he detected as the tendency of homosexuals to "glamorize" homosexuality, Bergler wrote that "there is no more glamor in homosexuality than there is in . . . a case of typhoid fever."[56] Irving Bieber adopted metaphors of physical disability, describing the homosexual as "a person whose heterosexual function is crippled, like the legs of a polio victim."[57] But when psychoanalysts described homosexuals as sick and homosexuality as an illness, they meant it literally as well. In 1964, the New York Academy of Medicine declared that "homosexuality is indeed an illness," or "in a strict sense . . . a symptom of illness."[58] And in 1970, Charles Socarides called for a national center for sexual rehabilitation, one that might respond to the "dread dysfunction" of homosexuality, "malignant in character, which has risen to epidemiologic proportions," with a "pooled program of research and treatment, similar to those for mental retardation, epilepsy, and alcoholism."[59]

In 1952, psychiatrists codified their understanding of homosexuality as a mental disorder. In that year, the American Psychiatric Association (APA) published its first edition of the *Diagnostic and Statistical Manual of Mental Disorders* (*DSM*), a catalog that standardized the field's nomenclature of mental illness.[60] While efforts undertaken by the U.S. Census in previous decades to track mental illness reflected the somatic orientation of early American psychiatry, the first edition of the *DSM* evidenced the mid-century ascendence of psychoanalytic perspectives. The *DSM* identified homosexuality and transvestism (alongside pedophilia, fetishism, and sexual sadism, and including rape, sexual assault, and mutilation) as pathological sexual deviations under the larger category of "Personality Disorders" in its first edition in 1952 and its second edition in 1968.[61] The *DSM* functioned (and continues to function) as a list of diagnostic codes for use by physicians and also as a reference used by courts, insurance companies, and social agencies as well as in public policy, and so its authority extended far beyond the clinic. The *DSM* also performed a territorial maneuver for psychiatrists, identifying and naming aspects of human life and behavior as illnesses or disorders and therefore as under the legitimate domain of psychiatry.

## Psychiatric Power

Why was the commitment to eradicating homosexuality, and the hostility that so often underlay that commitment, so central to psychoanalytic thinking and practice in the postwar United States? Historians have ventured a range of arguments to explain mid-century psychiatrists' striking antipathy to sexual and gender difference and their dedication to eradicating it, with most focusing on the psychoanalytic practice and thinking that so dominated American psychiatry in the 1940s through the 1960s. Some suggest that psychoanalysts' deep-seated antagonism toward homosexuality may have sprung from anxiety about their own association with matters sexual or that their performance of hostility was a strategy to ward off that association. Sex was unavoidably central to the psychoanalytic project, and so "the issue of libido was always palpably present, hovering over the enterprise, at once necessary to the entire conceptual framework and yet continually threatening to make the enterprise seem dirty and tawdry and trivial."[62] That anxiety might have been particularly acute for Jewish émigrés to the United States, who were already vulnerable to anti-Semitic stereotypes of sexual deviance.[63] As the pioneering psychoanalyst Ernest Jones wrote when reflecting on the conundrum of Jewish psychoanalysts in Europe, "A Jew was, so to speak, the wrong person to announce that the sexual instinct was a far more subtle and significant factor in mental life than had ever been supposed."[64] Psychologist Kenneth Lewes diagnoses the antihomosexuality of American psychoanalysts as a "projection of analysts' own alienated impulses." "It is as if psychoanalysis, having found refuge in a new homeland," Lewes writes, "sought to demonstrate its relief, gratitude, and worthiness by subscribing to and lending its weight to the consolidation of American values." Aligning psychoanalysis with the judgmental and stigmatizing ideas about homosexuality that began to intensify in the United States after the war may have offered refugee analysts some protection. Under the pressures of the postwar American context, one in which the state increasingly promoted heterosexuality as a national ideal and denounced homosexuality as a security threat, psychoanalysts abandoned their role as analysts and critics of social values and "took up roles as proponents of American values, American identities, American institutions."[65] Their diagnosis of homosexuality as a mental illness, both drawing on and contributing to a more general American heteronormative project, assisted in their assimilation and acceptance.

Psychiatry's internal professional politics and psychiatrists' struggles for professional legitimacy also surely contributed to their stance on homosexuality. Matthew Tontonoz speculates that American psychoanalysts' rejection of Freud's concept of universal bisexuality was part of a larger strategy to align the field more closely with medicine and science, and with the prestige of those fields.[66] Long associated with asylum custodial care of the elderly and the chronically mentally ill, psychiatrists had reason to be concerned about their own status.[67] Historian Ellen Herman describes America's "romance" with psychology in these years, charting the field's rise to power during and after the Second World War.[68] Psychiatrists' claims regarding scientific and medical expertise, and regarding homosexuality in particular, allowed them to pursue their ambitions beyond the asylum and to present that expertise as vital to postwar governance. After the Second World War, the federal government recognized psychiatry's new authority by passing the National Mental Health Act in 1946, which provided funds for the National Institute of Mental Health and made the mental health of Americans a federal priority.

Psychiatrists also staked their claims about homosexuality in the context of competition from rival practitioners and alternative sexual theories and methodologies. Psychoanalysts' anxiety about their own professional authority and cultural relevance grew, Herzog proposes, with the publication and immense popularity of Alfred Kinsey's reports on male and female sexuality, published in 1948 and 1953, and later with William Masters and Virginia Johnson's studies of human sexual response, published in 1966 and 1970.[69] It is hard to imagine a rivalry of more disparate diagnostic methods and metrics for determining the "truth" of sexuality than the psychoanalyst's exploration of an individual's unconscious, Kinsey's quantification of sexual experiences to orgasm from tens of thousands of amassed sexual histories, and Masters and Johnson's laboratory measurement of lubrication, dilation, heart rate, and erection. But in the view of psychoanalysts, they were competitors to be vanquished over the claim to expertise regarding sexuality.

Psychiatry's stance on homosexuality may have been born in part of professional anxiety; it was also born of ambition. Psychiatrists' claim to expertise and curative power regarding homosexuality was fortuitously timed, and perhaps strategically so, coming at a moment when homosexuality was of special interest and concern to the state. The years after the Second World War witnessed the elevation of the heterosexual family as a national model that might serve as a bulwark against communism and the concomitant condemnation of homosexuality as a threat to American vitality and security. Cold War rhetoric about "American values" and "enemies within" referenced anxieties about sexual difference as much as it did communism (and often an intertwined combination of the two). In the 1940s and 1950s, administrators of the "straight state" presided over the exclusion of homosexuals from the benefits of immigration and naturalized citizenship, from service in the military, from the social provisions of the GI Bill, and from employment in the federal government.[70] Psychiatrists' claims allowed them to forge strategic alliances with the state in these years, alliances that would substantially enhance their power and authority. As early as 1946, Chicago gay rights advocate Henry Gerber condemned the cooperative relationship between psychiatry and law, judging psychiatrists to be "mere assistant policemen . . . hired to uphold conventional sex 'morality' under the guise of 'science.'"[71] Gay activist Jim Kepner, too, comprehended the value of those collaborations to psychiatrists when he recognized that "analysts like Bieber do not spend all of their time at therapy sessions." Instead, he noted, "they spend a good deal of it as . . . 'authorities' in courts, state legislatures, licensing boards, prisons, parole boards, schools, and employment agencies."[72]

Psychiatrists received an enormous boost in status and authority, for instance, when they persuaded the federal government to incorporate psychiatric assessment in the screening of military inductees as part of the Selective Service Act of 1940. The First World War had brought a new awareness of the extent and tremendous cost of neuropsychiatric problems experienced by service members that came to be known as "shell shock," a term used to describe the stress disorders that afflicted people who experienced the trauma of combat. In late 1940, psychiatrist Harry Stack Sullivan was appointed as a consultant to the director of the Selective Service. He and Saint Elizabeths supervisor Winfred Overholser formulated guidelines for the Selective Service's psychological screening of military inductees in an attempt to weed out those who might be most vulnerable to the psychic stress of military service and combat. Although Sullivan's own unconventional clinical practice in the 1920s at the Sheppard and Enoch Pratt psychiatric hospital in Baltimore emphasized a depathologizing and sympathetic approach to homosexuality (and although Sullivan was himself in a lifelong and largely secret relationship with a man), the regulations that he helped draft and institute listed "homosexual proclivities" as a disqualifying factor for military service.[73] Psychiatrists also oversaw a shift in military policy whereby active-duty members of the armed service could be discharged for homosexuality. From 1941 to 1945, nearly ten thousand sailors and soldiers, most, though not all, of whom were men, were hospitalized for homosexuality in psychiatric wards and discharged as "mentally unfit" for service.[74] Overholser presented these measures as progressive and enlightened alternatives to the military's long-standing policy of criminal prosecution for sodomy. But as the historian Allan Bérubé points out, the system of screening inductees and discharging service members for homosexuality "was humane only to the degree that it saved some men from prison."[75] It also worked to project the understanding of homosexuality as a sickness into the public imagination.

Psychiatrists also made themselves useful to the state, enhancing their own influence and authority in the process, by offering their endorsement of sexual psychopath laws. Passed into law in twenty-six states and the District of Columbia, first in the late 1930s and in another wave in the late 1940s and 1950s, sexual psychopath laws were sparked by sensationalizing media reporting on sex crimes, usually involving the brutal and sexualized murder of a child. Bills criminalizing a range of sexual offenses were then promoted by grassroots citizens' groups, sponsored by state legislatures, and enacted into law.[76] While proponents of the laws most often cited the dangers posed by sexual psychopaths to children, they were used primarily to criminalize consensual sex between adult men.[77]

Psychiatrists were ambivalent supporters of sexual psychopath laws, and sometimes outright critics. As early as 1924, the distinguished psychiatrist William Alanson White proclaimed that the category of the psychopath had become "a sort of middle ground for the dumping of odds and ends" and was not a meaningful clinical category.[78] By the time sexual psychopath laws were first proposed in the 1930s, most psychiatrists had dismissed the diagnostic category of the "psychopath" as a "wastebasket diagnosis."[79] In their 1954 study of the treatment of sex offenders with group psychotherapy, psychiatrists Charles Cabeen and James Coleman clarified that "the term 'sexual psychopath' is a legal one and does not necessarily imply the psychiatric diagnosis of psychopathic personality."[80] Although Karpman was recognized as an expert in the study of the psychopathic criminal and authored some of the earliest work in the 1930s linking criminality to sexual deviance, in later years he came to the conclusion that "the terms 'sexual psychopath' and 'sexual psychopathy' have no legitimate place in psychiatric nosology or dynamic classification."[81] Likewise, the first edition of the *DSM* in 1952 did not include sexual psychopathy as a diagnostic category.

Psychiatrists were especially critical of the requirement under sexual psychopath laws that compelled defendants under penalty of law to answer questions asked by psychiatrists who were charged by the court with determining whether they met the statutory standard for sexual psychopathy.

As Overholser observed in 1948 about the District of Columbia's sexual psychopath law, known as the Miller Law after its sponsor, Nebraska Republican representative Arthur Miller, "You cannot expect to get the truth from [someone] when you are holding a club over his head."[82] Overholser expressed his reservations about the Miller Law's imperative that sexual psychopaths would be institutionalized until they were deemed "fully and permanently recovered."[83] Nearly a decade later, in 1956, psychiatric experts reported in a public forum on sex offenders that "neither a prison term nor surgery may make [someone] change his ways."[84] Such a determination of cure was especially difficult "if not impossible to render," psychiatrist Karl Bowman later claimed, in the case of homosexuals.[85] Still, psychiatrists overcame their hesitations and were rewarded with enhanced influence. As Overholser told members of Congress about sexual psychopaths, "It is an interesting group from a therapeutic point of view and we should welcome the opportunity to deal with them."[86]

Ultimately, psychiatrists' endorsement of sexual psychopath laws was key to their passage and psychiatrists' participation was crucial to the laws' administration. Willing to put their criticisms aside in exchange for greater authority and prestige, they agreed to serve as expert assessors of sexual psychopathy, oversaw the carceral institutionalization and treatment of people committed under the new laws, and certified the success of recovery and "cure" for safe release as required by law. Psychiatrists also provided the justificatory medical language of illness, treatment, and cure that at once authorized and mystified the laws' criminalization of nonnormative sex. In early drafts of the Miller Law, for example, sexual deviance was cast in criminal terms, emphasizing the law's punitive aims. In calling to order the February 20, 1948, hearing of the congressional Subcommittee on Health, Education, and Recreation of the House Committee on the District of Columbia, Representative Miller described the bill as one "to provide for the commitment, detention, and treatment of criminal sexual psychopaths."[87] But as the bill was discussed and revised, references to criminality, detention, and punishment were whittled away. The law's carceral aims and effects were masked in its final form, passed on May 20, 1948, and described in a slight but consequential change in wording as providing simply for "*the treatment of sexual psychopaths* in the District of Columbia, and for other purposes."[88] Advocates of the Miller Law succeeded both in expanding the criminalization of nonnormative sex and effectively cloaking that expansion through their use of the language of medicine. In accordance with the Miller Law's medicalized conception of sexual psychopathy, the person charged under its statutes was not referred to as "the defendant" or "the accused," but rather as a "patient." "This is in accordance with the theory that the title essentially provides treatment rather than punishment," its authors explained.[89] The virtue of the law, in Overholser's understanding, was in recognizing "a very large group of offenders as essentially sick people rather than vicious ones."[90]

The Miller Law's definition of the sexual psychopath as a "patient" rather than a "defendant" and its medical language of treatment instead of the legal language of criminalization, incarceration, and punishment had several important effects. Since it mandated the hospitalization and supported the rehabilitation of the sexual psychopath, it allowed supporters to characterize the law as progressive and humane. The description of the bill that went before Congress touted it as being "in conformity with the most up-to-date thinking in the fields of psychiatry and criminal law."[91] Minnesota Representative George MacKinnon, sponsor of the Minnesota sexual psychopath law passed nearly a decade earlier, described the Miller Law as "dealing in what you might call a more modern way with these psychopathic personalities."[92] Overholser praised the proposed legislation "as progressive, as practical, as indicating a closer union of the law with medicine, and as indicating that the law is ready to take advantage of the scientific knowledge concerning behavior."[93] Medical language aligned sexual psychopath laws rhetorically with modernity and progress.

The medicalization of the sexual psychopath had important juridical effects as well. In moving the determination of sexual psychopathy out of the courtroom and into the psychiatric clinic, the Miller Law effectively evaded the requirement of due process. While people formally defined as "defendants" were guaranteed a trial by jury, privilege against self-incrimination, and protection against double jeopardy, people defined as "patients" were not. "Since the proceedings here in question are not of a criminal character," MacKinnon stated, "the constitutional right to a jury trial does not apply to proceedings of this type."[94] This was the case even for what members of Congress and Overholser acknowledged would potentially result in lifelong carceral institutionalization. Commitment under most sexual psychopath statutes required neither a criminal charge nor conviction.

Among the most important results of sexual psychopath laws was to "cement the primacy" of psychiatrists in the criminal legal system and to establish and fund clinics attached to the courts that embedded psychiatrists firmly in that system.[95] A joint Committee of the American Bar Association and the American Psychiatric Association was established to work on "problems of mutual concern."[96] The court clinic, psychiatrist Manfred Guttmacher wrote approvingly, "brings psychiatry directly into the legal process," providing the sentencing judge with an evaluation of the personality of the offender that was founded on a psychiatric examination.[97]

Judges' deference to the authority of psychiatrists testified to the persuasiveness and power of psychiatry's insistence that homosexuality was properly understood as a sickness rather than a crime. Psychiatrists typically framed that shift from a legal understanding of homosexuality to a medical one and their motivation in facilitating it as humane and progressive. Psychiatrist Samuel Hadden explained that he wrote a book on homosexuality as a "treatable condition" "in the hope that it will contribute to having homosexuality regarded as a medical, psychiatric, and social problem and that those involved will no longer be treated, or thought of, as vicious criminals or moral degenerates."[98] But that claim to an enlightened stance masked the ways in which psychiatrists were deeply implicated in a criminal legal system that continued to criminalize consensual same-sex sex and gender nonconformity. The collaboration between psychiatry and the law meant that psychiatry operated as an arm of the state's disciplinary and carceral apparatus.

Psychiatry's claim to expertise regarding homosexuality proved useful to the postwar U.S. "straight state" even when psychiatrists themselves disavowed its application. In 1952, the same year that the APA published its first edition of the *DSM*, which listed homosexuality as a pathological sexual deviation, Congress passed the McCarran-Walter Act, revising U.S. immigration law by allowing people of Asian descent to immigrate to the United States and become citizens (even while upholding racist national origin quotas as the core principle for controlling immigration) and removing racial restrictions on naturalization. Alongside these purportedly liberal racial reforms, the new law also sharpened the language that allowed the United States to exclude or deport undocumented immigrants on the grounds of moral turpitude, adding a provision that called for the deportation and exclusion of those "afflicted with psychopathic personality."[99] Congressional sponsors made clear their intention to include homosexuality in that category. Some psychiatrists balked, again protesting the state's instrumentalization of the concept of "psychopathy," a clinical category they had long since discarded as meaningless.[100] In legal challenges to the enactment of the law, the courts affirmed psychopathic personality, and by extension homosexuality, as a legal construct rather than a medical one.[101] They did so, however, by retaining the authorizing use of medical language, thus licensing increasingly strict prohibitions against homosexuality and effectively leveraging psychiatric power without psychiatrists.

Pondering the relationship between the discipline of psychiatry and homosexuality, psychoanalyst Kenneth Lewes proposed that "the two are essentially and dialectically related, each requiring the existence of the other."[102] It is difficult to imagine the ascendence of psychiatric power in the mid-twentieth century without the productive and enabling utility of psychiatrists' claims to expertise regarding gender and sexual difference and their promises of conversion and cure. To those troubled by the increasingly visible phenomena of gender and sexual difference during and after the Second World War; to an American state increasingly invested in yoking citizenship, rights, and belonging to heterosexuality; and to people made to feel distress about their own desires and understandings of self, psychiatrists made an optimistic claim that obscured its inherent violence: We understand these problems. We are the experts on them. And we can fix them.

## CHAPTER TWO

# Fixing Queerness

Mid-century American psychiatrists were voluble about their theories of the etiology of homosexuality and the damage it did to individuals and the social order and boastful in their claims to be able to treat and cure it. They were considerably more circumspect when it came to the question of *how* to do so. For instance, the best-selling 1962 book by Irving Bieber and his coauthors, *Homosexuality: A Psychoanalytic Study*, devoted its 350 pages to detailed descriptions of the pathological permutations of family relationships that they believed caused homosexuality in men and not a single paragraph to the methods they claimed could successfully treat it.[1] The published works of psychiatrists, then, tell us a great deal about their understandings of the nature of sexual and gender difference but little about how they put those ideas into clinical practice.

Clinical practices to "treat" homosexuality and gender nonconformity were varied, and all were thoroughly integrated into American medicine, illuminating another pathway to psychiatric power. Rising to ascendency in the 1940s and 1950s, psychoanalysts dominated the psychiatric profession and innovated clinical approaches to homosexuality and gender variance. But psychoanalysis was not the only game in town. Psychoanalysts competed with other psychiatrists, neurologists, behavioral psychologists, and medical practitioners in allied fields, some of whom proposed to treat homosexuality and gender nonconformity with methods that targeted the body rather than the mind through shock and surgery.

Unlike psychiatric theories of homosexuality and cross-gender identification, psychiatric practice confronted psychiatrists with real people. Practice, then, was a messier and less manageable business than theory. Shifting our attention from theory to practice reveals the rough edges, compromises, and resignations involved in the psychiatric treatment of queer and trans people. A focus on practice also sometimes reveals psychiatrists' acknowledgment of the outright failures of their project of "curing" homosexuality and normalizing gender. A chronicle of their efforts lays bare, as well, the difficulty of distinguishing the clinical from the carceral and treatment from torture.

## The Psychoanalytic Fix

In the mid-twentieth-century United States, the treatment for homosexuality and gender variance that was most popular, most widely recommended, and most often pursued was psychoanalysis. Some promoted and practiced the classical and demanding form of analysis innovated by Sigmund Freud, requiring four or five sessions per week over the course of many months and often years, and others believed that less time-intensive and less orthodox psychoanalytically oriented psychotherapy was sufficient. At the core of psychoanalytic theory was the belief that people were motivated by unconscious thoughts, feelings, desires, and memories. The practice of psychoanalysis involved bringing the unconscious into consciousness. Repressed memories would surface in the course of free association, psychoanalysts believed, providing insight into the unconscious mind. Psychoanalysts used techniques including dream analysis and free association to help patients gain insight into how their past experiences informed their behavior and responses in the present day.

Neutrality on the part of analysts toward their patients, requiring a commitment to bracket their judgments and preconceptions and adopt a posture of benevolent impartiality, was a central tenet of psychoanalysis. Psychoanalysts were expected to be nonjudgmental guides, no matter where the patient's associations might lead. That suspension of judgment was especially important, they believed, for freeing their patients to express sexual or aggressive emotions that might cause them shame or embarrassment without self-censorship. Psychoanalysts understood that honesty about one's unconscious motives would not come easily, so they cultivated a practice of attentive listening, asking questions but refraining from offering advice or appraisal. In classic Freudian psychoanalysis, the patient lay on a couch with the analyst seated beyond their field of vision so that they might feel able to speak openly, freed of the self-consciousness, conventions, and expectations of face-to-face conversation.

However much psychiatrists valued a nonjudgmental stance in theory, though, many of them failed to deliver on that promise in practice when it came to their queer patients. As important as homosexuality was to psychiatrists' broader claim to authority in the mid-twentieth-century United States, the task of attempting to "cure" it led them to contort and pervert their own principles and methods. The antipathy with which many psychiatrists viewed homosexuality and their zeal for conversion were often readily apparent to their patients. Richard Isay, who undertook analysis in the early 1960s as part of his training as a clinical psychiatrist at Yale, recalled that his analyst "usually implicitly but sometimes explicitly conveyed his view that I was a neurotically inhibited homosexual." That therapist, who never called Isay by name in their sessions "because he felt it would interfere with the perception of his neutrality," congratulated him enthusiastically when he became engaged to his wife and sent a warm telegram to his synagogue on the occasion of their marriage the following summer.[2]

Psychotherapist Albert Ellis dispensed with the idea of therapeutic neutrality altogether. Ellis began his career with an interest in psychoanalysis, earning a PhD in clinical psychology at Columbia University in 1947 and later training at the American Institute for Psychoanalysis founded by the eminent German analyst Karen Horney. In his position as chief psychologist at the New Jersey State Diagnostic Center, Ellis used psychoanalytic methods to treat men classified as sexual offenders. But by the early 1950s, he had grown frustrated with what he viewed as the passivity and "inefficiency" of psychoanalysis, requiring "long, unhelpful silences" and years of restrained listening on the part of the analyst.[3] Drawing instead on the ideas of behavioral psychologists and learning theorists, Ellis developed a more "exhortative-persuasive, actively-directive" method that he called Rational-Emotive Behavior Therapy, an early form of cognitive behavioral therapy in which the therapist actively and sometimes aggressively intervened to combat their patients' self-defeating and irrational beliefs and persuade them to adopt beliefs judged to be more "rational."[4] Putting those theories to work in his private practice in New York City, Ellis became "more active" and assertive with his patients: "I tried to encourage, persuade, and impel them to do the things they were afraid of."[5] Taped and transcribed recordings of Ellis's sessions with patients document his aggressive and judgmental therapeutic style, in which he "attacked" his patients' sense of self and what he took to be their self-defeating beliefs and practices. Ellis understood his role as therapist not as a neutral guide, but as a "frank propagandist for a wiser, saner way of life."[6]

Mid-century American psychiatrists confronted competing ideas about the etiology of sexual and gender difference and a sexual and gender epistemology in flux. Many understood their first task and challenge in treating queer and gender-variant people as that of actively disabusing them of prior ways of thinking about themselves and winning them over to the idea that homosexuality and gender nonconformity were symptoms of mental disorder, which could be changed and eliminated through treatment. Ellis described this process as one of "de-propagandizing" or "de-indoctrinating" the people under his care, or of "deflating" homosexuals' "smug rationalizations" about themselves, which psychiatrists believed made them reluctant to seek psychotherapy and unwilling to commit to the hard work of change.[7]

Psychiatrists assailed both older and newer ways of thinking about the etiology and status of homosexuality and gender variance that patients brought with them and that conflicted with their own. Key among those ideas was the belief that homosexuality and cross-gender identity were somehow inborn or organic. Psychiatrists were frustrated by their patients' claims that homosexuality was immutable, incurable, or a biological inheritance over which they had no control—beliefs they characterized as self-serving and dismissed as relics of old-fashioned sexological thinking that had been overturned by modern psychiatry. Some people consulted with psychiatrists after having read the work of sexologists like Magnus Hirschfeld and Havelock Ellis, which convinced them that homosexuality was fixed and innate. In 1934, Austrian psychoanalyst Ernest Bien was rebuffed by a twenty-five-year-old clerk who "flatly refused to be treated because he believed, after reading Hirschfeld's works, that homosexuality is an inevitable fate."[8] Over three decades later, in 1965, Bieber claimed to be bewildered by the fact that "many homosexuals prefer to regard their condition as constitutionally determined," which he took to mean that "they more readily accept a view of themselves as biological freaks" than as mentally ill people suffering from a treatable disorder.[9]

Many cross-gender-identifying people, too, were convinced of the constitutional basis of their gender identity and firm in their resistance to psychiatric explanations of cross-gender identification as a neurotic symptom of a deeper psychopathology, one that psychiatrists often attributed to an underlying and core homosexuality. Trans people professed their belief in the authenticity and immutability of their gender and usually articulated their longing for physical rather than psychic transformation. Raymond Shea, who was tried for desertion by the U.S. Navy in the late 1930s, discharged for "transvestism," and committed to Saint Elizabeths after attempting suicide, described a plan of trans-becoming to psychiatrist Benjamin Karpman, hatched at the age of fourteen, to "save my money and some day live by myself in some out-of-the-way place in the country where I could let my hair grow like a girl. I intended to live there for about a year wearing nothing but feminine attire. The reason for this isolation was that it would give me a chance to change my entire nature to that of a girl. . . . Then I intended to go back to New York and live and work as a woman." Shea charted a path to transition beyond the clinic; they also wrote of a hope, decades before gender-affirming surgery was available in the United States, "that perhaps doctors could operate on me and after the removal of my testicles, graft the clitoris and ovaries of a woman to me." Refusing Karpman's psychoanalytic explanation of transvestism, Shea insisted that "whatever your theories are, I honestly think that perhaps I am a woman."[10] Another of Karpman's patients, Kate Stewart, lamented "the bitter accident of sex" that resulted in her female embodiment. Karpman diagnosed the roots of Stewart's feelings of "'really' being a boy" and dreams "of changing into a boy" as "buried in the unconscious," perhaps in "some completely forgotten aspect of infantile sexuality." But he pronounced Stewart "an extremely difficult subject for psychoanalysis because she is completely resistive to all psychoanalytic approach" and because Stewart claimed that "all the psychoanalytic theories fail to explain the strong psychic feelings of masculinity which to me were always primary."[11]

Gender-variant people often drew on narratives of intersex embodiment to argue for an understanding of their gender difference as organic in origin. "Have you ever thought that sexual aberrations such as mine might be caused by glandular disturbances?" Shea asked Karpman. "That this might be more than mental?" To support their theory, Shea noted that Danish painter Lili Elbe, whose autobiography *Man into Woman* was published in 1933, had been diagnosed with "rudimentary female organs which gave out female hormones instead of only male."[12] Intersex explanations helped Shea and others make sense of a gender identity so deeply felt that they believed it must have a biological basis. After 1952, following the extraordinary publicity surrounding Christine Jorgensen's transition, the articulation of transgender identification as constitutionally based was no doubt shaped as well by initial reports in the media that Jorgensen had been diagnosed with a mixed-sex condition. Jorgensen professed her belief in her own physical bisexuality in interviews and her autobiography. "My body was not only slight," Jorgensen wrote, "but . . . the sex organs that determined my classification as 'male' were underdeveloped." Believing that her femininity "might in some way be related to glandular disturbances," Jorgensen first consulted an endocrinologist but was disheartened when he referred her to a psychiatrist who proposed a minimum of thirty psychoanalytic sessions.[13] She found an answer that made more sense to her in her readings in endocrinological texts, and then in Denmark, where endocrinologist Christian Hamburger told her that "perhaps my body cells, even my brain cells, were female." To prepare her family for her return to the United States as a woman, Jorgensen told them that she had initially feared that she suffered from a "horrible illness of the mind," one "not as yet accepted as a true illness," but was relieved when doctors were able to "clear" an "imbalance" in her glands. "Nature had made a mistake, which I have had corrected," she wrote, "and I am now your daughter."[14] Jorgensen's story, along with those of earlier trans autobiographers, gave hope to others longing for gender transition rather than psychiatric treatment. Reading about Jorgensen while institutionalized in a veterans' hospital, Jane Fry wrote that she "had always felt that my troubles were physiologically based" and that "the article in the paper expressed that point of view."[15] The fact that for decades in the United States, gender-affirming surgery was only accessible to those with demonstrable intersex physiologies also no doubt inclined people to locate the origin of their gender difference in their bodies.[16]

Psychiatrists combated arguments that homosexuality and cross-gender identity were innate or constitutional; they also dismissed claims made by some of their patients that homosexuality was an "esthetically superior" or more exciting and glamorous way of life or a marker of genius.[17] Psychiatrist Edmund Bergler emphasized the necessity of "deglamorizing" homosexuality in the eyes of one of his gay patients, who was convinced of "the superiority of his kind over all others."[18] For Bergler, this process required "stripping the neurotic disease of its aura of false allure."[19] Psychologist Robert Harper likewise underlined the need to combat the notion "that the homosexual life is more exciting, more romantic, more exhilarating, more wonderful, more 'out-of-this-world' than anything that can be offered by the dull, drab, dreary, deadly world of heterosexuality."[20] Of a man institutionalized at Saint Elizabeths who "numbers himself . . . among the homosexual great," Karpman conjectured that "this is probably typical of the compensatory efforts of the aesthetic homosexual . . . to identify homosexuality with genius, and to seek moral support from half the great names in the history of art and literature."[21] While psychiatrist Samuel Hadden conceded that "many extremely talented homosexuals have made great contributions to the arts and sciences," he noted derisively that "homosexuals would have us believe they are *all* Platos, Andre Gides, or at least, Oscar Wildes."[22]

Sometimes, Hadden found, gay men could be induced to "depropagandize" each other. One of the leading innovators and theorists of group psychotherapy in the late 1930s, Hadden first integrated individual gay men into therapy groups of heterosexual patients, but he observed that they dropped out when "the nature of their problem was revealed," often in the face of hostility from other group members.[23] Concluding that gay men "lacked sufficient ego strength" to be in groups with straight people, Hadden began leading therapy groups comprised entirely of gay men in his Philadelphia practice in the 1940s through the 1960s. A "beneficial effect" of such groups, he boasted, was "the speed with which the group breaks down the rationalization of its component members."[24] "I have never observed a group in which homosexuality, as a way of life, was not fiercely attacked when a member tried to present it as desirable."[25] Hadden was gratified when the gay men he treated expressed "little tolerance for the obvious homosexual, 'The Fairy'": "He is frowned upon and vigorously rejected unless his conspicuous dress and mannerisms are quickly altered." When a member of the group displayed "gay mannerisms" or wore "conspicuous gay clothes," Hadden relied on other group members to demean and ostracize him. "They tell him that none of them want to be seen leaving the building with anyone dressed the way he is," an admiring *Time* magazine journalist wrote of Hadden's program in 1965.[26]

Hadden encouraged psychotherapeutic groups of gay men to police one another's gender expression and flamboyance; he also relied on gay therapy groups to neutralize articulations of a political critique that located the source of psychological distress in a hostile and discriminatory society rather than in family pathology and individual psychic structures. Hadden forced members of his therapy groups to reckon with what he called their "abnormality" in discussions that he initiated about brutal crimes allegedly committed by gay men, gay men's high suicide rates, and "the loneliness and the ostracism" of gay life. In one session, Hadden exploited a local news story of the murder and dismemberment of a sailor by a gay man purportedly known to some of the members of his group to underline the perverse brutality and sadism that he believed to be characteristic of homosexuality. One group member claimed to know a young gay man who had "recently disposed of his parents by poisoning." The group went on to search for an explanation of "why homosexuals committed such violent crimes." By the end of the first session, Hadden noted, "they were in agreement that homosexuals were not as gentle and artistic as they appeared."[27] After these exchanges, group therapy participants would "soon discard any beliefs that they are an especially gifted and unique group" and "no longer denounce society or its harsh attitudes toward the homosexual." Instead, he observed approvingly, they would recognize themselves as "sick" and "encourage each other in the efforts to change."[28]

Belief in the constitutionality, and sometimes the superiority, of homosexuality was antiquated and antiscientific, mid-century psychiatrists held; it was also, they believed, troubling evidence of the influence and appeal of "homosexual propaganda" disseminated by an emerging gay rights movement and its cultivation of a civil rights imaginary among gay men and lesbians. By the 1950s, as psychiatrists became increasingly confident in their ability to cure homosexuality, they confronted the challenge of some gay activists' claims that homosexuality was a normal variation of human sexual expression. Bieber contrasted Alcoholics Anonymous, the mutual help organization for alcoholics founded in 1935, in which "members must recognize that alcoholism is an illness," with "the homosexual organization" that regrettably "consolidates and more deeply entrenches the psychopathology of its members."[29]

Early gay activists revived nineteenth-century sexological arguments about the innateness of homosexuality; they drew inspiration and political ammunition as well from more contemporary sex research, especially from Alfred Kinsey's explosive findings demonstrating that same-sex sex was a relatively common phenomenon rather than a rare psychiatric condition. In his 1948 bestseller *Sexual Behavior in Human Males*, Kinsey reported that nearly 40 percent of American men had engaged in same-sex sex as adults. "This is more than one male in three of persons that one may meet as he passes along a city street," Kinsey added for emphasis.[30] His figures for women of around 13 percent, published a few years later, were lower but still shocking to many.[31]

Kinsey was interested in documenting the range and frequency of human sexual acts rather than adjudicating questions of sexual identity, and he argued that sexuality was best understood as a continuum of "endless gradations" rather than a homosexual-heterosexual binary. In 1952, Kinsey gently criticized Edward Sagarin, author (pseudonymously, as Donald Webster Cory) of *The Homosexual in America: A Subjective Approach*, for limiting his attention to "two kinds of persons, the more or less exclusively and overwhelmingly homosexual and the persons who are primarily heterosexual," while neglecting the majority, who "lie in a middle ground."[32] Still, early gay rights advocates put Kinsey's findings to identitarian purposes to argue for strength in numbers and for the recognition of homosexuals as comprising an oppressed minority group. "One out of five, or ten, or even twenty!" Sagarin exclaimed. "Every thinking person must realize that his brother, his child or unborn grandchild may be one of this large group who is being cast out."[33] Gay leftist Harry Hay credited Kinsey's work as among his inspirations in founding the Mattachine Society in Los Angeles in 1950. Hay dedicated Mattachine's first meeting to a discussion of Kinsey's *Sexual Behavior in Human Males*.

Kinsey's effort to determine what was "natural" as opposed to what was purportedly "normal" in human sexuality launched a powerful critique of the moralistic claims of both psychoanalysis and religion. Insisting that the "mammalian background" of human beings conditioned their sexual response, Kinsey argued that while "it may be true that heterosexual contacts outnumber homosexual contacts in most species of mammals," it would be "hard to demonstrate that this depends upon the 'normality' of heterosexual responses, and the 'abnormality' of homosexual responses."[34] Psychoanalysts were among the loudest critics of Kinsey's methods and findings, attacking him for including the sexual histories of prisoners, outcasts, and "neurotic volunteers" in a data set that they believed inflated the incidence of homosexuality.[35] Charging Kinsey with being an "involuntary dupe of the highly efficient homosexual propaganda machine," Bergler castigated him as "a naïve propagandist for his own preconceived notion that in sex anything goes" and speculated darkly that Kinsey's research was perhaps also tainted by his own unconscious sexual conflicts.[36]

Bergler criticized Kinsey for being overly influenced by the claims of early gay activists. He and other psychiatrists responded to the challenge of early gay rights claims more broadly by pathologizing them and folding them into their diagnostic profile of homosexuality, characterizing gay men's and lesbians' recognition of discrimination as itself a neurotic symptom associated with homosexuality. The critique of a heteronormative, hostile, and discriminatory social order was for Bergler evidence of the "psychic masochism" that was part of the neurotic disorder of homosexuality.[37] "Every homosexual is an exquisite injustice collector," Bergler wrote, driven by a "wish to suffer." "These people always construct and provoke situations in which they feel themselves unjustly treated," an impulse that Bergler argued led them to "pity themselves masochistically."[38] Injustice collecting, Bergler explained, "means there are people who constantly construct or misuse situations in which they are badly treated, humiliated, rejected."[39] Bergler's stance could be breathtaking in its callousness. Speaking to a teacher who was forced to resign because of his "homosexual record" and ordered by the court to undergo analysis, Bergler asked, "Has it occurred to you that you yourself, masochistically, created your own trouble?"[40]

For some psychiatrists, "de-propagandizing" their queer patients involved assigning "homework" that required them to pursue heterosexual courtship and sex as part of their therapeutic treatment. One man in analysis with Irving Bieber in the mid-1950s recalled that Bieber "would repeat—more times than I could even begin to estimate—one sentence . . . : 'There is no shortage of beautiful women.'"[41] Ellis was more explicit and interventionist in his heterosexual instruction. Assuming that "fixed deviates" had "failed to gain the knowledge and practice of petting methods that most heterosexuals gain during their adolescence and early adulthood," Ellis educated his gay male patients in female anatomy and trained them in sexual technique. In tutoring one man in the aggressive heterosexuality expected of mid-century white American men, Ellis urged him to first put his arm around a woman and then try to kiss her. If she resists, he said, "you can just stop for a little while and go back to it later." If she "cooperates," Ellis told him, "start taking off some of her clothes." "I've never found a homosexual who couldn't do it with girls, when he really tried," he asserted. "Obviously you're able to fuck a girl when she'll let you. And one of these days," he assured him, "one of them is going to let you."[42] Some gay men felt guilty about using women to "try out" heterosexuality as part of their therapy. M. P. Moore found it "hard to face the fact that I am going to have to use a woman as my guinea pig" (with Karpman's encouragement).[43] Charles Silverstein heeded his psychiatrist's advice to date women "in the hope that something would take," but he ended up feeling that they were "being used." "Afterwards I realized how unfair it was to these women, all of whom cared for me a great deal," he recalled.[44] "None of the women I dated knew that they were filling a prescription from my therapist."[45]

The therapist must deindoctrinate the patient, Ellis wrote; he must then "reindoctrinate" them with psychiatry's "new idea" about homosexuality.[46] That new idea was that homosexuality was not organic in its etiology, not something people *were* or a kind of human being, but rather, for psychoanalytically oriented psychiatrists, a neurotic symptom born of family pathology or preconscious trauma. Modern psychiatrists, Bergler claimed, "have proven conclusively that the allegedly unchangeable destiny of homosexuals (sometimes even ascribed to nonexistent biological and hormonal conditions) is in fact a therapeutically changeable subdivision of neurosis."[47] American psychiatrists in this period almost invariably used *homosexual* as an adjective that modified something else—tendencies, drives, impulses, leanings, feelings, habits—and rarely as a noun identifying a kind of person. In doing so, psychiatrists went against the grain of what has been taken as the twentieth century's steady march toward understanding homosexual sex as irrefutable evidence of homosexual identity. They did so, importantly, at the moment at which modern gay identity was taking shape. "There *is* homosexual behavior," psychiatrist Robert Stoller acknowledged; "there is no such *thing* as homosexuality."[48] Hadden made clear to his gay group therapy participants that "we do not consider them as 'homosexuals' but as neurotics whose preference for sexual experience with the same sex is one of their symptoms."[49] Psychiatrists worked to get their patients to abandon their understanding of homosexuality as fated, as biologically ordained, or as an identity or quality of self, and instead to recognize it as a mental disorder that could be treated and cured. "I do not believe you are a homosexual or a lesbian in the popular sense of the word," Karpman told a woman hospitalized at Saint Elizabeths in 1941 who had only had relationships with women.[50] "There is no such thing as congenital homosexuality or homosexuality due to glandular disturbance," he assured her. Instead, homosexuality was "an acquired neurosis" resulting from "psychological accidents."[51] When Warren Goldfarb's psychiatrist submitted a letter to the draft board to support his application for exemption from conscription during the Vietnam War, he documented Goldfarb's "chronic and acute anxiety" but not his homosexuality, because, Goldfarb recalled, "he didn't believe there were such things as homosexuals."[52]

Some took comfort in their psychiatrists' pronouncement that they were not "really" homosexual. After two hospitalizations for depression and suicide attempts, Betty Berzon was relieved when a psychiatrist told her, "I don't think you're homosexual at all." On hearing those words, she recalled, "the sun came out and the birds began to sing again, and I came back to life," at least until the next time she was confronted with her desire for women.[53] When psychiatrist Lionel Ovesey asked a patient why he did not list homosexuality in his initial life history as "one of the symptoms he wished to have corrected," the man told him that "it had never occurred to him that homosexuality was a neurotic symptom, nor that one went to a psychiatrist to have it cured." When Ovesey responded that he considered homosexuality "a psychiatric illness which could be treated by psychotherapeutic means," the patient "seemed generally confused, anxious, and yet delighted."[54] Another man was relieved by Karpman's assessment that he was bisexual and that his "heterosexual component has been suppressed, bringing forth a strong homosexual bent."[55] "True homosexuality," Karpman wrote, "does not exist," because "in the history of every homosexual we find a bisexual period, which may cease early or even persist throughout life."[56]

While some people were reassured and relieved by psychiatrists' skepticism about the existence of homosexual identity, psychiatrists' understanding of homosexuality as artificial, fleeting, and symptomatic put them at odds with many others in treatment with them. For many queer people, the understanding of same-sex desire as an integral and constitutive feature of their identity made the idea of "cure" or conversion to heterosexuality difficult to conceive of, much less pursue. Because Edward Sagarin understood desire to be a core feature of selfhood, accepting a reorientation of the direction of desire amounted to willful self-annihilation. To contemplate conversion to heterosexuality, Sagarin suggested, would be to obliterate an essential sense of self. As a consequence, he wrote, homosexuality "is virtually as ineradicable as if it involved the color of one's skin or the shape of one's eyes."[57] Sometimes he entertained the wish "to be normal," Sagarin confessed, "just for a brief period," so that he might "know the freedom from the anxiety of being the outcast." Yet even his "wildest flights of fancy" did not allow him to imagine being heterosexual. "If I were not what I am," he wondered, "what pursuits would occupy my pen, what problems would occupy my mind?" "I know that I cling to my entire personality," he wrote, "and that sexuality is basic in this personality and can never be relinquished."[58]

Countering psychiatrists' belief in the symptomatic, ephemeral quality of homosexuality, some of those in psychiatric treatment affirmed the centrality of homosexuality to their personhood. When Karpman asked his patient Rex Cronin, "Can you live without homosexuality?" Cronin replied, "I would exist—not live."[59] "My whole way of life is colored by this," another of Karpman's patients wrote, "as I might say it is my whole soul. Even if I were able to live my whole life again, with all the trials and tribulations I have gone through"—trials that in his case included a lobotomy and over a decade of institutionalization at Saint Elizabeths—he insisted that he would still be homosexual.[60] When Kate Stewart became aware of her attraction to women, she "was not at all sorry to see this development" because "it was in keeping with my own feelings about my basic nature." She knew that she would experience "lots of troubles on account of my 'difference,'" but at the same time she felt that "it was utterly unthinkable that I could be, or try to be, anything but what I was."[61]

Psychiatrists tried to dissuade people from believing that their homosexuality or gender variance were constitutionally based, a benign form of human difference, more glamorous and exciting than heterosexuality, or evidence of genius. They were also critical, though, of patients who expressed what they took to be overly harsh ideas about homosexuality and gender variance, which psychiatrists judged as archaic or "puritanical" attitudes rooted in old-fashioned and moralistic ideas, attitudes overly influenced by religion rather than science. A secular Jew and dedicated practitioner of the science of psychoanalysis, with its insistence on the motivating force of human sexual impulses and desires, Karpman was critical of patients whose feelings about themselves seemed overly influenced by their religious upbringing. "Homosexuals are not degenerates," Karpman corrected one patient's answers to his questionnaire. "Professional psychiatrists object very strenuously to such terms."[62] Karpman was troubled that another patient had been "conditioned to associate homosexuality only with that which was base, sordid, and bestial."[63] To a patient's wife who wrote to Karpman about her shock on learning about her husband's cross-dressing, Karpman chastised her for a response that was, in his judgment, "a bit too dramatic." "Transvestism is much less a perversion than a neurotic condition rooted in unconscious psychological complexes," he informed her.[64] When Rodney Frank, a married man diagnosed with "homosexual panic" and committed to Saint Elizabeths by his wife, wrote in response to Karpman's questionnaire that "a queer to me is the lowest form of animal life," Karpman asked, "WHY do you make this statement? Have you read anything of a scientific nature about homosexuality? Have your ideas on the subject undergone any change or modification since your hospitalization?" (In a private memorandum, Karpman judged Frank "dumb" and found "nothing abo⏹

is the least bit interesting.")[65] Frank confessed that he had characterized homosexuality in this way because "that's the way the majority of society thinks" and also "to make you believe that I'm an honorable person who abhors homosexuality."[66] After months at Saint Elizabeths in treatment with Karpman, he learned to parrot psychoanalytic ideas, writing dutifully that "I have learned that homosexuality is common to everybody at certain ages. In children it's considered wrong for a child not to be homosexual and a little while after he reaches the age of puberty he has to change and start having heterosexual drives. Apparently homosexuality is the result of not making these changes in drives."[67]

## Adjustment

Psychoanalysts like Bergler, Bieber, and Socarides grabbed the attention of the public and appealed to the state with their claims to be able to "cure" homosexuality. Turning our attention from psychiatrists' bold assertions in their published writing and public proclamations to what we can glean about their practice, though, reveals evidence of the considerably more modest goals that many pursued with their patients in these years. Some scaled back their curative ambitions in the face of their widespread failure to convert gay men and lesbians to heterosexuality. A few acted out of a more sexually progressive and compassionate stance toward queer patients in their private practice than they felt willing or able to commit to in public or in print.[68]

Contrary to psychiatry's stated goal of *cure*, at least some psychiatrists in the 1940s, 1950s, and 1960s pursued the goal of *adjustment*, working to help people accept their homosexuality rather than convert to heterosexuality. The psychological language of adjustment circulated widely at mid-century, and some queer people took it up themselves to articulate their own goals.[69] Samuel Steward, a novelist, poet, tattoo artist, and dedicated diarist, wrote that since his graduation in the early 1930s, "I have been trying to make a more mature adjustment to my condition." For Steward, that meant that "I have stopped pretending that I am normal," and also learning "not to look upon every good looking boy I meet as a possible lover."[70] One man in Karpman's care at Saint Elizabeths who first sought the advice of an army psychiatrist found the therapeutic experience "strengthening," but he noted that "in the final analysis he only helped me accept, a little more fully perhaps, what I already knew. I was homosexual." In accommodating himself to that fact, he found "peace—the capacity to be comfortable in life."[71] Historian Jonathan Ned Katz entered into analysis "with the idea that my 'problem' was my homosexuality, and my goal a heterosexual 'cure.'" He later counted himself lucky to have happened on a therapist "who did not view my 'problem' as I did myself" and who instead helped people "find and be themselves."[72] After poet Allen Ginsberg was released from a New York City psychiatric hospital in 1950, he found his way to a "lady psychiatrist" who "called up my father and told him my parents must accept the fact that I like men."[73] Charles Silverstein was familiar enough with the psychotherapeutic goal of adjustment to know that he did not want it—a familiarity that suggests that the concept of adjustment was well known. For Silverstein, "the idea of being 'adjusted' burned a hole in me." He entered therapy pledging to himself that "under no circumstances would I 'adjust' to homosexuality."[74]

Karpman's sympathy for his patients led him to embrace the treatment goal of "adjustment," at least for some, which meant prioritizing self-acceptance over heterosexual conversion. For instance, Karpman expressed concern to Marina Harris "not so much with your homosexuality or heterosexuality as such, but only with your comfort and happiness." Heterosexuality, Karpman made sure to note, was an easier path because it was granted "social approval and that means a great deal to most of us." But "if I should find that you can be happier as a homosexual," he told Harris, "I shall help you to find yourself that way."[75] To a man struggling with "a choice between heterosexuality and homosexuality" in 1944, Karpman told him that "we are not so much concerned with the nature of your choice as with your acceptance of it in mental comfort and with no sacrifice of normal efficiency."[76] Likewise, he judged a married man of sixty-two to be too old to be cured of his homosexuality, and so "the best that was expected was to help him adjust comfortably to the situation, which was done."[77]

Perhaps the most remarkable example of Karpman's commitment to helping his patients "adjust" to their homosexuality was his therapeutic work with Hal Richardson. A twenty-eight-year-old man who had worked as an elevator operator, Richardson was admitted to Saint Elizabeths in 1932 for "hysterical neurosis" and homosexuality following multiple arrests for soliciting sex with men in parks and public restrooms. Richardson traced his own mental breakdown to contracting gonorrhea: "It made me nervous and I couldn't sleep. I lost weight, and finally I broke down."[78] For reasons that are not clear from his files, he spent at least the next two decades at the hospital, at one point attempting suicide.

Several years into Richardson's institutionalization, Karpman arranged for him to spend weekends away from the hospital with one of his former patients, an older gay man who identified himself in correspondence with Karpman as "Mr. X." (That insistence on anonymity in print speaks, probably, to the man's desire to conceal his own homosexual identity in the written record; it may also have offered him protection as a participant in Karpman's unorthodox treatment plan). In regular progress reports to Karpman, Mr. X wrote of sharing his collection of physique magazines with Richardson and sharing "affectionate intimacy" as well, which occasionally included sex. Mr. X understood his role as that of a tutor in respectable homosexuality, taking Richardson to the "legitimate theater" and modern dance recitals and encouraging him to read novels "of a high type." When Richardson asked Mr. X "why it was that so many homosexual persons 'aren't nice, like you,'" Mr. X told him that "'nice' homosexual persons" were "not to be 'picked up' in public toilets and parks."[79] "I am more inclined to believe now that the psychotherapy will achieve in his case a definite result in the elevation of the general level of consciousness," Mr. X wrote to Karpman, "and that the sordid and absurd encounters which have been so large a part of his past program will gradually give place to something more resembling a 'safe and sane' sexual celebration."[80] Mr. X's tutelage, under Karpman's supervision, then, can be understood as a project in training Richardson in the cultural, aesthetic, and sexual practices of homosexual respectability that might make him less vulnerable to arrest, rather than attempting to convert him to heterosexuality. Richardson's "adjustment" was successful in Karpman's view. "Gradually under the influence of his mentor," Karpman wrote, "he acquired a changing sense of values and his promiscuous homosexual activities became steadily fewer in number."[81]

At the same time, Mr. X recognized that the discrimination written into U.S. law and the stigma and exclusions rooted so deeply in mid-century American life meant that homosexual respectability would only take one so far. Mr. X made clear to Karpman that Richardson would not be able to truly elevate himself "until the social status—or at least the legal status—of homosexual people is made tolerable."[82]

One organization in New York City quietly committed itself to the project of the psychiatric adjustment of gay men with the aim not of "curing" them, but instead of reforming their behavior to make them less likely to get in trouble with the law. In 1946, Quaker reformers who had been working with conscientious objectors during the war approached psychiatrist George W. Henry about a project to assist men who had been arrested for sexual offenses or had been incarcerated and released on parole. In 1948, Henry founded the George W. Henry Foundation, naming himself psychiatrist-in-chief and his longtime collaborator Alfred A. Gross as executive secretary.[83] A closeted gay man who had worked closely with Henry in the 1930s on the Committee for the Study of Sex Variants and later in studying working-class and indigent gay men in New York City, Gross was committed to a sympathetic approach to gay men in legal difficulty.[84] The Henry Foundation chartered with the state of New York and set up shop in the University Settlement House on Manhattan's Lower East Side, dedicating itself to helping those who "by reason of psycho-sexual deviation are in trouble with themselves, the law, and society" and arranging with New York's criminal and municipal courts to refer cases of gay men who had been arrested and convicted to the foundation. Henry and Gross then referred them to psychiatrists (for "those who can pay"), psychologists (for "those who can pay somewhat less"), and clinically trained clergy members (for "those who cannot even pay the fees charged by the clinics").[85] The foundation also functioned as "an unofficial employment agency," helping gay men who had been arrested or incarcerated to find jobs.[86] Gross explained the foundation's project as helping gay men "rid themselves of . . . guilts and giving them reassurance of their own worth as persons."[87] Such men, Gross wrote in 1963, need to "be taught to grow up and recognize the limits that society places upon the freedom of action of its members."[88] "We seek to help men come to terms with their sexual maladjustment."[89] "That does not mean that these men are 'cured' of their homosexual interests or even activities," Gross clarified. Instead, the foundation aimed to bolster their self-esteem and coach them in self-control so that "they seem no longer obliged to seek companionship in places constantly under police surveillance and . . . under especially sordid circumstances."[90] Gross was even more candid in his personal writing, characterizing the aim of the Henry Foundation's work as helping the homosexual "'live with his neurosis,' avoiding promiscuity and cheapening himself."[91] Of a young man referred to the Hartford, Connecticut chapter of the foundation in 1966, Gross noted that "we reduced his overt homosexual behavior" and "have given him a better image of himself."[92] Gross compared psychiatric adjustment to the physician's palliative rather than curative treatment of chronic conditions: "I can see a certain parallel between my doctors making me as comfortable as they can with my angina," he wrote in 1969, "and our Foundation undertaking to make those who come to it as comfortable as they can with their handicapped position."[93]

In their public writing, Henry and Gross made sure to cloak the foundation's work in the conventional psychoanalytic argot and assumptions of the day by underlining the "immaturity" and "maladjustment" of the homosexual.[94] The foundation "regards homosexuality . . . as symptomatic of a deep-seated personality disorder," as stated in the 1955 annual report.[95] At the same time, the foundation's offer of what was euphemistically termed "practical assistance" and "realistic treatment" went strikingly against the grain of the psychiatric orthodoxy of the day in emphasizing adjustment over cure. Gross's definition of adjustment also lodged an implicit but cutting political critique of the conditions of life for queer people in postwar America: "One has to get along, somehow," Gross wrote, "with a world in which escape is impossible."[96] Recognizing the risk that the foundation took in pursuing an agenda of adjustment, Gross made clear that the foundation saw "no need for publicity," but rather preferred "to hide its light under a bushel."[97] "What needed to be done was done quietly and unobtrusively," Gross wrote.[98] Because "we are dealing with an unknown climate of opinion," Gross counseled the Hartford chapter of the Henry Foundation in 1967 to "satisfy themselves with small beginnings," as "there is always the danger of going too far."[99]

## Somatic Treatments

In the 1940s, 1950s, and 1960s, at the same time that an ascendant American psychoanalytic community promoted treating disorders of sexuality and gender using dynamic therapies of the mind, neurologists, psychologists, and other psychiatrists developed alternative treatments focused on the body. For somatic as well as psychoanalytic practitioners, the middle decades of the twentieth century were a time of experimentation, an ambition to cure homosexuality and gender variance, and optimism about their ability to do so. The treatment modalities they developed, featuring the use of shock, surgery, and aversive conditioning, would reverberate in queer historical memory as forms of torture.

The first of the somatic treatments harnessed what was understood to be the therapeutic power of shock. Though neurologists and psychiatrists confessed that they did not understand the mechanism by which shock treatment worked to relieve the symptoms of depression or mania (and they still do not), many hailed it as a breakthrough, especially in cases of schizophrenia. The first shock treatment, developed by Austrian physician Manfred Sakel in 1934, employed the use of insulin. Over a period of five or six weeks, patients received insulin injections to lower their blood sugar to near-fatal levels and then were revived from hypoglycemic coma to consciousness with a glucose solution. One man, who was hospitalized at Saint Elizabeths in the 1940s for homosexuality and treated with thirty insulin-induced shock treatments over the course of seven weeks, testified to his "tremendous fear" of the therapy, which he found "torturing and hellish." "From the first to the last treatment," he wrote, "I dreaded the experience."[100] Other physicians employed metrazol, a circulatory and respiratory stimulant that in large doses induced grand mal seizures, in early shock treatment.

In 1939, Bellevue Hospital psychiatrist Paul Schilder described the effects of metrazol on patients, who on injection felt the sensation of electricity "playing all over their body," followed by "the feeling as if they would be destroyed completely."[101] By the 1940s, virtually every hospital, sanitarium, and mental institution in the United States included shock therapies in their armamentarium.[102]

In the 1940s, drug-induced shock was largely replaced by the use of electric current. First developed in Italy in the late 1930s, electroconvulsive shock treatment became popular and widespread in U.S. hospitals in the 1940s. Saint Elizabeths Hospital superintendent Winfred Overholser noted his preference for electric shock "for the reason that metrazol caused so much . . . emotional distress in the patients."[103] Insulin- and metrazol-induced convulsions could also result in fractures of the vertebrae, whereas shock via electric current could be more carefully calibrated and controlled.

Shock therapy was prescribed most widely for schizophrenia, depression, and epilepsy. Because psychiatrists believed homosexuality and gender variance to be closely and even causally linked to the first two of those conditions, many queer and gender-nonconforming people were treated with electroconvulsive shock, often under the guise of treatment for something else.[104] But some physicians experimenting with these new modalities targeted queer people more directly. Atlanta psychiatrist Newdigate Owensby reported in 1940 on treating homosexuality in men and women with metrazol shock, based on the assumption that homosexuality was a symptom of "an under developed schizophrenia which was arrested at the particular phase in its psychosexual development where the libido became fixated and that metrazol liberates this previous fixation of the libido and the psychosexual energy becomes free once more to flow through regular physiological channels."[105] Psychiatrist George N. Thompson reported on treating six patients with electroshock in the late 1940s, among them a thirty-two-year-old man unable to hold a job because he was "different, sissified, and queer," a twenty-five-year-old man and former Boy Scout troop leader arrested for "committing sexual perversions upon young boys," and a twenty-year-old man depressed about his homosexuality. Thompson concluded reluctantly that "no benefit was obtained in any of the cases in altering the homosexuality or other form of sexual psychopathy."[106] In 1955, psychiatrists Russell Dinerstein and Bernard Glueck reported on subjecting men incarcerated in New York's Sing Sing Prison who suffered from "acute anxiety attacks" based on "homosexual conflicts" with insulin at doses too low to cause a coma but enough to cause "moderate hypoglycemia."[107] "The amount of time available for individualized therapy is . . . limited" in this carceral setting, Dinerstein and Glueck explained, necessitating the use of somatic treatments and the development of therapeutic techniques "requir-ing a minimum amount of individual psychotherapy."[108]

Psychiatrists also turned to shock therapy in the effort to treat what they termed "transvestism." In 1944, psychiatrist Samuel Liebman published a report of his treatment of a twenty-three-year-old Black patient hospi-talized in the Norwich State Hospital in Connecticut and suffering from what Liebman described as a combination of "homosexuality, transvestism, and psychosis." The patient was delivered by the police to the hospital in November 1941 "dressed in a very effeminate manner," wearing mascara, rouge, and powder and with manicured and painted fingernails and "a woman's silk chemise and skirt" under "male sport clothing."[109] Liebman characterized them as having "a defensive, persecuted sort of attitude which bordered on perpetual sullenness" and "an inflated opinion of himself."[110] The patient made "a general spectacle of himself," he wrote, underscoring their gender transgression of going to beauty parlors to request permanent waves, wearing their hair in curlers, presenting "a generally feminine make-up," and walking the floors of department stores "as though he belonged there," a judgment that likely betrayed Liebman's sense of their racial trans-gression as well.[111]

Liebman administered eight courses of electroshock treatment within days of the patient's admission to the state hospital. He reported that the treatment jolted the patient into mortification about their feminine presen-tation, quoting them as saying afterward, "What on earth ever made me act like I did before I came here? No wonder they locked me up, I must have been crazy. Imagine me in Fox's trying on furs and evening gowns!"[112] On discharge from the hospital, Liebman reported confidently that the patient "seemed more manly."[113] However, when they were arrested the following year on a charge of "idleness" and reinstitutionalized at Norwich, they con-fessed to still having "homosexual desires." Liebman credited electroshock with "repressing completely his transvestism but only partially his homo-sexuality."[114] The patient was recommitted to the hospital for a third time a month later, in November 1942, given thirteen additional electroshock treatments, and then discharged to the police and reincarcerated. This per-son's racialized and criminalized queerness and transness propelled their transit through and among the various regulatory sites of psychocarceral power in this period and compelled their subjection to one of the most vio-lent of psychiatric modalities.

At the same time that shock treatment came into prominence in psy-chiatric hospitals in the United States, a revolution in psychosurgery was occurring as well. First introduced by Portuguese neurologist Egas Moniz in 1935, the prefrontal lobotomy was understood initially to be a treatment of last resort but one of great promise for people who failed to respond to other treatments, especially in cases of debilitating mental illnesses like schizophrenia, psychosis, and profound depression, which often resulted in long-term institutionalization. In lobotomy, the nerve fibers that connected the frontal lobes of the brain were severed. As with electroshock, physicians were uncertain about why this procedure would ease the symptoms of mental illness and psychic distress. Some theorized that the destruction of nerve connections between the lobes "divorces psychotic ideas from accompanying emotional components" and interrupted the fixations and obsessions that tormented people.[115] At a time when state hospitals suffered from overcrowded conditions and treatment options for debilitating mental illness were few, psychiatrists promoted lobotomy as providing a way to relieve people of their worst symptoms and allow them to leave the hospital and go home.

American neurologist Walter Freeman and neurosurgeon James Watts introduced psychosurgery to the United States in 1936. Initially prohibited from performing lobotomies at Saint Elizabeths, where Freeman was the director of laboratories (superintendent William Alanson White believed lobotomy to be a "'spurious and irresponsible' treatment" and a "mutilating operation"), Freeman and Watts received permission from White's successor, Winfred Overholser, to perform psychosurgery on a limited number of Saint Elizabeths patients.[116] They performed lobotomies as well at other Washington, DC, hospitals and clinics, most notoriously the surgery in 1941 that left Rosemary Kennedy permanently disabled and institutionalized for the rest of her life.

Freeman was especially enthusiastic about a less invasive transorbital lobotomy technique, developed in the mid-1940s, which utilized the eye socket as a surgical pathway to the frontal lobes rather than drilling through the skull. Freeman proclaimed the transorbital lobotomy so simple that it could be performed by physicians without surgical training or certification and in the physician's office rather than the sterile field of a hospital operating room. Neither did the new method require anesthesia, Freeman insisted. Instead, he used a series of electric shocks to induce unconsciousness, a procedure he valued for its amnesiac effects on anxious and fearful patients as well as its general availability to psychiatrists because of the ubiquity of electroshock devices in clinics in the 1940s. Rather than recovering in a hospital, patients were provided with sunglasses to conceal their blackened eyes and sent home in a taxi an hour after a procedure that took less than ten minutes. (Freeman and Watts's partnership would come to an end over Watts's disapproval of Freeman's transorbital procedure and his insistence that "any procedure involving the cutting of brain tissue was a major operation and should remain in the hands of the neurological sur-geon.")[117] Freeman was evangelical in his advocacy for lobotomy and the-atrical in promoting the procedure: he posed for photographs using a car-penter's mallet and ice pick rather than surgical implements to showcase its ease and ordinariness; later, he traveled around the country in a car he dubbed "The Lobotomobile," performing thousands of lobotomies at state hospitals and on children as young as four. Initially recommending the sur-gery for long-suffering and chronically mentally ill people, Freeman later advocated its use for a much wider range of conditions, including anxiety, phobias, and obsessive thoughts.[118]

From the late 1940s through the 1950s, lobotomy was a mainstream psychiatric practice performed on tens of thousands of people across the United States in state hospitals, private clinics, and university medical cen-ters. Freeman and Watts initially expressed doubt about the use of lobot-omy as a treatment for homosexuality, believing that the operation "cannot be expected to alter the fundamental deviation of the individual," even as references to perversion saturated their description of the procedure as in-activating the "perverted activity" of the frontal lobes, which produced "de-viation in behavior."[119] At the same time, they agreed with psychiatrists that homosexuality was often prevalent in schizophrenics and perhaps a root cause of schizophrenia, and so while they professed a reluctance to operate on patients "whose homosexual drive was openly expressed," they did in fact perform lobotomies on many queer people.[120]

One of Freeman's gay patients was Benjamin Miller, a twenty-nine-year-old Washington, DC, resident who sought Freeman's services in 1948 after suffering a series of depressive episodes that he attributed to his homo-sexuality. Miller had enlisted in the army, but he was discharged after two months "on a suspicion of homosexuality." He worked in hotels, restaurants, and nightclubs and participated in DC's vibrant gay social world. In 1943, he married a woman who worked at the nightclub where he worked in the hope that he might "leave the homo-sexual life behind me" and "make the grade of being a husband" (even as he approached the altar hoping that "one of my homo-sexual friends would break into the church and come running down the aisle and tell everybody that this boy was queer and not meant for married life"). But he "couldn't get over my feeling of admiring handsome men, and seemed to be obsessed with that feeling." After consulting with the DC Office of Vocational Rehabilitation, Miller was referred to Freeman, who performed a transorbital lobotomy on him at Casualty Hospital, a fa-cility in the Capital Hill neighborhood that was founded to provide care for those unable to pay for their treatment. Miller "seemed to feel a little better for awhile" after the procedure, but his depression returned within months, as did his desire for men. "In the beginning, I left my wife under the impression that the operation had cured me of homosexuality," he explained, but after returning to sex with men, he admitted he "couldn't stand the guilt feelings." Freeman arranged for Miller to be institutionalized at Saint Elizabeths, where he came under the care of Karpman. Karpman diagnosed Miller's "outstanding difficulty" as one of "sexual maladjustment" and his "homosexual background" as the cause of his "subsequent social and mental trouble" and pronounced him "a pretty hopeless case."[121]

Miller was not the only gay patient Freeman operated on, his professed reluctance notwithstanding. Two years later, in 1950, Freeman and Watts documented their performance of a lobotomy on another man who attributed his suicidal depression to his homosexuality, reporting that two years after the operation the patient stated that "there had been no recurrence of the urge and that sex as a whole meant little to him."[122] Two decades later, in 1970, Freeman stated in a press conference that he had "'severed the frontal lobes' of a number of homosexual inmates at Atascadero," a maximum-security institution in California for people designated as sex offenders and those committed as "criminally insane."[123] In 1973, Freeman claimed that "many instances of latent homosexuality have been relieved of their preoccupations and ideas of reference"; he added that "homosexuality is of little practical importance after frontal lobotomy."[124]

Clues in the published literature and psychiatric case studies on lobotomy suggest that when psychosurgery was performed on queer and gender-variant people, it was probably used more often as a managerial measure than as an even aspirationally curative one and was often performed in carceral or semicarceral institutional settings to make people more tractable. In 1955, physicians Moses Zlotlow and Albert Paganini were able to identify and study sixty postlobotomy patients with "homoerotic or autoerotic manifestations" in one institution alone, Pilgrim State Hospital, located in Brentwood, New York, the largest state-run psychiatric institution in the country. All were given lobotomies because "they constituted severe management problems" for the institution, including problems of same-sex sexuality and masturbation as well as what was characterized as "aggressiveness."[125] However, after their lobotomies, Zlotlow and Paganini reported that many patients continued to pose "management problems," including sexual behavior that became even "more obvious."[126] One example was the case of a patient identified as E.R., a twenty-three-year-old committed to Pilgrim State Hospital in 1933, who "admitted that he had become a 'fairy'" as a teenager and had "consorted with men in Greenwich Village." In 1951, he was given a prefrontal lobotomy, and despite initial "improvement in behavior," he displayed "an increase in his sexual manifestations after the operation."[127] Shock treatment, and the threat of it, were used as a form of control and punishment as well: "You were threatened with it all the time to keep you in line," a lesbian institutionalized in the 1950s recalled. "That kind of treatment was used as punishment."[128] Black patients in the segregated Searcy State Mental Hospital in Mt. Vernon, Alabama, reported in 1967 that "if you talk back to an attendant or sass them, . . . you are given a shock treatment. All the attendant has to say is, 'I want this patient shocked,' and the patient is taken in for a treatment."[129]

## Behavioralists and Aversion Treatment

Psychoanalysis and the somatic therapies of the 1940s and 1950s would seem to be fundamentally at odds and are often posed as opposing trends in mid-twentieth-century psychiatry. Psychoanalysts understood mental disorders to derive from psychic traumas of infancy and early childhood, while advocates of psychosurgery believed that many psychiatric illnesses were organic in origin. Historian Mical Raz calls into question the binaries often invoked in histories of psychiatry: neurology versus psychiatry and somatic versus dynamic psychotherapeutic approaches to mental illness.[130] "Psychosurgery and psychoanalysis enjoyed a surprisingly close relationship in the 1950s," Raz finds, and were viewed by patients and many doctors as "complementary treatments with shared goals."[131] Like American psychoanalysts, practitioners of somatic methods like electroshock and lobotomy countered what they characterized as therapeutic nihilism or pessimism with optimism about treatment.

If psychoanalysis was understood to be compatible with somatic treatments in the mid-twentieth century, with one modality complementing and reinforcing the other, psychoanalysts faced more serious competition from behavioral psychologists, who were indebted not to Freud but to learning theorists like Russian physiologist Ivan Pavlov and Harvard psychologist B. F. Skinner. Rather than plumb the depths of the unconscious to analyze human motivation, learning theorists understood behavior to be learned and determined by environmental stimuli, both positive and negative. At the turn of the twentieth century, Pavlov famously used experiments with dogs to demonstrate the principles of what he called classical conditioning, a learning process that occurs when an unconditioned stimulus (e.g., food) is paired with a neutral stimulus (e.g., a bell) to elicit a conditioned response (in the case of Pavlov's initial experiments, salivation). Once "learned," Pavlov showed, the response could be induced by the stimulus alone. Behavioralists built on those basic concepts to explore how behavior was acquired through conditioning and how they might intervene in that process. In the 1930s, developing ideas about learning that he termed "operant conditioning," Skinner demonstrated that behavior could not only be induced or strengthened by positive reinforcement but could also be avoided and even extinguished by what he called negative reinforcement delivered along a continuum of severity, and ultimately through the application of punishing shocks. If behavior followed by pleasant experiences was repeated, Skinner reasoned, behavior followed by unpleasant consequences would likely be avoided.

Pavlov and Skinner developed their theories of learning through experimentation with dogs, pigeons, and rats. In the 1960s, psychologists began to extrapolate from these theories of animal learning to human behavior. One of the leading behavioralists in this period, South African psychiatrist Joseph Wolpe, postulated that what psychoanalysts diagnosed as neuroses were simply maladaptive behaviors akin to any bad habit. When subjected to the experimentally established principles of learning, Wolpe proposed, neurotic symptoms could thus be unlearned. "Unadaptive habits are weakened and eliminated" through proper conditioning, he wrote, while "adaptive habits are initiated and strengthened."[132]

Drawing on these principles, psychologists and psychiatrists began to develop new therapeutic methods, deploying the use of negative or aversive stimuli to counter "maladaptive" desires and behavior. The first formal use of aversive therapy was conducted at the Leningrad Psychiatric Hospital by physician N. V. Kantorovich in 1929, with the aim of treating alcoholism. Kantorovich gave patients painful electric shocks after they smelled or drank alcohol, and although he reported that the majority avoided drinking after the treatment, most of them relapsed months later.[133]

Despite the disappointing results in treating alcoholism with aversive techniques, psychologists pressed on, turning next to sexual disorders, including impotence, voyeurism, fetishism, exhibitionism, and pedophilia, and targeting homosexuality and transvestism in particular. In 1935, British psychiatrist Louis Max published a short description of his treatment of a homosexual man using aversive conditioning, instructing the patient to fantasize about "the attractive sexual stimulus" while he administered an electric shock. Max initially used "low shock intensities," but when they seemed to have little effect, he applied shocks "in intensities considerably higher than those usually employed on human subjects in other studies." After four months of aversive conditioning, Max wrote, "that terrible neurosis has lost the battle, not completely but 95 per cent of the way."[134]

After a decline in interest in aversion treatment in the 1940s and 1950s, psychologists returned to the practice with new enthusiasm in the 1960s.

By this time, queer and gender-variant people had become privileged sub-jects of treatment by therapists who used aversive methods to weaponize people's own bodies and sexual desires. The first aversion therapy trials for homosexuality and "transvestism" used drugs to induce nausea as the aver-sive stimulus. Physician and sexologist Kurt Freund began experimenting with this method to treat homosexuality in Prague in the 1950s. He injected patients with apomorphine, an emetic drug that induced vomiting; when the effects began to take hold, he showed the patient slides of attractive men. In the second phase of the treatment, the patient was shown images of attractive women in combination with injections of testosterone, with the aim of inducing a heterosexual response. Freund reported disappointing findings, however: of the twenty patients he treated, only three "achieved any kind of heterosexual adaptation and in no case did this continue for more than a few weeks." In a follow-up two years later, none of the patients "could claim complete absence of homosexual desires. . . . Clearly these results do not encourage . . . optimism," British psychologist M. P. Feld-man concluded in a critical review of aversion therapy.[135] But a record of well-documented failures did not deter others from using this painful and humiliating form of "treatment" to attempt to "cure" homosexuality.

People diagnosed with what psychiatrists and psychologists referred to as "transvestism" were also targeted by behavioral psychologists and psy-chiatrists who believed they were able to offer a cure for a disorder that they agreed with psychoanalysts was essentially "fetishistic" in nature.[136] In 1961, a team of researchers in Surrey, England, subjected trans people to aversive conditioning "based on the hypothesis that the aberrant behavior has been acquired as a learned response, and must be abolished along the lines dictated by the laws of learning."[137] It was crucial "to prepare the con-ditioned stimulus carefully," they noted, "so that it corresponds exactly to the patient's perversion." Since their patient was "not excited by the texture or feel of women's clothes" but instead by dressing in front of a mirror, they projected photographs of the patient in various stages of female dress and played a tape recording of the patient's own narrative of pleasure in dress-ing, so as to "insure the presence of the stimulus even when the patient's eyes were closed during vomiting."[138] In 1963, newspapers around the coun-try described the treatment of a patient who had "since childhood experi-enced strong desires to dress in female clothes." Standing on an electric grid in a small room—a rubber mat stapled with copper wire and attached to a generator—the person was instructed by the doctors to put on their favorite clothes while a "sharp electric shock" was delivered to their bare feet. This treatment was repeated seventy-five times a day for six days, resulting in an experience "so unpleasant" that doctors reported that the patient "neither desired nor indulged in any transvestite behavior" six months later.[139]

Behavioral psychologist Michael Serber described a technique that exploited the aversive effects of humiliation and that he dubbed "shame aversion therapy," which was developed as an accidental discovery in the process of photographing a patient cross-dressing in order to prepare slides to be used in conventional aversion therapy with electric shock. When Serber instructed the patient to begin dressing, he noticed that they were embarrassed and "ashamed to be observed." Theorizing that humiliation and shame might be substituted for pain as the aversive stimulus, Serber reported that a twenty-five-minute photographic session "had completely 'turned [the patient] off'" and had "changed his entire feeling about cross-dressing." In later sessions, in which Serber required the patient to cross-dress in front of him and two assistants, they "hesitated, cried, and asked to stop" and reported having nightmares and "intermittent anxiety" between shame aversion sessions—signs of profound trauma that, to Serber, signaled success. Another patient of Serber's, a thirty-four-year-old "voyeur-exhibitionist," "showed disassociated thought-content" during a shame aversion session and had to be placed on tranquilizers for several weeks afterward.[140]

One report on the treatment of cross-gender identity by a team of psychiatrists at the University of Mississippi Medical Center in 1973 revealed the psychiatric desire for the wholesale eradication of gender and sexual difference and the destruction and reconstruction of personhood that was at the heart of the behavioralists' project. The patient was seventeen years old, too young to be considered for the gender-affirming surgery they wanted and requested, and who agreed instead to enter a behavior modification program "on the premise that it might at least make him more comfortable" and might sufficiently modify their behavior so as to ward off the bullying and torment they experienced in high school. In what the psychiatrists touted as "the first successful change of gender identity in a diagnosed transsexual," they described in detail their development of a treatment plan based on their analysis of "male and female components of sitting, standing, and walking," as well as vocal pitch, intonation, and sexual orientation. Over the course of a year, they reported, the patient's entire comportment was changed from feminine to masculine through the use of behavior modification techniques.[141] When, after several months, the patient "behaved like a man, felt like a man, and thought as a man does" but was still sexually attracted to men, the psychiatrists turned to aversion therapy with electric shock to attempt to extinguish same-sex desire. "These data suggest that complex role behavior such as masculinity or femininity can be defined, broken down into its components, and changed piece by piece," the psychiatrists wrote, "producing clinically important changes."[142] The behavioralists' project, then, and by their own account, involved the psychic disassembly of a person and their reconstruction along normative lines.

Psychologists and psychiatrists pressed on in experimenting with aversion therapy to treat homosexuality and gender nonconformity, attempting to fine-tune the process by deploying different aversive stimuli and varying the timing of their delivery. Some attributed Freund's poor results in early trials to his use of emetic drugs. Because people metabolized emetics differently, the drugs were unpredictable in their onset and effect, making it difficult for the physician to time the induction of nausea to coincide precisely with the attractive stimulus, as dictated by learning theory.[143] Nausea-inducing drugs were also "highly unpleasant," behaviorists acknowledged.[144] Chemical aversion required an arduous hospital stay over many days. The treatment regime induced fear, hostility, and sometimes aggressive resistance on the part of patients. Emetics could also have harmful and potentially lethal side effects. When a psychologist subjected a patient diagnosed with transvestism to chemical aversion in 1961, he had to reduce the dose after they fell into "a semi-collapsed condition."[145] After seventy-two emetic trials, the aversion had to be terminated when "the patient succumbed to the rigors of the treatment," suffering from impaired coordination and dangerously elevated temperature and blood pressure. British psychiatrist Basil Jones described a case in 1962 in which he had to terminate an aversive treatment trial because the patient developed acetonuria, a potentially lethal concentrate of acetone in the urine caused by the administration of nausea-inducing drugs over the course of thirty-two hours.[146] Emetics were also distressing for the staff administering them, and drug-induced aversive nausea placed great demands on the nurses responsible for cleaning up after patients. "It is not uncommon for attendants to object to participating in this form of treatment," psychologist Stanley Rachman reported, "and there can be no doubt that it arouses antagonism in some members of the hospital staff."[147] A student nurse who helped administer aversion therapy in England in the 1960s described a patient's room as "comparable to a zoo: there was feces, vomit, and urine everywhere."[148]

For these reasons and more, electric shock became the aversive stimulus of choice for most behaviorists. Psychiatrists and psychologists valued it for its more precise control, which made it possible to administer in closer association with the behavior to be modified. This fetishized claim to precision was emphasized to the point of redundancy by Rachman, who wrote that the therapist using electric aversion therapy "is in a position to administer a discrete stimulus of precise intensity for a precise duration of time at precisely the required moment."[149] Unlike chemical aversion, electric shock allowed for frequent repetition of the association between the unwanted behavior and the aversive stimulus. Psychiatrists and psychologists shocked patients up to seventy times a day for many days in a row over the course of several months—a long-term, high-intensity regimen that they referred to as "massed practice."[150] Aversion therapy using electric shock also offered the advantage of being able to be administered in a clinic rather than a hospital and by a single therapist rather than requiring a medical team. As with nausea, "most people have a fear of electric shocks," a response that therapists believed made the stimulus usefully frightening but less physically dangerous.[151]

Behavioral therapists administered shock to patients at intensities intended to be, in medical euphemism, "distinctly unpleasant" and that were, in a more honest assessment, "extremely painful."[152] (As one psychologist noted, "avoidance learning improves at higher shock intensities.")[153] One early technique was to place the patient in a small, darkened room, the floor of which consisted of an electrical grid that delivered shock to the feet. As they refined the technique, most psychologists came to rely on a battery-powered apparatus with electrodes that attached to the patient's forearm or calf. Some aversive shock devices were small and portable enough that patients could administer shocks to themselves in their own homes, to "reinforce the patient's conditioning when he is away from the protective confines of the office or institution."[154] Farrall Instruments, the leading manufacturer of equipment for aversive conditioning, advertised the "Take-Me-Along," a "personal shocker" that was "easily concealed and unobtrusively operated by the patient so that he can administer shock to himself whenever he encounters, in real life, stimuli associated with his disorder." Despite its small and unassuming appearance, the ad promised that "the apparatus has a very aversive shock" of up to eight hundred volts.[155]

Behaviorists experimented with a range of treatment protocols using electric shock. In some instances, patients could avoid the shock by instructing the therapist to change the slide with the "homosexual stimulus" within a sufficiently short period of time; other therapists made shock inevitable regardless of the patient's response, with the aim of compounding its aversive effect.[156] In violation of their purportedly scientific method, many clinicians improvised elements of the treatment plan as they went along. In a critical review of aversion therapy, Feldman charged that "very few of the techniques . . . have been derived in any logical way from the general body of the experimental psychology of learning."[157]

While behaviorists shared some views with psychoanalysts about the challenge of treating homosexuality, they operated under different assumptions about what homosexuality and gender nonconformity, in essence, were. While psychoanalysts understood them to be regressive and neurotic adaptations to family pathology and early trauma, behaviorists conceptualized them instead as bad habits—forms of "maladaptive behavior" acquired by learning and thus susceptible to unlearning, or what one behaviorist tellingly called "the extinction process."[158] Patients undergoing aversion therapy were told, in simple and straightforward language, "We view this type of problem as a bad habit that has been picked up over the years and we are going to try to break that habit."[159] Some behavioral psychologists intended this language to shift the understanding of homosexuality and gender nonconformity away from sickness and cure. As psychologist J. G. Thorpe wrote in 1963, "If we regard homosexuality as a learned behavior pattern and not as a disease, then the medical concept of cure is also inapplicable."[160]

In place of the language of normality and abnormality, behaviorists referred to adaptive and nonadaptive behaviors. Still, the language of disorder and cure inevitably crept into their accounts. Judgment about sexual and gender difference featured prominently in aversion therapy, often in ways that behavioralists instrumentalized in their therapy. Some combined aversive shock or emetics with "hectoring condemnation," playing taped recordings that "stressed the 'disgusting and unpleasant' nature of the patient's deviation."[161] Psychologist David Barlow described this aspect of treatment in grotesque detail: the patient was encouraged to visualize approaching his boyfriend's apartment. As he got closer and then opened the door to see his boyfriend lying naked on the bed, the administering doctor told him, "You can sense that puke is filling up your stomach and forcing its way up to your throat." As the patient visualized walking toward his boyfriend, the doctor told him, "You can taste the puke, bitter and sticky and acidy on your tongue, you start gagging and retching and chunks of vomit are coming out of your mouth and nose."[162] A variation of this scene, other therapists noted, "might involve the patient finding the homosexual contact rotting with syphilitic sores, or finding that the contact had diarrhea during the sexual encounter."[163] Psychiatrist Michael Miller believed that because gay men, "like females," were disproportionately sensitive to sensations of smell, touch, and taste; tended to be "fastidious"; and were "often averse to a lack of cleanliness and personal hygiene on the part of their sexual partners and often compulsive about their own cleanliness," it was possible to "exploit such sensitivities and aversions by regressing these individuals back to the time of their most disturbing disgust reactions" and to connect those reactions to the male body.[164] These efforts to cultivate the feeling of disgust and exploit its aversive effects, of course, depended on the belief that disgust was a commonsensical response to same-sex desire and could be expected to chime in some shared response in the patient.

In spite of their differences, psychoanalysts and behavioralists shared an understanding of homosexuality as based, in large part, on a fear of heterosexuality. Consequently, many practitioners paired aversive conditioning with therapeutic procedures intended to increase heterosexual responsiveness. At the most basic level, aversion therapists hoped that simple relief from electric shock or nausea, when paired with images of attractive heterosexual partners, would spark heterosexual desire. Some injected gay men with testosterone while showing them images of attractive women, and sometimes they encouraged men to masturbate to them. Some made use of a plethysmograph, an instrument that measured men's erectile response, in an attempt to empirically verify evidence of heterosexual attraction. Others went further, supplementing aversion treatment with social training in "heterosexual skills."[165] To be treated for homosexuality in the aversion therapy program at Temple University, overseen by psychiatrist Joseph Wolpe, patients were required to have "a cooperative (female) partner" with whom they could have sex.[166] Behavioral therapists staged role-playing sessions, teaching their patients "courting skills . . . from the beginning right up to intercourse."[167] Inculcating heterosexual desire in gay men turned out to be one of the most difficult tasks for aversion therapists. Indeed, one psychologist who surveyed the literature found that "there is no evidence that aversion relief increases heterosexual responsiveness."[168]

As with electroconvulsive shock treatment and lobotomy, aversion treatment was also used beyond the clinic in more explicitly disciplinary, punitive, and carceral contexts.[169] At the Atascadero State Hospital, a man convicted of sex with adolescent boys described undergoing aversion treatment with electric shock. "You're sitting there, and you catch yourself tripping about a kid or something. And bap! The shock right on the inside of the wrist."[170] Some men incarcerated at Atascadero and other prisons who were deemed "incorrigible," rebellious, or uncooperative, as well as those designated as "sex deviants," were subjected to a particularly abusive and dangerous form of aversive conditioning, injected with the drug succinylcholine, which paralyzed the person's muscles, temporarily stopping their breathing and producing a sensation of suffocation and drowning. "Although the effect of death is only a few seconds," one observer wrote, "the impression is enormous."[171] "The patient feels as if he had had a heavy weight on his chest and can't get any air into his lungs," psychiatrist Walter Nugent reported. "The patient feels as if he is on the brink of death."[172] One reporter estimated that more than one hundred Atascadero patients were treated with succinylcholine between 1966 and 1969.[173] Electric shock was used as well at Atascadero, Vacaville, and other prison hospitals, and "many of the prisoners receiving electrotherapy have been gays," the *Berkley Barb* reported in 1975.[174]

Behavioralists matched and in some cases surpassed their psychoanalytic competitors in optimism about their ability to cure expressions of sexual and gender difference, boasting higher success rates with shorter and less expensive treatments. The behavioral therapy team at the Temple University Medical School, for instance, claimed a success rate of 80 percent, contrasted with the 30 to 40 percent purported to be achieved by traditional psychotherapy.[175] "Behavior shapers are an optimistic bunch," an article in the *Los Angeles Times* reported in 1973. "Evangelism sparks in their eyes when they talk about their science."[176]

Psychiatrists' boasts of high cure rates, however, were often accompanied with caveats about who was most likely to be "treatable" and "curable." Conversion to heterosexuality was much more easily accomplished, psychiatrists and psychologists acknowledged, with people who otherwise conformed to conventional gender norms. Many conceded that "overt" or "committed" homosexuals, usually identified as such by their gender nonconformity, were beyond their ability to cure. In the case of men, psychiatrist Judd Marmor observed, treatment was more effective on those with "a relatively intact masculine gender identity" than those "who are obviously effeminate or swishy."[177] While some psychiatrists and psychologists held that normalizing a patient's gender through psychiatric treatment might be possible if they were diagnosed with "transvestism," which they understood to be a fetishistic attachment to cross-dressing, most admitted that it was unlikely to be effective for those with cross-gender identification and a desire for gender-confirming surgery (ironically so, given psychiatrists' promotion of psychiatric treatment for trans people over surgery and hormones). Bieber boasted of his ability to cure homosexuals, "with the possible exception of effeminate transvestites."[178] Of her experience treating lesbians, Claudia Wilbur wrote that "the 'dyke' rarely seeks treatment" and was largely impervious to it and that the lesbians who came to see her were "usually of the 'feminine' type."[179] The gender-variant and queer figures that had been the focus of such intense preoccupation in earlier decades—the fairy, the pansy, the bulldagger, the butch—were all but written off by psychoanalysts in their search for curable homosexuals.

Motivation was also crucial. Psychiatric treatment only worked when the person truly wanted to change, most psychiatrists acknowledged, so genuine commitment on the part of the patient was a key requirement. "Alienation from homosexuality," psychiatrist Lawrence Hatterer observed, was linked to a "highly favorable prognosis."[180] Therapy to reorient sexual orientation to heterosexuality was less likely to work with people who had never had heterosexual sex. It worked better on younger people than older ones, who were judged by many psychiatrists as too set in their ways to change (Hatterer found that people over the age of thirty-five had "a poor prognosis").[181] People who "have the greatest choice to change," Hatterer summarized, were those who "have been least *homosexualized*."[182] Not surprisingly, "alienation from homosexuality" led to a "highly favorable prognosis" for conversion.[183]

The number of people on whom psychiatric treatment could *not* be expected to work, then, by the admission of psychiatrists themselves, was strikingly high. One might have expected that mid-century American psychiatric optimism would be dampened by psychiatrists' many provisos and bracketed exceptions about their ability to treat and "cure" homosexuality and their own admissions of low "cure" rates and outright failures, but it was not. On the contrary, psychiatric enthusiasm for "cure" amplified over time, as psychiatrists expanded their jurisdictional claim over matters of gender and sexual nonconformity and extended their reach into new institutional and clinical venues, the criminal justice system, and popular culture.

## CHAPTER THREE

# Psychiatric Power and Queer Life

Edmund White, a novelist, memoirist, and gay man who came of age in the 1950s American Midwest, opens his autobiography *My Lives* with a chapter titled "My Shrinks." In so doing, he identifies an encounter with psychiatry (in his case, encounters with multiple psychoanalysts over the course of nearly a decade and a half) as foundational to his own relationship to his sexuality. White was in his mid-teens in the mid-1950s when his mother sent him to a psychoanalyst in the Chicago suburb of Evanston, Illinois, in an attempt to cure him of his homosexuality. That was the first of many such efforts through the late 1960s, when, White reflected, "I was still a self-hating gay man going to a straight psychotherapist with the intention of being cured and getting married."[1]

White's experience was shaped by the privileges of gender, race, and class. Psychoanalysis, especially in its orthodox, expensive, and time-intensive form, was no doubt more central to the experience of men, who could more often afford it, than to women, and certainly more so to white people than to people of color. That fact has led historians to conclude that the reach of psychiatry's institutional and epistemological sway and pathologizing effects were limited to white men of privileged backgrounds in northeastern coastal cities.[2] But the influence of psychiatry's understanding of sexual and gender variance as forms of treatable mental illness extended far beyond those who could afford private analysis. To be queer or gender nonconforming in the United States in the middle decades of the twentieth century was to live in a culture saturated with psychiatric power. The world that psychiatrists made during the height of their professional prestige—one in which they leveraged institutional, cultural, and state power in large part by defining gender and sexual difference as treatable mental disorders—would be one that many if not most queer and gender-nonconforming people would have to navigate.

It is true that if we restrict our understanding of psychiatry to psychoanalysis, the dominant intellectual trend in psychiatry at mid-century, and if we understand an "encounter" with psychiatry to require a face-to-face clinical relationship, our story will be limited to mostly white men of means, most of whom lived in big cities. Psychiatrist Benjamin Karpman acknowledged that psychoanalytic treatment was typically "prohibitive for economic reasons to everyone except the wealthy."[3] Fees for analysis varied—by psychiatrist, by region, and over time—but some expendable income was a base requirement. Writer Patricia Highsmith paid her Manhattan analyst fifteen dollars an hour in 1948. "Of course need to find work to pay for all of this," she wrote in her journal.[4] A former patient of Irving Bieber recalled that Bieber charged five dollars an hour in the early 1950s—a low fee for the time that was probably offered on a sliding scale, but when multiplied by three times a week, an expense that "placed a prohibitive strain" on the fifty dollars a week he earned as a writer.[5] Martin Duberman paid his analyst twenty dollars a session while an undergraduate at Yale in the early 1950s.[6] Being middle class, Jewish, New York raised, and Ivy League educated, Duberman was careful to particularize an experience with psychiatry and psychiatrists from the 1950s through the early 1970s that he speculated he shared with "many other privileged young middle- and upper-class big city white men of the pre-Stonewall generation who, like myself, had internalized the reigning medical model of homosexuality as pathology, who could afford the fees of the talking cure."[7]

Some among Duberman and White's educated and left-leaning demographic were no doubt drawn by what historian Barbara Taylor would characterize decades later as the "prestige-value" of psychoanalysis. "I was infatuated with psychoanalytic theory," Taylor wrote in her account of her own institutionalization in the 1980s. Along with other members of the British "left-wing intelligentsia," she "read it voraciously, talked about it incessantly, formed strong opinions on ego-psychology, Jung, Lacan. Freud was my god, I read him devotedly." "Hovering on the edge of this world, listening to people comparing analysts, swapping couch gossip, I yearned to join in," Taylor recalls, "or so I thought."[8]

From its introduction in the early twentieth century, psychoanalysis captivated intellectuals, activists, and academics in the United States as well. When anarchist and political organizer Emma Goldman heard Freud lecture in Vienna in 1896, she "grasped the full significance of sex repression and its effect on human thought and action" for the first time, and was led to "understand myself, my own needs."[9] Literary critic and Smith College professor Newton Arvin, who grew up in Valparaiso, Indiana, with a sense of "radical difference" as a "girlish small boy" and experienced his first relationship with a man as an undergraduate at Harvard, wrote to his childhood friend David Lilienthal in 1920 to ask, "Are you 'up' much on Freud?" Arvin had "read several of his things this year," and as a consequence was "obsessed (literally) with the desire to be psychoanalyzed."[10] That attraction grew with the expanding influence of psychoanalysis in the United States in the 1940s and 1950s. "Read lots of Freud," Highsmith recorded in her diary in June 1943, "which brings my heart joy!"[11]

Despite the pathologizing judgment, and in some cases outright hostility, that many mid-century American analysts brought to their treatment of queer people, it is not difficult to understand the particular attraction that queer and trans people felt to psychoanalysis as "the first great theory and practice of 'personal life,'" one that put sexuality at its center and understood human behavior as motivated by sexual impulses beyond one's conscious control.[12] "In the middle decades of the twentieth century," Duberman writes, psychoanalysis was "the elective choice of the moment, *the* certified path to self-knowledge."[13] "Psychoanalysis gave voice to this sense of a unique, idiosyncratic intrapsychic life," historian Eli Zaretsky writes, an idea that surely appealed to people eager for self-knowledge and anxious or curious about motivations and desires that put them at odds with the society around them.[14] "There was now a way to discover hidden factors from the past that caused sexual problems," writer Dan Wakefield recounted in his memoir and cultural history of life in New York City in the 1950s, and "the name of this seemingly magical, but certifiably scientific process was psychoanalysis."[15] For queer people, the psychoanalytic emphasis on the power of the unconscious and its critical appraisal of the normalizing demands of civilization may have held out a special appeal. "Homosexuality inclines one to introspection," Edward Sagarin wrote under the pseudonym of Donald Webster Cory in 1951. "All homosexuals feel that they are forced to seek the origins of their sexual temperaments," and consequently turn to "self-analysis."[16] "Why am I this way?" wondered Frances Elliott, institutionalized at Saint Elizabeths in the mid-1940s following an alcoholic binge, the dissolution of her marriage, and her recognition of her attraction to women.[17] Elliott and other queer people searched for answers to what historian Jennifer Terry terms "questions of the self," questions "by which the subject must account for herself as an anomaly: 'Who am I?' 'How did I come to be this way?' 'How and why am I different?' 'Is there something wrong with me?'"[18] Psychoanalysis offered a purportedly scientific method, one with considerable cultural cachet, to address those questions for people who puzzled or despaired about sexual desires or gender difference characterized as deviant.

## Pathways to Psychiatric Scrutiny

The intellectual attractions of psychoanalysis notwithstanding, gay men had a reputation among mid-century psychiatrists for avoiding psychiatrists unless they were under some form of coercion.[19] Lesbians were even less likely to pursue psychiatric treatment on their own initiative, psychiatrists believed. Los Angeles psychiatrist May E. Romm conjectured that "because society is not so alert in discovering and censoring the sexual preferences of homosexual women, such women have less anxiety about their inversion and therefore seek psychiatric help less frequently than do male homosexuals."[20]

"Very few homosexuals ever seek treatment," psychiatrist Samuel Hadden noted in 1955, "until either the law or their families force them into doing so."[21] Queer and gender-nonconforming people often ended up in psychiatric treatment as a result of external compulsion or coercion, whether familial or legal. A father's rage about his daughter's love life was the animating force behind the case that inspired one of the first psychoanalytic texts on homosexuality, Sigmund Freud's "The Psychogenesis of a Case of Female Homosexuality," published in 1920. Freud's analysis of the young woman was initiated by her father, who "boiled over with anger" when he learned of his eighteen-year-old daughter's passionate infatuation with an older woman. "It was evident that this one interest had swallowed up all others," Freud reported. "The girl did not concern herself with any further educational studies, placed no value on social functions or girlish pleasures, and kept up relations only with those friends who could help her in the matter or serve as confidantes." When she attempted suicide, her father pressed Freud to take her on as an analysand, entrusting him "with the task of bringing their daughter back to the normal."[22]

Freud felt uncomfortable about treating someone under his care only as the consequence of parental pressure, as he believed that "the ideal situation for analysis is when someone, otherwise master of himself, is suffering from an inner conflict which he is unable to resolve alone, so that he brings his trouble to the analyst and begs for help." Entering into treatment under the compulsion of others, Freud felt, was "unfavorable for psycho-analysis."[23] But he apparently overcame his skepticism and conducted a brief analysis of eleven weeks with the young woman.

In the decades that followed, psychiatrists and psychoanalysts would likewise put aside their discomfort with treating people who came to their offices and clinics at the behest of others rather than of their own volition.

Indeed, many psychiatrists depended on that coercion for their livelihood. Parents continued to pressure their children into psychiatric treatment, and their authority over sons and daughters was especially striking in autobiographical accounts and case studies of queer and gender-nonconforming people. "I have seen a number of homosexual people who came in here with a bayonet up their backs, from their families," one New York City psychiatrist reported. "They were found out, so they were dragged in to see me."[24] Romm recalled treating a twenty-year-old woman whose parents threatened her with "dire consequences" if she did not see a psychiatrist to cure her of her lesbianism.[25] Barbara Gittings, who would become one of the leading activists in the fight for the declassification of homosexuality as a mental illness, had several unproductive sessions with a psychiatrist at her father's insistence in 1954, after she failed her classes at Northwestern University and her father discovered her copy of Radclyffe Hall's *Well of Loneliness*. In a fascinating correspondence between Gittings's father and her psychiatrist, Dr. Paul J. Poinsard, one in which neither referenced Gittings's lesbianism directly, Poinsard wrote, with regret, that he had "few specific suggestions to make of things that might help Barbara toward a more happy adjustment in the future" because she was "resistant to the idea of changing the way that she is in terms of her feelings and attitudes towards people and life in general."[26] Gittings's father pushed back, pressing Poinsard for "a suggestion for a practical and inexpensive programme, outside of psychiatric treatment, towards overcoming this trouble." But Poinsard replied that there was "no effective means" of resolving her "conscious and unconscious conflicts" "other than continuing psychiatric treatment."[27]

Some parents and spouses went so far as to have family members committed to mental hospitals for homosexuality or gender variance. The process of involuntary psychiatric commitment varied by state, but in the 1930s and 1940s, reforms were enacted across the country that were intended to make commitment a medical process rather than a legal one and to transfer decision-making power from judges and juries to psychiatrists.[28] Superintendents and psychiatrists at Saint Elizabeths, for example, campaigned to end the mandatory jury trials under which people had long been committed in the District of Columbia, arguing that they were harmful and humiliating. They succeeded in 1938 in replacing commitment by jury with review by a panel of nine psychiatrists, to be convened by a newly formed Commission on Mental Health. Commitment to Saint Elizabeths required the petition and affidavits of two "responsible residents" of the District of Columbia alleging that the person was "of unsound mind, unable to manage his affairs," not fit to be "at large," and "in need of treatment."[29] If the commission determined a person fit that definition, they were sent first to the psychiatric ward at a nearby municipal hospital for observation and assessment. If the ruling was affirmed, they were committed to Saint Elizabeths.

Throughout the nineteenth century, most commitments to mental institutions were initiated by immediate family members.[30] That dynamic continued through the twentieth century and was especially evident in cases of young people discovered by their parents to be queer or gender nonconforming. Rex Cronin, a college student living in Washington, DC, was committed to Saint Elizabeths by his parents in the mid-1930s after he invited his boyfriend home with him. "They would sit at the table eating and mincing over their food," his mother reported, "talking 'love talk,' with their arms about one another."[31] His parents first employed the upper-class strategy of separating their son from his lover by sending him to Europe, but when time and distance failed to dissolve their relationship, his mother arranged for her son to be hospitalized at Saint Elizabeths.[32]

Case files, hospital records, and psychiatrists' writings are full of such stories of parental coercion. When a nineteen-year-old college student in Philadelphia began to cut his classes, "plunged into the 'gay' life of the community," and feared he would be suspended from school, he confessed "the nature of the problem" to his parents and they had him committed to a private sanitarium for eight months.[33] When another young man lashed out physically at his father on being discovered dressed in women's clothes, he was sent to a private psychiatric hospital in White Plains. "I don't think I wanted to kill him," the patient reflected later, or even to hurt him, but rather, driven by "hellish burning shame" on his exposure, he intended "to create some diversion to take the crux of the situation away from the female clothes."[34] The superintendent of Pilgrim State Hospital, one of the eight state hospitals for the mentally ill in New York and the largest mental institution in the United States, reported in 1962 that the hospital admitted around a hundred homosexual patients a year, many of them teenagers committed by their parents.[35] When Margaret Deirdre O'Hartigan's parents learned of her enrollment in the University of Minnesota's gender identity clinic in the 1970s, they moved to hospitalize her "for electroshock treatment."[36] Husbands and wives also committed their spouses or pressured them into psychiatric treatment. In 1956, a woman whose spouse had traveled to Europe for "an emasculation . . . for purposes of 'sexual transformation'" had her committed to a state hospital. Her spouse was later referred to the University of Illinois Neuropsychiatric Institute, where psychiatrists diagnosed her decision to transition as "a defense against homicide directed especially toward the mother figure and mother-surrogates."[37]

By the late 1960s, gender-affirming medical care began to be available in a few university clinics. But strict rules and restrictions governing access to that care, requiring evaluation by a psychiatrist, added another form of compulsion for people who sought medical transition. Indeed, it was impossible for people desiring access to legally prescribed hormones and surgery to avoid psychiatrists since they effectively established themselves as the arbiters of admission to medical gender transition.[38] Historian Jules Gill-Peterson observes that what is now called "conversion therapy" and transsexual medicine were "developed in tandem," with psychiatrists working as gatekeepers to medical transition and with a "failed bout of conversion therapy" serving as a "prerequisite for transition."[39] Many psychiatrists shared Charles Socarides's view, stated in 1970, that "the fact that a transsexual cannot accept his gender is a sign of emotional and mental disturbance." "It is the emotional mental disturbance which must be attacked through suitable means by psychotherapy," Socarides maintained, "rather than amputation or surgery."[40] For these reasons, if "given a choice," Nancy Hunt wrote in her account of her transition in the 1970s, "a transsexual would never consult a psychiatrist in the first place except for the fact that a psychiatrist's recommendation is usually required for surgery; few doctors will operate without it." Thus gender-nonconforming people, too, were likely to seek psychiatric treatment in the context of coercion, if only in the effort to get "permission to attain the salvation of surgery."[41]

Queer people, and gay men especially, were also compelled into psychiatric treatment by force of law. By the 1950s, psychiatrists had thoroughly embedded themselves in the criminal legal system, a relationship bolstered by their claims to expertise regarding homosexuality. "In this area," psychiatrist Manfred Guttmacher wrote from his position as chief medical adviser to the Supreme Bench of Baltimore, "psychiatry must be of the very greatest assistance to the courts."[42] Psychiatrists and psychologists staffed the new court clinics funded by sexual psychopath laws, served as expert witnesses, delivered psychiatric assessments of people charged with criminal offenses, made recommendations for sentencing, and oversaw probation and parole. That relationship grew more lucrative for psychiatrists in the 1950s and 1960s as the policing and criminalization of queer people intensified.[43] Queer people could be arrested under an array of public order statutes that targeted a range of behaviors and subject positions defined as "lewd and lascivious," or for loitering, solicitation, public exhibitionism, contributing to the delinquency of a minor, the capacious crime of vagrancy, laws against cross-dressing, and, less frequently, through laws against sodomy (though arrests for sodomy increased dramatically in these decades as well).[44] New York state criminalized gay cruising as a form of disorderly conduct (sometimes referred to as "degenerate disorderly conduct," or simply "degeneracy").[45] Vagrancy laws often included under their sweeping definition "lewd and dissolute" persons, a charge used so often that such people were referred to by police and the courts in California as "vag lewd." As historian Risa Goluboff summarizes the legal landscape for queer people at mid-century, "Vagrancy laws criminalized the status of being lewd, and law enforcement officials understood homosexuality, by definition, to be lewd. This made gay men and lesbians vagrants, and that made them criminals."[46]

Anti-cross-dressing laws, passed in more than forty municipalities across the United States, in both big cities and small towns, provided another tool to police gender nonconformity and another opportunity for collaboration between psychiatry and the criminal legal system. Increasingly, over the course of the twentieth century, cross-gender expression was understood to be both a public offense and evidence of mental disorder.[47] Growing up as a young Black trans woman in Chicago in the 1950s, Miss Major Griffin-Gracy recalled that "wearing a dress could get you sent to jail immediately. And not really jail," she qualified. "Cause they didn't put us in jail at that time. They felt that if you were a different gendered person in attire that didn't suit your birth gender then you were a crazy person. And they would take you to . . . [the] mental hospital!" Miss Major was institutionalized "several times," in Chicago and later in Bellevue Hospital in New York City.[48]

Psychiatrists did not merely assist courts with assessing criminality, determining proper sentencing, and weighing the possibility of rehabilitation. Their affiliation with the courts and involvement in legal processes also *drove* the criminalization of sex offenses, homosexuality primary among them. Collecting data from courts in Baltimore, where he directed the court clinic, Guttmacher found that sex offenders formed about 20 percent of the total number of cases referred to the Baltimore Court Clinic for psychiatric evaluation from 1952 to 1954. That number, he observed, represented a sharp increase from the 3 to 5 percent of sex offenders referred to the clinic twenty to twenty-five years earlier. That marked increase "is not due to any significant increase in sex offenses tried in our courts," Guttmacher acknowledged; instead, and boastfully, he attributed it to the fact "that judges have come to recognize sexual criminality as an area of social pathology to which psychiatrists can contribute understanding and counsel of value."[49]

Same-sex-desiring men were the target of this enhanced surveillance, policing, and criminalization in the postwar United States, but the law's application (and by extension, the reach of psychiatric power) was determined by race and class. Guttmacher encapsulated the way that the consequences for "homosexual offenses" followed race, class, and social hierarchy in his summary of the fates of three people arrested and convicted of "homosexual offenses" in Baltimore in the 1950s. A "48-year old Negro" man who "masturbated in a public park in daylight" was given a six-month jail sentence. His sexual partner, a "deteriorated chronic alcoholic," presumably white given that his race went unremarked on by Guttmacher, was committed to a state psychiatric hospital. And finally, "a soldier and a law student," also racially unmarked and therefore presumably white, was arrested for having sex with a man in a parked car and was granted "probation without verdict" and required to pursue treatment with a psychiatrist to protect him against future disbarment and dishonorable discharge from the army.[50] Guttmacher laid out these varied outcomes for similar "crimes" to support his claim about the value of judicial discretion informed by psychiatric knowledge. That knowledge underwrote and legitimized a racialized sorting and shuttling of people in and among the linked institutional sites of regulation—the prison, the psychiatric hospital, and the clinic.

Some gay people who were arrested and convicted of crimes submitted themselves to psychiatric treatment on the order of the court in lieu of jail time, in exchange for a shorter sentence, or as a condition of parole—a practice with origins in the Progressive Era and facilitated by judicial discretion in the lower criminal courts, which handled misdemeanors and lesser felonies. The connections forged between those courts, psychiatrists, and state-run psychiatric clinics created a courtroom-to-clinic pipeline.[51] Because the policing of queer people intensified over the same decades that psychiatry gained great power and influence, that pipeline was a robust one. For some psychiatrists, court referrals probably accounted for the majority of their patients (and therefore the majority of their income). Hadden reported that most of his gay patients came to group therapy after having been arrested and taking judges up on their offer of psychiatric treatment over jail time. "Proof that they are seeing a psychiatrist regularly is all that is necessary," Hadden wrote.[52]

Psychiatrists conceded that patients compelled to seek treatment by the court were not inclined to be strongly motivated to change. To the contrary, Hadden noted, "They may be initially hostile to a situation which seems punitive rather than helpful."[53] "More than once I have been called upon by an officer of the court to give a note to the effect that I have been seeing certain homosexuals who were simply fulfilling the letter of the court's requirement, with no real motivation for treatment."[54] But that skepticism did not discourage psychiatrists from accepting as patients people ordered by the court to undertake psychiatric treatment. Some people undergoing court-ordered psychotherapy seemed more concerned with the length and cost of treatment than its efficacy. Thomas Johnson, a forty-four-year-old married man, was fired from his teaching job in a suburban Maryland high school and ordered to undergo psychiatric treatment after he was arrested for having sex with men. While in treatment with Karpman, Johnson was anxious about the financial strain of analysis: "I have been coming to you for treatments for 14 months now," he wrote, "and can not afford to go on indefinitely," adding that paying $50 a month for analysis "is a lot to a poor school teacher like myself."[55] Another man in treatment with Karpman after having been arrested for public exposure in a theater in 1956 also complained about the cost of psychotherapy, which, after a year, he thought was taking much too long: "I know that I have tried to be as cooperative with you to the utmost to make a quick ending of this case," he wrote to Karpman. "I know that I never wanted it to linger, as the expense has been terrific for me, as I am a poor man."[56]

Psychiatrists' collaboration with the courts meant that psychiatric power and authority extended far beyond those who entered into treatment of their own volition, and therefore far beyond the middle- and upper-class white men that historians usually feature in discussions of psychiatric authority over queer people. A survey conducted in 1960, which estimated that 30 percent of gay men and 12 percent of lesbians had arrest records, offers a sense of the wide reach of the law's impact on sexual minorities.[57] The possibility of arrest loomed so large, for gay men especially but also for some lesbians, that the Mattachine Society printed up wallet-sized cards explaining "What to Do in Case of Arrest."[58] The Daughters of Bilitis authored a guide under the same title and invited an attorney to speak to members on the topic in 1956.[59] Queer and gender-nonconforming people who undertook psychotherapy under legal compulsion were often those also criminalized by poverty, transience, homelessness, unemployment, and alcoholism. And so while private psychoanalytic therapy may have been largely limited to white men (and some white women) of means who lived in metropolitan areas where most psychoanalysts practiced, psychiatric treatment for sexual and gender difference when mandated by judges was prescribed for a much wider demographic. Among the participants in a New York City therapy group in 1959, for instance, was Alfred, a thirty-two-year-old married Black man referred to the clinic by the Probation Department of the Court of Special Sessions following his arrest for soliciting sex in a subway restroom.[60] Baltimore psychiatrist Lino Covi's psychotherapy group of thirty patients, many of whom were there as a condition of their sentence, included eight white women, five Black men, five skilled and unskilled manual workers, and five people who were unemployed.[61]

People convicted under state sexual psychopath laws, which were passed over the same decades in which psychiatry was gaining great influence, were among those for whom the law was a route to psychiatric scrutiny and treatment. While historians have characterized gay men as the collateral victims of mid-century sexual psychopath laws that targeted violent sexual crimes against children, the congressional debate on the District of Columbia's Miller Law reveals consensual sex between adult men to have been a deliberate and even primary target. The Miller Law increased the punishment for sexual offenses with minors, as well as for sodomy. But the aspect of the law that most radically enlarged its purview was its inclusion of behavior characterized sweepingly as "inviting for the purpose of immorality."[62] Although the imperiled child was the privileged subject of community outrage and media reporting on sex crimes and has been characterized by historians as the instigating motor of these laws, Minnesota representative George MacKinnon identified the primary focus of the Miller Law as the man who "is a constant menace to society, particularly to younger boys and young men." That person was particularly dangerous, MacKinnon insisted, in contexts of hierarchical relations among men such as the military and the workplace: "They go around and they may not force them, but the fact that they may have a superior rank, they may be a chief petty officer where the boy is in a subordinate capacity; and the same thing exists out in the ordinary, everyday life where somebody may be an employer. . . . And while it is true there is no act of force, such a person is a substantial menace to society."[63] The virtue of the Miller Law, in the eyes of its proponents, was in criminalizing such acts of "social menace" that were not captured by existing criminal law but were newly understood as indicative of dangerous sexual psychopathy. Psychologist Blanche Baker, a counselor at Mendocino State Hospital in northern California, observed in 1959 that to her "utter amazement," a large number of the cases referred to her were "plain, garden variety homosexuals who were sent there on a sexual psychopathology charge."[64]

That fact was apparent in the case files of Saint Elizabeths Hospital as well, where those determined to be sexual psychopaths in the District of Columbia were committed to indefinite sentences. When George Raymond was brutally beaten by two men whom he and a friend picked up for sex in 1949, he ran toward the road, hailed a car, and asked to be taken to the police. "I don't recall why I did this," he stated, "for later I had every reason *not* to call the police." Rather than chasing down his assailants, the police took Raymond to jail; there, "one of them hit me and gave me a black eye."[65] He was later evaluated by two psychiatrists, who, when they learned of his sexual history with men and adolescent boys, determined him to be a sexual psychopath as defined by the District of Columbia's Miller Law. So diagnosed, and without a criminal charge or conviction, he was committed indefinitely to Saint Elizabeths.

Historians have noted that fewer men of color than white men were diagnosed as sexual psychopaths under the new statutes of the 1930s and in the following postwar period. Rather than being subject to psychiatric diagnosis and treatment, some speculate, Black men were more often treated as criminals and incarcerated in prisons rather than hospitalized as patients.[66] Stephen Robertson argues that mid-century psychiatrists viewed sex crimes that would have been a sign of dangerous sexual pathology for white men as dangerously criminal (and "normal") for Black men.[67] But while Black men may have been less dramatically disproportionately represented among those determined to be sexual psychopaths than they were in incarcerated populations more generally, they did not escape the psychiatric-carceral net created by sexual psychopath legislation and were still disproportionately committed under sexual psychopath statutes.[68] Some left traces in the archive beyond the simple fact of their institutionalization. Twenty-six-year-old Samuel Archer claimed to have been falsely accused of molesting children with another man. When he was arrested, the police "said they would squeeze it out of me till I did confess." Then, he reported, "they tightened up on me and did things I won't relate." He was taken to Gallinger Hospital for an evaluation; after being judged to be a sexual psychopath, he was given an indefinite sentence at Saint Elizabeths Hospital. Archer maintained his innocence of the charge and was confused by his hospitalization: "I am not feeling sick or bad in any way. I am not out of my mind."[69]

In 1963, Arthur Alston, a twenty-seven-year-old Black man from Baltimore identified in his case file as an "unskilled laborer," was arrested and convicted for assault with a deadly weapon. Alston was diagnosed by a court-affiliated psychiatrist with "emotional immaturity reaction" as well as "sexual deviation, homosexuality," with the latter evaluation earning him a designation as a "defective delinquent" and an indefinite sentence at the Patuxent Institution in Jessup, Maryland, a maximum-security facility designed to house the state's most dangerous and "psychopathic" criminal offenders.[70] Alston appealed his sentence to Patuxent's director, arguing that he had not been convicted of a sex crime. When his appeal was denied, Alston wrote to Frank Kameny, a gay activist and founder of the Washington, DC, chapter of the Mattachine Society, to ask for help. "Should I be convicted of this," Alston wrote, "I am afraid . . . I'll be here for the rest of my life because of my personal life."[71] Kameny corrected what he took to be Alston's misunderstanding of the law, responding, "I do not understand your being 'convicted' or committed for BEING *a homosexual*. There is no such crime. To be a homosexual is against no law. No state can put you in prison or otherwise restrict your freedom for this."[72] While Kameny's claim may have been technically true, Alston better understood the ways in which his own criminalized racialization worked along with sexual psychopath legislation to authorize his perpetual incapacitation. Legal and psychiatric power were intertwined and mutually reinforcing. In Alston's case, psychiatry's entanglement with the carceral state, along with the long-standing association of blackness with criminality, resulted in his indefinite institutionalization on the grounds of his homosexuality.

## The Pull of the Normal

While many people underwent psychiatric treatment under the compulsion of family members and the court, the more diffuse but still powerfully coercive force of a hostile culture was sufficient reason for many others to seek treatment with the hope of a cure. In psychologist Albert Ellis's view, the need to adapt to the world as it was—in the mid-twentieth-century United States, one that harshly penalized and stigmatized homosexuality—was the principal reason for queer people to pursue psychotherapy and cure. An outspoken champion of sexual liberalism and sexual pleasure, Ellis had little patience for arguments against homosexuality (or other nonnormative sexual expressions, including sex between siblings and sex between adult men and underaged girls) based on moral judgments and what he considered the "puritanical sex attitudes" of American culture.[73] But "whether you like it or not," Ellis told one of his patients, "we live in contemporary Western civilization, and not in ancient Greece nor in any other culture where homosexuality is fully accepted." "However foolish it may be for our society to ban homosexual relations between consenting adults," Ellis went on, "the fact remains that it presently *does* punish homoeroticism." That meant that people were "unjustly jailed, fined, fired from jobs, and otherwise ostracized for engaging in sex acts with members of their own sex."[74] To another patient, a voice teacher and a married man, Ellis reminded him that "in this society, in your position in life, with your wife, with your pupils, you could get absolutely ruined." Conversion from homosexuality to heterosexuality was necessary, Ellis told him, "not because homosexuality was 'wicked or wrong,'" but because it was "stupid to do it while it is against the law."[75] Ellis assured another patient that the "urge to handle a man's genitals" was "a perfectly good thing," but when he felt that urge, to remind himself that "my goddamn society doesn't allow it, therefore I can't do it." Ellis compared the urge to have sex with men with the urge to steal, telling his patient that while he might be tempted to reach out and take the "bank notes piled up behind the teller's window," he was able to stop himself "because you know you can't get away with it."[76] If the patient lived in ancient Greece, Ellis told him, "you would have no trouble. You would have been screwing boys, having a great time, and then marrying, having a wife, and also screwing girls in the market place." "But you weren't raised in ancient Greece," he reminded him. "You were raised in this society," with its punishing laws that made homosexuality, in Ellis's view, an irrational and self-defeating lifeway.[77] In a context in which homosexuality was policed and harshly penalized, Ellis argued, it was incumbent on people to seek treatment. Resistance to psychiatric cure was simply more evidence of mental instability, since "anybody who defeats his own ends," Ellis reasoned, "is obviously crazy."[78]

The hostility of the broader culture and fears about the potential consequences of sexual and gender difference—the prospect of arrest, the fear of public exposure, the possibility of the loss of a job, the threat to a marriage, or the fear of the wrath of parents—did indeed motivate many people to consult a psychiatrist. Eugene Davis, a Black man in his early thirties who aspired to run for public office, sought treatment at Saint Elizabeths when a relationship with another man "was spreading to other boys and because it was undermining my efficiency." "Instead of going up, advancing, I find that I was going down. . . . Instead of going up the ladder," he wrote, "here I am indulging in homosexual practices, an evidence of mental degeneracy and deterioration, and I find that I was getting further away from my goal . . . instead of approaching it." "I cannot describe the remorse I have been under since this thing came into my life," Davis added.[79] He explained his reason for coming to Saint Elizabeths as "chiefly to keep from being arrested."[80] He was not alone in seeking psychiatric treatment in order to avoid arrest, which to many men seemed a nearly inevitable consequence of queer life. When one of Ellis's patients was arrested for cruising, it convinced him "that I may be incapable of remaining out of serious trouble unless I was in therapy."[81] Another sought help from Ellis in 1966, writing that his "problem" was "getting to a place that it would soon destroy me or my life completely."[82] One man told psychiatrist Charles Socarides that he had become "increasingly fearful of exposure and the ensuing legal and social consequences" of homosexuality and wished to enter into treatment with the aim of "develop[ing] a heterosexual personal life."[83] Another of Karpman's patients, a married businessman, had been blackmailed by a man who solicited sex from him in a public restroom. That experience, combined with his confession to his wife about his desire for men and "talk of separation," led to his first hospitalization at Saint Elizabeths in the late 1930s and treatment with insulin-induced convulsive shock. A decade later, in 1948, feeling depressed and fearful "that strangers were talking about his homosexuality," he was institutionalized again, certain that homosexuality was "the real source of my trouble and unhappy experiences," and with the "intense desire for the cure of my homosexuality."[84]

Others were concerned about the threat of exposure as queer to their jobs or professional ambitions. One person wrote to Ellis from Vietnam in 1966, expressing their concern that their life was "dominated with transvestite fantasies," which threatened their successful career as a Foreign Service officer. Aware of the U.S. government's "not entirely unjustified attitude toward this sort of thing," they wrote to Ellis "against every blind instinct of self-preservation" to ask for help.[85] Fear of exposure was not limited to people in high-status professional careers, or to men. Marijane Meaker, who wrote a popular account of lesbianism in 1955 under the pseudonym Ann Aldrich, introduced Iris, a male impersonator who went by the name "Rick" "in gay circles," who went to a psychoanalyst to be "cured" out of "fear of old age." "What'll become of me when I'm forty or fifty?" Rick asked. "How long can I hold a job where I can wear these clothes? . . . The future scares the hell out of me!"[86] Sex researchers William Masters and Virginia Johnson treated over one hundred men and women for homosexuality between 1968 and 1977 and found that the dominant motivating factor for those who sought "conversion" to heterosexuality was "social pressure." The men who came to their institute worried about "public identification" and "the concomitantly implied social threat to their job security"; the lesbians who applied for treatment did so, they reported, out of concern for the fate of their marriage.[87]

For some queer people, a sense of exclusion from what one psychiatrist called "the heterosexual human family" was enough to propel them into psychiatric treatment. "It is . . . this motivation," psychiatrist Albert Abarbanel-Brandt wrote in 1966, "this yearning to be normal," that compelled people to seek treatment.[88] Historians committed to documenting examples of queer courage and resistance have tended to downplay the profound unease in the face of the challenges of queer life that many people felt and their longing for normalcy. But that emphasis on queer defiance and celebration of the flouting of norms requires that we read the historical record very selectively and ignore evidence of the deep effects of stigma and exclusion on queer and gender-nonconforming people. In the late 1930s, one man feared that his homosexuality would make him "a disgrace to my family" and committed himself to Saint Elizabeths. "It is one of my greatest desires to overcome what homosexuality I have as much as possible," he wrote, "so that I may lead a normal, practical heterosexual life with a wife and children in a home of our own."[89] Albert Wright entered into psychoanalysis with Karpman in 1951 because his homosexuality "causes me to feel lowered," and because he couldn't "see anything but unhappiness in being a homosexual."[90] When Betty Berzon entered into her first relationship with a woman in 1951, she initially felt "deeply involved and thrilled by it," but later felt "excluded from the mainstream of life, and corrupted and ashamed." "Out of those feelings," Berzon recalled, "I tried to destroy myself." She was committed to a psychiatric ward after a suicide attempt. "I was 23 years old and I felt doomed to this shadow existence," she explained.[91] Hadden described a man who entered into group therapy with him in 1964: "He reported that he was depressed and disgusted by his . . . promiscuous homosexual life," which involved spending every night "in gay bars, Turkish baths, and in liaisons with men he had known for years." Disillusioned, he "could see no future in his homosexual existence."[92] A lesbian in psychoanalysis with Karpman in the mid-1940s told him that "my soul feels like a pig-sty sometimes when I think of this Homeric maggot in me."[93] "The intolerable feeling of being different" led another lesbian to undertake psychiatric treatment while in college in the early 1960s.[94] A team of Boston-based psychiatrists described a thirty-two-year-old married man with a fourteen-year history of "homosexual experiences," "usually in public toilets," who had recently fallen in love with a man, a relationship that threatened his marriage and "motivated him to seek treatment."[95] Charles Silverstein went to a psychiatrist with the goal of curing his homosexuality, motivated by "the shame it would represent in the family; the feeling of being a pervert; being a criminal; losing all my friends; not being able to get married and have children."[96] Martin Duberman recalled the way that the "incantatory psychoanalytic rhetoric" echoed in his mind, leading him to consult psychiatrists in search of cure: "Homosexuality, by its very nature, meant a lifetime of wrong connections, the impossibility of nurturing commitment."[97]

Some people invoked the language of disease and disability to describe the sense of pain and shame that drove them to psychiatric treatment. Accepting the psychiatric establishment's judgment that he was "a disabled person," "defective," and "crippled in my affective life," Duberman characterized the promise of "conversion" to heterosexuality as "my only hope for a happy life."[98] "I am a homosexual woman," one woman in treatment with Karpman wrote. "A half-masculine freak. What can I do about it?"[99] Another woman, writing in 1945, referred to her "dazed, choking realization of my homeric tendencies—like an unhealthy, cancerous growth which I cannot throw off."[100] One man's "growing state of panic" led him to seek psychiatric treatment with Karpman in 1948. After a sexual experience with a man at a bathhouse, he had "a feeling that something horrible had been indelibly burnt into me."[101] Edmund White sought out therapy, he recalled, "because I was in such terrible pain, driven by desires I wanted to eradicate because I felt they were infantile, grotesque, damaging, and isolating."[102]

It is important to keep in mind the context in which people made these comments and the audience they addressed them to. Some surely framed their understanding of their sexual or gender difference in terms they thought a psychiatrist might want to hear, and others did so in retrospect, from the vantage of years of reflection and with the intention of contrasting the attitudes of an earlier time, one that psychologist John Money characterized as an "era of the shame of being," with a more progressive present day.[103] At the same time, it is impossible to discount the evidence of distress and even trauma that many people felt about their sexual and gender difference in the middle decades of the twentieth century. That evidence speaks to the underexplored power and extent of stigma in queer history and the importance of what French philosopher Didier Eribon terms "insult" in modern gay subject formation. "A gay man learns about his difference through the force of insult and its effects," Eribon writes; and "this wounded, shamed consciousness becomes a formative part of my personality."[104] In his classic work on stigma, published in 1963, at a time when pathologizing psychiatric explanations of homosexuality were in full force, sociologist Erving Goffman linked homosexuality with other "blemishes of individual character," including mental disorder, imprisonment, and unemployment, and likened the psychotherapy to cure homosexuality to the plastic surgery pursued by a "physically deformed person."[105]

## Psychiatry and Mid-Century American Culture

While many queer and gender-nonconforming people entered into psychiatric treatment in the 1940s, 1950s, and 1960s—whether compelled to do so by family members or a judge, swayed by the coercive pressures of a hostile society, forced to do so in an effort to access gender-affirming health care, or drawn by their own interest and curiosity or by shame and distress— many more surely learned about psychiatric ideas about gender and sexual difference through less direct means. In the middle decades of the twentieth century, at the zenith of psychiatrists' power and influence, psychiatric ideas exerted authority far beyond the clinic and the hospital. Psychiatrists promoted ideas about homosexuality and gender difference that traveled beyond their publications in specialized and often arcane journals into the broader public discourse via their own, more popular writing; its translation in best-selling books, magazines, and mass-market paperbacks and by journalists; and its uptake in postwar American culture more generally.

Many people who were curious, confused, or distressed about their own desires consulted the published writing of psychiatrists in an attempt to understand their gender or sexual difference. "As a young homosexual you feel alone," activist Gary Alinder wrote. "You need answers but there's no one to talk to. So you read books."[106] Indeed, accounts of defining and often life-changing encounters with psychiatric ideas about homosexuality through reading are repeated so often in the writing and recollections of queer people in this period as to constitute a foundational experience of queer self-knowledge. While in high school, sensing that "there was something radically wrong with me," Raymond Shea read works by Freud, Carl Jung, Stekel, Havelock Ellis, and Hirschfeld to find the "cause" of their cross-gender identification. That reading led Shea to feel that "[I] had an unnatural attraction toward my father," but "I never found out how to cure it."[107] In 1949, as a first-year student at Northwestern, Barbara Gittings cut her classes to spend time in the library "reading about myself in categories such as 'Sexual Perversion'—and wondering and worrying."[108] As an undergraduate at Stanford in the early 1950s, Betty Berzon recalled that the "trip to the library was nerve-wracking." "I looked all around before I pulled out the little wooden drawer marked 'H,'" she admitted. Catalog cards directed her to books that "told me that homosexuals were perverted, diseased, social outcasts, and pitiful creatures." For Berzon, that knowledge was reassuring: "Whatever my feelings for women might be," she wrote, "they had nothing to do with the awful condition described in those books."[109] Others felt more implicated by what they read. "The prevailing psychoanalytic theory was that the cause of homosexuality was an overprotective mother and a hostile, distant father," Charles Silverstein learned. "Had these authors been peeking through the windows of my home?"[110] Ron Gold had more distance than Silverstein on the psychiatric texts he read, "but something always seemed to ring true. . . . I almost believed Dr. Bergler's notion that my persistence in going to bed with men was nothing but 'self-created troublemaking' caused by my 'unconscious wish to suffer.' I began to think that my love was 'childish' and 'sick.'"[111] Black trans woman Cei Bell recalled "reading psychiatry books" as an effeminate teenager and learning that "a favored treatment for homosexuality was electroshock therapy."[112]

Writer Samuel Delany also testified to the power of psychiatric texts in influencing his own ways of thinking about and representing himself. After "a kind of breakdown" in 1964, at twenty-two years old and newly married, Delany was hospitalized in New York City. At the time, Delany recalled, "homosexuality was a 'mental problem' if not a 'mental illness,'" and it was an issue he felt obligated to discuss in his group therapy. Fearful but determined, Delany "launched in" with "the most abject of confessions": "I had this problem—I was homosexual, but I was really 'working on it.' I was sure that, with help, I could 'get better.'" But when he was alone that night, Delany reconsidered his own contrite explanation of himself. "I'd talked like someone miserable, troubled, and sick over being gay; and that just wasn't who I was." To the contrary, Delany realized, his "actual feeling" was that the "gay aspects of [my] life" were "the most educational, the most supportive, the most creative, and the most opening part of my life." "Where had all the things I'd said that morning come from?" he wondered. Answering his own question, he attributed his ideas about homosexuality to "a book by the infamous Dr. Burgler [*sic*]" that he had read as a teenager and "that had explained how homosexuals were psychically retarded." Delany came to realize that books like Bergler's create a "public language," one that he took up unthinkingly; in the process, he came to understand, he had "betrayed" his own experience.[113]

It was not necessary to go to college or have access to a medical library to learn about psychiatric thinking about homosexuality and gender difference. Others read about the work of psychiatrists or the writing of psychiatrists themselves in more popular forms. Bergler's book, *Homosexuality: Disease or Way of Life?*, published in 1958 and announcing "the fact that homosexuality can be cured" to "diversified groups of people," was a bestseller, which was reviewed widely and positively through seven editions.[114] Albert Ellis authored columns for *Playboy* magazine, *True* magazine (also known as "A Man's Magazine"), and *Pageant* and published more than seventy-five books, many of them bestsellers. He was also a regular contributor to the homophile publications *ONE* magazine and the *Mattachine Review*. There, subscribers could read about his claims that "exclusive" homosexuality constituted a dangerous neurosis that could be cured.[115] Many people requested treatment from Ellis or asked him to refer them to a psychiatrist after reading his popular 1965 book, *Homosexuality: Its Causes and Cure*. One man wrote to Ellis in 1969 from Puerto Rico about the possibility of moving to New York to enter into treatment with him. "I read in a magazine an article in which you explain the way you cured a homosexual with a special method you have developed," he told him.[116]

Others learned about psychiatric thinking about homosexuality and gender variance through reading published inquiries to popular advice columnists and their responses. The influential Protestant clergyman Norman Vincent Peale used an advice column in the popular biweekly magazine *Look* to answer a young man's anguished question about homosexuality in December 1956. Their published exchange exposed the magazine's more than three million readers to the understanding of homosexuality as a mental disorder and the possibility of psychiatric "cure." "You are suffering from an emotional sickness," Peale wrote to the nineteen-year-old. "If you want to get over your trouble . . . I feel sure you can become a normal person."[117] In reviewing 130 letters from men and women to Peale expressing anxiety about same-sex desires, historian Rebecca Davis finds that Peale's correspondents "largely accepted his description of homosexuality as a disease and found hope in the prospect of a cure."[118] Davis proposes that psychiatric thinking about homosexuality fit neatly within Peale's liberal Protestantism and its optimistic assessment of human nature, as well as his belief that happiness "required marriage and a family."[119] That appeal might have been at work as well for Martin Luther King Jr., who wrote a monthly column, "Advice for Living," for *Ebony* magazine from 1957 to 1958. King was no doubt moved as well by what historian Thaddeus Russell describes as an understanding "that the attainment of full citizenship for African Americans required the creation of a heteronormative black culture."[120] In January 1958, *Ebony* published the letter of a young man who wrote to King to say that he felt "about boys the way I ought to feel about girls" and who asked, "What can I do? Is there any place where I can go for help?" King reassured him that his problem was "not at all an uncommon one" but that it was "culturally acquired" rather than "an innate tendency," and he instructed him to "see a good psychiatrist who can assist you in bringing to the forefront of conscience all of those experiences and circumstances that lead to the habit."[121] The fact that the religious leaders King and Peale called on the language of psychiatry rather than that of religion and morality testified to the persuasive power of psychiatry's medicalized understanding of homosexuality at mid-century.

By the 1960s, Ann Landers and Abigail Van Buren began to publish letters about homosexuality with some frequency in advice columns that were widely syndicated in newspapers across the country. Ann Landers, a pen name created by a *Chicago Sun-Times* columnist in 1943 and taken over by Esther Pauline "Eppie" Lederer in 1955, promoted a sympathetic approach to people whom she characterized as lonely and "tortured" and whom, she reported, she often "counseled . . . through the mail."[122] She also told readers in 1964 that homosexuality was a "gross symptom of a serious psychological disturbance" and described it as "unnatural," a "sickness," and a "dysfunction."[123] Landers repeated that framing nearly ten years later, in 1973, the year the American Psychiatric Association removed homosexuality from the *Diagnostic and Statistical Manual of Mental Disorders*, telling readers that homosexuality, "in spite of what some psychiatrists say," was "a sickness—a dysfunction."[124]

The popular column Dear Abby, founded in 1956 by Lederer's twin sister Pauline Phillips under the pen name Abigail Van Buren, also often featured letters and responses about homosexuality. In a column in 1969, Abby wrote to a woman who had recently learned that her husband had had a past relationship with another man that her "authorities on this subject tell me that homosexuality is 'learned' and can be 'un-learned' IF . . . the patient is properly motivated. . . . Your only hope," she concluded, "is to insist that he see a psychiatrist."[125] Landers and Van Buren responded to questions from people about gender nonconformity as well, taking care to distinguish "transvestism" from homosexuality. "Though it may seem unbelievable to you," Abby wrote to a woman whose husband liked to wear her underwear, "a transvestite is NOT necessarily a homosexual. So when you describe your husband as something 'less than a man,' you may be doing him a disservice."[126] Likewise, in answer to a woman whose boyfriend liked to wear her clothes, Landers reassured her that he was "not a homosexual." "If you want to marry a man who enjoys wearing your clothes and getting passes from men," she wrote, "go ahead. But please urge him to get professional help right away."[127] To the parents who found women's lingerie in their eighteen-year-old son's gym bag, Landers said they should "get him to a doctor at once."[128] When a mother wrote to Landers in 1970, distressed that her child wanted to undergo gender transition, Landers responded that "individuals who so desperately desire to be of another sex that they are willing to have their bodies mutilated are severely disturbed."[129]

Read by millions, advice columns circulated psychiatric ideas about homosexuality and gender variance to a broad reading public. At the same time, advice columnists proved to be less than reliable translators of the postwar psychiatric understanding of homosexuality in all its aspects. Although both Landers and Van Buren communicated to readers the belief that homosexuality was a form of mental illness (Van Buren changed her mind on this question by the mid-1970s; Landers held on to it until 1992), neither was sanguine about the possibility of cure. In 1967, Landers responded to a woman in distress about her daughter marrying a gay man, "The chances for 'curing' a homosexual are slim, even when the sick one wants desperately to live a normal life."[130] In 1968, Landers reported that cure rates were "something under 5 percent."[131] In 1970, Van Buren wrote that "almost all my mail from homosexuals themselves says that the most they can hope for is understanding on the part of others, and the ability to accept themselves as they are, and learn to live with it."[132] Contrary to the insistence of psychiatrists that homosexuals were paranoid "injustice collectors," whose efforts to identify and protest discrimination were properly understood as a symptoms of their neurosis, and in spite of her own pathologizing views, Van Buren located the roots of the mental illness that purportedly manifested in gay people in oppression and stigma rather than family dysfunction. When one reader asserted that "the homosexual is a crippled personality in other ways than sex," Van Buren asked, "Who can blame him? All his life he's heard that he's a 'sick, perverted, abominable, loathsome creature,' or some kind of freak. He has had to live like a criminal much of the time—for fear someone would find out about him."[133] In answer to another correspondent's insistence that homosexuality was "a form of mental illness," Van Buren wrote that "much of the maladjustment seen in homosexuals is due to the rejection, persecution, and guilt imposed upon them by intolerant and ignorant contemporaries."[134]

The question-and-answer form of the advice column, encouraging readers to comment on each other's queries and weigh in on the columnists' responses, showed both the uneven uptake of psychiatric ideas and their vernacular translation. Van Buren's increasingly sympathetic posture invited a letter from a mother of a gay son who thanked Abby for her "kind words in defense of homosexuals" and explained that "most homosexuals feel that they were born that way and are not the product of their environment." "Please ask any one of your medical experts how easy it would be for him to turn himself into a homosexual if society demanded it," she requested. At the same time, the mother concluded with a hope and prayer "that some day there will be a medical cure for these poor persecuted individuals.[135] Many of Landers and Van Buren's correspondents echoed the psychiatric assessment of homosexuality as an illness, but their deployments of "sick" as an epithet (with variations including "sicko," "twisted," and "wacko") exposed the judgment and contempt at the heart of a diagnosis that claimed to be objective, scientific, and humane.

By the 1960s, readers of popular magazines also learned about homosexuality from feature stories in popular magazines, most of which affirmed the expertise of psychiatrists and their belief that homosexuality was a mental disorder. In 1964, *Life* magazine published an article titled "Homosexuality in America," which concluded with a section on "Medical and Psychological Aspects."[136] In another article published in *Life* later that year, journalist Ernest Havemann worked to disabuse readers of the antiquated understanding of "our great-grandfathers," who "believed that homosexuality was inherited: some men were just born 'queer,' with a woman's disposition in a man's body." This view, Havemann told readers, had been countered successfully by psychiatrists, who "believe that homosexuality represents a form of arrested development."[137] In 1965, *Time* magazine announced in the title of one of its articles that "Homosexuals Can Be Cured," which included an interview with psychiatrist Samuel Hadden.[138] Journalists often translated psychiatric ideas for a broad audience in language that brought to the surface the hostility that was often more muted and implicit in psychiatrists' writing. In "The Homosexual in America," a two-page essay published in *Time* magazine in January 1966 and featured on the magazine's cover, readers learned that homosexuality "is a pathetic little second-rate substitute for reality, a pitiable flight from life" that deserved "compassion . . . and, when possible, treatment," but "no glamorization, no rationalization, no fake status as minority martyrdom, no sophistry about simple differences in taste—and, above all, no pretense that it is anything but a pernicious sickness."[139]

Black popular magazines of the same period were typically more circumspect in their coverage of sexual and gender difference and sensitive to associations of blackness with deviant sexuality.[140] But there, too, readers could learn about psychiatric ideas about homosexuality and gender transgression. In 1952, *Jet* magazine published "Is There Hope for Homosexuals?," an article that identified homosexuality as "the biggest psychological problem of modern times," one studied by psychiatrists who "have viewed homosexuals as sexually immature, often guilt-ridden, maladjusted persons." The best hope for cure, *Jet* concluded, was to be found in the work of Benjamin Karpman, who "claims that he has cured 32 such persons, many of them Negroes."[141]

Popular print culture extended the influence of psychiatric thinking on homosexuality to wide and diverse audiences. For many more people, screening for induction into military service would be another site of encounter with psychiatry and psychiatric thinking about homosexuality as a mental disorder, one serious enough to disqualify people from service. Psychiatrists warned government officials of the "psychopathic personality disorders," homosexuality among them, that they believed rendered men unfit to fight. When appointed as consultants to the Selective Service, psychiatrists devised procedures of psychiatric screening for military inductees. Those standards and methods were often diluted or deformed in translation by local draft examiners and the demands of a mass practice undertaken by over six thousand local draft boards staffed by people untrained in psychiatry and unable to adopt the individualized approach recommended by psychiatrists. But beginning in 1941, the integration of psychiatry into the process of military screening meant that the eighteen million American men who were examined at induction stations and draft boards during the Second World War encountered some version of the medical model of homosexuality and the concept of homosexuality as an undesirable and disqualifying personal trait, even if only in the rushed and abbreviated form of formulaic questions from a draft board examiner.[142]

Queer and gender-variant people in the middle decades of the twentieth-century United States encountered psychiatric thinking and authority in a range of direct and indirect ways. Some sought psychiatric treatment out of personal distress or curiosity, some were compelled or coerced to submit to it by family members and courts, and no doubt many more learned about psychiatric ideas about sexual and gender difference as part of the air and water of postwar American life and culture. Psychiatric authority was not total, however, nor were queer and gender-nonconforming people simply the passive recipients or victims of their encounter with it. Psychiatry and modern homosexuality may each have required the existence of the other, as Kenneth Lewes proposes, but both were transformed by their encounter.[143]

## CHAPTER FOUR

# Psychiatric Encounters

"Total institutions" are "the forcing houses for changing persons," sociologist Erving Goffman asserted. "Each is a natural experiment on what can be done to the self."[1] Goffman made this claim in *Asylums*, his classic work on the social world of mental patients, based on a year of participant observation fieldwork at Saint Elizabeths Hospital in 1955 and 1956. With these words, Goffman conjured the adaptive transformations wrought by institutional regimentation, the "abasements, humiliations, and profanations of self" that attended life in the psychiatric hospital.[2]

Goffman intended his observations of the asylum to extend to other closed worlds—the prison, the boarding school, the convent, the concentration camp. But Saint Elizabeths was more than a convenient case study for his reflections on the transformative effects of sequestered institutional life. Beyond the hothouse ecosystem of the psychiatric hospital, mid-century psychiatry more generally declared itself a "forcing" technology dedicated to "changing persons." Nowhere was that project more explicit than in psychiatrists' curative approach to homosexuality and gender variance.

Psychiatrists were optimistic about the transformation they hoped to effect in their queer and gender-variant patients. However, reading their published work against the grain, alongside writing by people in psychiatric treatment, tells a more complicated story of the changes wrought by that treatment. Psychiatric encounters were radically asymmetrical in their balance of power, and some people subjected to psychiatric treatment learned to understand themselves according to the language and logics offered by psychiatrists or were compelled to make their desires and self-understandings fit psychiatric narratives. At the same time, psychiatric encounters, especially those structured by the practice of psychoanalysis, were dialogic and improvisational, marked by performance, negotiation, subterfuge, and sometimes outright resistance. Some people in psychiatric treatment took advantage of those opportunities, exploiting the possibilities in what Foucault termed the "microphysics of power" that circulated between psychiatrist and patient to push back against pathologizing ideas and articulate new understandings of self and new critiques of a hostile world.[3] Others forged a collaborative relationship with psychiatrists, a collaboration that left its mark on psychiatric practice and psychiatric knowledge as well as on modern queer subjectivity and politics.

## Shame and Subjection

Historians of marginalized groups have understandably been drawn to stories of resistance. The history of the encounter of queer people with psychiatry offers up such stories, to be sure. But it should not surprise us that for many people who came under psychiatric scrutiny, psychiatric thinking and treatment instilled, compounded, and consolidated a sense of shame. After his admission to Saint Elizabeths in 1933, one man wrote that he "answered something like three, four, or five hundred questions," many of them focused on homosexuality, which "giv[es] one a feeling of being some kind of monstrosity."[4] Falling in love with another man for the first time as a Harvard undergraduate in 1920, Newton Arvin wrote incandescently about the "very beautiful, very fine, and very precious thing that has come into my life, and very nearly changed the whole seeming of existence to me."[5] But two decades later, after years of psychotherapy, several hospitalizations, and a series of electroconvulsive shock treatments, Arvin's internalization of the psychiatric understanding of homosexuality led him to understand himself as beset by a "loathsome affliction."[6] Hospitalized at Saint Elizabeths in the early 1940s, Marina Harris wrote that after months in psychotherapy with Karpman, "my homosexual tendencies are now ugly and revolting to me."[7] Three months at the Payne Whitney Psychiatric Center in New York City convinced a trans woman that she was a "humanoid, a freak."[8] "Everybody saw me as a 'case,'" Jane Fry wrote after spending three years in intensive psychotherapy and months in psychiatric wards in the 1960s for her cross-gender identification. "It's like, 'Look, Joe, we've got a real live one now. I only read about these things in books, now we've got one.'" "It didn't make me feel good to be so odd," Fry explained.[9] "Almost all of us bought into the straight notion that there was something really wrong with us," Alan Helms wrote in his memoir of gay life in New York in the 1950s and 1960s. "We knew that . . . we were beyond the pale of what was considered acceptably human." A sense of shame, Helms recalled, "was pervasive in our lives, and I don't know anyone of my gay generation who's ever been able to shake it."[10] Karl Bryant's experience as a research subject in psychiatrist Richard Green's study of feminine boys in the late 1960s at the University of California, Los Angeles, in a gender clinic established to normalize the gender of queer and gender-variant children, made him "feel that I was wrong, that something about me at my core was bad, and instilled in me a sense of shame that stayed with me for a long time afterward."[11]

Psychiatric thinking about homosexuality carried so much authority in mid-century America that even those who publicly challenged the psychiatric paradigm of mental disorder and ventured more affirmative arguments for queer existence seemed to feel required to acknowledge and endorse at least some of psychiatry's claims. Edward Sagarin advanced the novel argument that homosexuals were an oppressed minority worthy of civil rights in his groundbreaking 1951 book (published under the pseudonym Donald Webster Cory), *The Homosexual in America*. And yet he echoed psychoanalysts' claims when he enumerated the "causes" of homosexuality in "broken homes, divorces, early deaths, frigid parents, unequal love," and especially the "unbalanced love of a boy for his mother."[12] Writing under the pseudonym Ann Aldrich, Marijane Meaker intended her 1955 book *We Walk Alone* to be the lesbian counterpart to Sagarin's sweeping account of gay men. But Meaker, too, opened her largely affirming insider account of lesbian life with the question of etiology and an implicit acknowledgment of pathology. In a chapter titled "How did She Get that Way?," she cited fear of sex with men and a search for "mother substitutes, child substitutes, and substitute sisters" as among the causes of lesbianism.[13] Meaker concluded her book with a chapter that asked "Can a Lesbian Be Cured?," agreeing with mid-century psychiatrists that heterosexual conversion was possible for those who truly desired it.

Some gay men incorporated the psychiatric understanding of homosexuality as a mental disorder into camp humor. Of gay social life in New York City in the early 1960s, Edmund White recalled that "there was never a gathering that dissolved before one of us felt the other's head for a fever and declared, 'But pet, you're not a well woman,' making light of the effeminacy we feared and the mental illness we could not deny." "We wilted into stylized attitudes of illness," White wrote, "mock[ing] our low self-esteem without in any way elevating it."[14] Mart Crowley's 1968 play, *The Boys in the Band*, about a gathering of gay friends in New York City to celebrate a birthday, opens with a canceled appointment with an analyst. In the course of a long and boozy night, the characters banter about their neuroses, their shrinks, and their experiences in analysis. "Christ," the party's host, Michael, muses, "how sick analysts must get at hearing how Mommy and Daddy made their darlin' into a fairy." Toward the end of the play, Michael ventures a utopian hope as he ponders the transformation that might come "if we could just *learn* not to hate ourselves quite so very much." But in the play's most famous line, Michael answers his own question with a cutting joke: "You show me a happy homosexual and I'll show you a gay corpse."[15]

Some people were moved through encounters with psychiatry and psychiatrists to understand themselves according to psychoanalytic logics and recast their own lives in psychoanalytic terms. Some of Karpman's patients, for instance, reproduced the genre of the psychoanalytic case file in writing about themselves as "cases," sometimes in the third person.[16] An encounter with psychiatry compelled many people to analyze and diagnose themselves, borrowing ideas and terms they learned from psychiatry. Terry Willis wrote to Karpman in 1949 that he suspected that his "mother's influence" might have "caused homeric tendencies in me" by making him do "women's tasks" in the house, such as dusting and vacuum cleaning.[17] In an appeal to Albert Ellis for treatment for transvestism, one letter writer assured him they had determined that they were "a fairly common type of sex variant, not a freak," and had "already written an analytical outline of my psychological history, running 120 handwritten pages, in an attempt at self-treatment."[18] People searched through their own family histories for clues to the origins of their difference. One man attributed his homosexuality to the fact that he had grown up without a father. "I may be wrong in my opinion as to the cause of my homosexuality," he wrote to Karpman, "but I have thought of this 'cause' for many years."[19]

Some of this ventriloquizing of psychoanalytic understandings was surely self-justifying, self-interested, and self-preserving. One man, institutionalized at Saint Elizabeths in the mid-1950s under court order after multiple arrests for sexually molesting children, came to explain his attraction to the genitals of young boys as a substitute for his mother's breast. After several months of analysis with Karpman, he wrote, "I always felt a longing and hunger that was up until now unexplainable." He was "not nursed very much by mother," he reported, and he speculated that his rejection by his mother and his thwarted desire to breastfeed were "the beginning of my turn from normalcy." [20] In psychoanalysis, he wrote, "I found the key to my whole problem."[21] "At long last we have come to a point where . . . we know why I like little boys."[22] Karpman identified this patient's self-diagnosis as self-serving: "From his point of view, he knows which side his bread is buttered," he wrote, "and is not going to tell anything that in his opinion might jeopardize the possibility of his being discharged in the near future, which is what he hopes for." Karpman also judged him as limited and deficient in his understanding of psychoanalytic concepts. "To knock into his head the meaning of the term repression is a heroic job that would take the stoutest heart," he wrote.[23]

Karpman's notes exposed the extent to which psychiatrists and psycho-analysts endeavored to instill in their patients their own theories and as-sumptions about homosexuality and gender variance. Karpman's question-naires, which opened with the question, "What are the basic psychological causes of homosexuality?," steered patients pedagogically to psychoanalytic conclusions. "Do you feel that most homosexuals have a mother-complex?" he asked one patient in 1942.[24] Some patients dutifully repeated those con-cepts back to him. "I don't know whether 'most' homos have a mother-complex," one replied, "but I think very many have."[25] Psychoanalytically oriented psychiatrists taught their patients about the Freudian concept of constitutional bisexuality and about homosexuality as a stage of human development. Benjamin Rogers confessed that until he was in psychiatric treatment with Karpman, he "had never heard the theory that everyone of both sexes has some homosexual component," and he said that the concept reassured him.[26] Harold Crowe, a thirty-six-year-old man institutionalized at Saint Elizabeths, learned through psychotherapy that "it was natural for everyone to have a varying percentage of homosexual tendencies."[27] Eu-gene Reed, a married man in his sixties who was hospitalized at Saint Eliza-beths for a suicide attempt after being blackmailed by a man who solicited him for sex in a public restroom, wrote to Karpman that he believed he had "a very clear understanding of these phases of sexual life. In infantilism," he explained, "every human is bi-sexually constituted, but as adult life devel-ops, the normal course is heterosexual." Thus far in his own life, Reed wrote, he had "not overcome the homosexual content," and so he considered him-self "bi-sexually constituted."[28]

## Challenges to Psychiatric Authority

For some people, the encounter with psychiatry instilled and compounded stigma; others called on the language and concepts of psychiatry and psychoanalysis to describe (and sometimes to absolve) themselves. For oth-ers still, that encounter could be the site of resistance to psychiatric ideas. Paul Murphy, a thirty-five-year-old man hospitalized after a breakdown in 1946, questioned whether Karpman was "stressing a little too much on sex as one of the basic causes of my 'Neurosis,'" and went on to wonder, "Who originated the origin of dream symbols and what proof is there that those dream symbols . . . are correct? Is scientific proof available?"[29] In response to Karpman's interpretation of his dreams, he pushed back, writing, "I'm goddamned sick and tired of these so called father and mother and fam-ily fixations I'm supposed to have."[30] Another of Karpman's patients protested the psychoanalytic privileging of sex as the key to understanding human motivation, writing that "after all there are other things in life besides sex, sex, SEX, continual SEX."[31] One man questioned Karpman's speculation that his homosexuality was caused by an unconscious attraction to his brother. "I cannot understand how, if I have been strongly attracted to my brother, that this attraction could have remained entirely on the subconscious level and never broken through to my consciousness."[32] Of a lesbian under his care, Karpman wrote that "as usual, her associations are not helpful, and she persists in her ridicule of all Freudian ideas."[33] When Martin Duberman's analyst conjectured that his "unconscious resistance" to sex with women stemmed from a "breast complex" and asked him if he had "reacted violently to being weaned," Duberman "laughed and said I couldn't remember as far back as yesterday's movie, let alone my experiences in the crib."[34] A man in treatment with Irving Bieber could not accept his analyst's conviction that his desire for men was based on hostility, an idea that made no sense to him, given "the profoundly affectionate, warm, life-enhancing emotion I felt for men with whom I have fallen in love."[35]

Psychoanalysts anticipated resistance on the part of patients as a predictable and even productive stage of their treatment that could alert the therapist to uncomfortable memories or especially revelatory aspects of a person's past. But some people expressed a more wholesale disinterest in being cured of homosexuality or gender variance and a more overarching disdain for the psychiatric enterprise. One woman wrote matter-of-factly to Karpman in the mid-1940s, "I do not want to be normal and I do not want to fall in love with a man. Men bore me," she clarified, and "I have no taste for that." Instead, she explained, "I like this freedom of being able to have love with a beautiful, talented, brilliant, strong, and accomplished woman." "Can this not be my cure," she asked Karpman, "instead of making me normal?"[36] Of another lesbian in analysis in 1950, Karpman documented what he called "her profound skepticism with respect to all psychoanalytic findings and her intense resistance to all forms of psychic therapy." "If people tolerated homosexuality openly, so that I were more free to experiment and seek companionship," she wrote to Karpman, "I would not be neurotic at all."[37] "Actually she does not want therapy," Karpman acknowledged. "What she wants is either a social revolution which will permit her neurosis to be accepted, or a secret means of securing sexual gratification."[38] A young college student hospitalized by his parents to separate him from a lover wrote to Karpman, explaining, "I want to know nothing about homosexuality. . . . I do not of it want to be cured."[39] Later diagnosed as schizophrenic, he wrote in response to a detailed survey presented by Karpman, "My imagination is attacking your questions."[40]

Cross-gender-identified people were typically forceful in their resistance to the prospect of psychiatric "cure." In 1953, psychiatrist Hyman Barahal recounted his work with a patient hospitalized at Pilgram State Hospital on Long Island, New York, for what Barahal termed "female transvestism." The twenty-two-year-old factory worker, who since childhood had had an "ungovernable desire to be a boy," had sought psychiatric help for anxiety and headaches but explicitly not for treatment of their gender variance. "As much as I want to be helped," Barahal's patient explained, "I don't want you to change me so that I will begin to wear dresses." Barahal diagnosed the etiology of the patient's "transvestism" in psychic masochism that "demands that she be ridiculed and made to suffer," but he noted that "analysis was carried on with considerable difficulty because of strong character resistance" over the course of months.[41]

Gender-variant people also often professed their disinterest in psychiatrists' theories of the etiology of their gender identification. "I spent three years searching for psychological reasons and other kinds of reasons, because I was expected to," Jane Fry reported to sociologist Robert Bogdan in the late 1960s, after having been institutionalized in five different psychiatric facilities. "I'm not interested in reasons anymore. I don't give a damn what caused it."[42] Bogdan noted that Fry was "particularly annoyed by professional theories that point to early trauma or an abnormal childhood with parental deprivation as the root of her feminine feelings."[43] Christine Jorgensen, who would introduce the American public to the concept of transsexuality in 1952, declared simply that "results seemed to me of greater importance than the cause."[44]

Among the most striking refusals of the psychiatric goals of curative heterosexuality were from those who had same-sex sex while institutionalized for treatment for homosexuality. At least as remarkable was the fact that so many wrote and spoke about their sexual adventures, without apology, to their psychiatrist. Patients institutionalized at Saint Elizabeths found sexual opportunities in wards, in hydrotherapy rooms, and in quiet spots around the hospital's massive, wooded grounds. One man described having sex with another man, a much younger sailor, for the first time while in the hospital: "The patient seemed so dropped in my lap by fate," he told Karpman, "that I was afraid to let the opportunity pass."[45] Marina Harris, hospitalized for alcoholism, a drug overdose, and depression following the end of her marriage, also had the first chance to pursue her attractions to women at Saint Elizabeths. Among them was her ward-mate Muriel, who "walked and talked like a man," was "aggressive and self-confident" and "a hot lover" who "makes passes at any woman on the ward," and "made love to me as a man would to a woman." After Harris was transferred to another ward, "We had little opportunity for expression of our passion for each other. . . . We would hurriedly kiss and feel each other in the box room and bath rooms."[46] Harris and Murial read together, listened to radio programs, and dreamed of traveling west, where Murial "was to dress as a man" and work as a milkman. Though Harris confessed to some guilt when she reported these liaisons to Karpman ("I know it is all wrong but I do not want to be otherwise"), it did not keep her from pursuing attractions to women while hospitalized or from telling her analyst about them.[47] The patient who reported the most active sexual life at Saint Elizabeths was a twenty-nine-year-old man hospitalized in the late 1940s following a transorbital lobotomy that failed to cure him of his depression or his desire for other men. "Many opportunities to engage in homo-sexual relationships have presented themselves here at the hospital," he reported openly to Karpman.[48] He described having sex with other patients in the movie theater, in the ward, and on the wooded grounds. He was especially proud of his liaison with a male nurse.

Others expressed themselves sexually in art. Tucked into Karpman's case files of his Saint Elizabeths patients is an envelope containing what is described as "a collection of erotic reproductions, drawings, cartoons, news pictures, montages, etc. by a female Pt depicting female homosexual, heterosexual, and mixed activities."[49] The unidentified artist seems to have worked in a range of media and the collection includes a number of her collages, composed of photographs of nude women cut out and rearranged into sexual scenes (figures 4.1 and 4.2).

Collage was part of the art therapy program that Saint Elizabeths staff used to treat and occupy patients; it is also an aesthetic form and practice that art critics and historians have identified as queer, involving appropriating found images; decontextualizing and rearranging them to create new fantasies, possibilities, and imaginaries; and "constructing new worlds and identities from the same materials as everybody else."[50] This Saint Elizabeths patient-artist employed the medium of the collage to produce lesbian erotic representation out of materials presumably marketed to heterosexual viewers, thus aestheticizing and celebrating forms of desire that the institution, and psychiatry more broadly, were trying to eradicate.

This same artist sketched hundreds of drawings in pencil on the blank back of Saint Elizabeths Hospital Daily Statement forms—forms that aides and nurses used to chart the status of patients on the ward: the number of patients and bed capacity, which patients "eloped" (or escaped) and which ones returned, who had needed to be restrained or secluded, who was "untidy," who had "city" or "ground" parole privileges, and other indices of institutional life (figure 4.3). Perhaps the forms were given to her as scrap. The institutional form bled through the blank side of the page, rendering

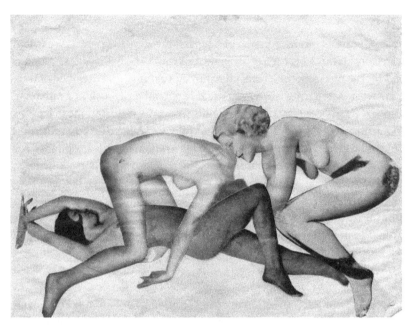

FIGURE 4.1. Collage, unidentified artist, Saint Elizabeths Hospital, Benjamin Karpman Papers, Jean-Nickolaus Tretter Collection in Gay, Lesbian, Bisexual, and Transgender Studies, University of Minnesota, Minneapolis, MN.

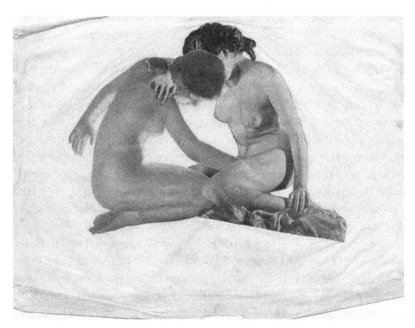

FIGURE 4.2. Collage, unidentified artist, Saint Elizabeths Hospital, Benjamin Karpman Papers, Jean-Nickolaus Tretter Collection in Gay, Lesbian, Bisexual, and Transgender Studies, University of Minnesota, Minneapolis, MN.

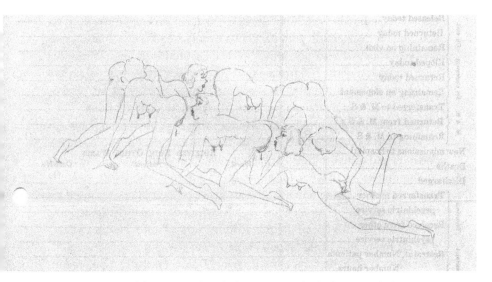

FIGURE 4.3. Pencil drawing, unidentified artist, Saint Elizabeths Hospital, Benjamin Karpman Papers, Jean-Nickolaus Tretter Collection in Gay, Lesbian, Bisexual, and Transgender Studies, University of Minnesota, Minneapolis, MN.

the artist's drawings as a kind of reverse-image or negative of that document and registering a powerful dissent to the psychiatric project of sexual normalization. Drawing on the back of those forms, the artist also created a counterarchive of queer pornography out of institutional efforts to document and exercise management and control.

Both popular and historical understandings of the responses of queer and gender-variant people to psychiatric treatment prime us to expect either shamed submission or heroic resistance to psychiatric ideas. But many encounters were more ambivalent and complex. Some patients framed their relationship with their psychiatrist as a collaboration (though one freighted with the dramatically unequal power of its participants). Karpman's unusual analytic practice of requiring his patients to write and his active engagement with their writing often elicited this understanding.[51] Karpman asked people in treatment with him to write autobiographies, record their dreams, respond to detailed questionnaires, and keep diaries. "In answering the questions submitted," Karpman instructed, "please remember . . . to go into every detail." When describing a masturbatory episode, for instance, he encouraged his patients to "tell where you were, how you were clothed, or whether you were nude, exactly how you masturbated, and describe in detail the phantasy which accompanied the process."[52] "We are not only concerned with what you did, but with how you felt," Karpman wrote to

George Raymond in 1943. "Your doubts, fears, hopes, disappointments, re-grets, etc. in connection with particular events are of as much interest as the events themselves, if not more."[53] When Raymond was less forthcoming than his analyst wished, Karpman told him that while the material he had written so far was interesting, it was "much too deficient in detail," and he asked him for "a more detailed account of your emotional reactions."[54]

Karpman's patients referred to the writing assignments they did for their analyst as their "work," some with a sense of great purpose and ex-citement and others with frustration. One complained that Karpman was "piling on too much work for me to do."[55] Another who wrote gleefully about Karpman giving him his "first assignment" later berated himself for his own "laziness": "I have deliberately let whole days go by without doing any work at all."[56] A "passion for rewriting" slowed down another's prog-ress. He reported writing "about 4½ pages per day, not nearly enough."[57] A few days later, he scolded himself again: "Due to the distractions and in-terruptions of the day room, I wrote, crossed out, and threw away twelve pages before I wrote three I could keep."[58] A number of patients wrote auto-biographies, some several hundred pages long. One man who was Karp-man's patient in the early 1950s wrote three hundred short essays describing every man he had had sex with, titling each one with a descriptor, such as, "CCC Boy," "Blonde Curly Haired Soldier from 9th Street," "Trade at the Carlton," "Sailor at Biloxi," "Boy Who Took My Wallet," and "Bill the Anthropologist."[59]

For patients who were institutionalized in particular, writing for Karp-man could offer a welcome distraction from the monotony of hospital life. Others chafed at the time and labor required by Karpman's iterative method, in which he used patients' responses to his questionnaires to de-velop new, more refined versions, seemingly ad infinitum. (For Karpman, of course, this was precisely the value of his questionnaire method. He noted "the immense number of questions that one can ask and keep on ask-ing a patient, modifying, enlarging, amplifying, and so on before the mate-rial is exhausted.")[60] Walter Moore, hospitalized at Saint Elizabeths in the mid-1950s after multiple arrests for sex with minors, lost his patience with Karpman's endless back-and-forth questionnaires, fearing that the analyst would never "no [sic] enough to let me go."[61]

The dynamics of collaboration between patient and psychiatrist were also at work in Karpman's analytic practice of having his patients read and respond to psychiatric texts. For some, that assignment encouraged them to accept psychoanalytic ideas about homosexuality and provided them with a new language to describe themselves. One woman recognized her-self in Freud's account of the tendency of the "neurotic" to feel a sense of satisfaction in the failure of their analysis and thus to "resign himself to his condition with an easy conscience," knowing that "he has done everything possible he can." "I have many times wondered if this is not just exactly what I am doing," she wrote.[62] After reading a text titled "The Homosexual Neurosis," Harold Crowe wrote that "it bears out Dr. Karpman's opinion that I am bisexual, but my heterosexual component has been suppressed, bringing forth a strong homosexual bent." The book also "gives me the impression that my family played a very important part in my mental content," he wrote.[63] From reading Freud's *A General Introduction to Psychoanalysis*, another patient of Karpman's gleaned that "sexual instincts must be subdued to fit in with the mandates of society."[64]

Some patients' reviews of psychiatric texts were rote and obedient, repeating back to Karpman what they took to be the meanings of the texts he assigned them to read. Others, though, took the opportunity to stage a critique and write their way into a new kind of knowledge and authority. Karpman's assignment could become an invitation to speak back to a stigmatizing medical model, and for some patients, to become producers rather than objects of psychiatric knowledge. Perhaps the most striking example was that of Benjamin Rogers, hospitalized in the mid-1940s for alcoholism. At Karpman's invitation, Rogers undertook a review of George W. Henry's 1941 study, *Sex Variants: A Study of Homosexual Patterns*, a massive work based on a six-year study of the life stories of eighty queer men and women.[65] But Henry's medical credentials and the imposing heft of his two-volume study's eleven hundred pages were not enough to persuade Rogers of his expertise on a topic that Rogers felt better qualified by his own experience and identity to speak on. "When you think of how eminent the authors are," he concluded, "and then you think how often they have failed to understand things that the simplest little homosexual ribbon counter clerk would grasp at a glance—you are tempted to conclude that homosexuality will never receive a satisfactory scientific study *until a psychiatrist who is a homosexual himself investigates it*."[66] In a scathing review that ran over a hundred pages in length and took Rogers months to write, drafted "in a tempest of rage and rebellion" and submitted to Karpman with "exquisite pleasure," Rogers assailed Henry's study for its "hopelessly confused terminology" and "conventional point of view." He criticized Henry's belief in the explanatory power of gender inversion to explain homosexuality, which he argued left Henry confounded by masculine gay men and feminine lesbians. He blasted Henry for his imprecision about gender and sexual roles in gay relationships: "There are no words that must appear more often in a work of this kind than masculine and feminine," he wrote, "but to what do they refer?" He likewise assailed Henry for organizing his taxonomy of homosexuality around the binary of "active" and "passive": "With all my exhaustive knowledge of my own case," he wrote, "I don't know whether I am active or passive. At one time I am one, at another time the other."[67] As for Henry's inquiry into the physiological difference of homosexuals, Rogers wrote, "The whole question of the physical characteristics of homosexuals is to me so simple that all this elaborate research seems a little silly."[68] At the end of his lengthy review, Rogers concluded that he had come to believe "that the homosexual has his place in the scheme of things, and that his salvation lies rather in developing his own peculiar gifts than in trying to imitate those of a heterosexual." "This is to reject both the theory that the homosexual is mentally ill," he clarified, "and that he is a person who has failed to reach adulthood."[69]

Karpman's own lengthy review of Henry's *Sex Variants*, published in the *American Journal of Psychiatry* in 1943, quoted liberally from Rogers's review and borrowed ideas from his critique. Karpman echoed Rogers's review in criticizing Henry's reliance on "active" and "passive" to describe homosexual men. He took Henry on as well for his "descriptive" approach, which Karpman judged to result in "superficial" conclusions, and for what Karpman took to be his neglect of psychoanalytic understandings of homosexuality. Crediting "a rather lengthy but very pertinent statement made by one of my homosexual patients" for some of his ideas, Karpman also plagiarized directly from Rogers's review.[70] Using Rogers's arguments and verbatim language without attribution, Karpman exposed the intellectual labor performed by patients and the reliance of psychiatry on their expertise as well as the exploitative and parasitic nature of psychiatric knowledge production. At the same time, it is clear that Karpman and Rogers conceived of their relationship and work together as collaborative, complicating any expectation of an inevitably antagonistic relationship between queer patient and psychiatrist.

Queer and gender-nonconforming people were transformed by their encounter with psychiatry; psychiatry and psychiatrists were transformed in turn by their encounter with queer and gender-nonconforming people. Psychiatrists claimed expertise regarding homosexuality, but they learned much about queer life from patients and were indebted to them for knowledge about gender and sexuality. Karpman regretted Marina Harris's early departure from Saint Elizabeths because "she was a veritable gold mine of information," which helped him understand lesbianism and what he believed to be its link with alcoholism.[71] Knowledge gleaned from patients, which was sometimes solicited directly by psychiatrists, was often more ethnographic than psychiatric. Benjamin Miller wrote a three-page essay on "Homeric expressions" at Karpman's request in 1950, defining words like *cruising*, *gay*, and *drag party* and translating other terms: "lavatory = tearoom; a homosexual who flaunts his nature = Belle or Queen." Sometimes, he informed Karpman, homosexuals "refer to themselves individually as 'YOUR MOTHER.'"[72]

The influence of queer patients on the work and thinking of psychiatrists is evident over the course of Karpman's long career, which began in the early, heady days of the introduction of psychoanalysis in the United States in the 1920s and stretched into psychiatry's "golden age" of power and influence in the 1950s and early 1960s. Soon after he started working at Saint Elizabeths, in the mid-1920s, Karpman traveled to Vienna to "see what was going on with psychiatry."[73] There he attended seminars and meetings of the Freud group and underwent analysis with Stekel, a psychoanalytic maverick and former pupil of Freud. He returned to Washington, DC, eager to put his new knowledge into practice. In his early days at the hospital, Karpman struggled with the challenge of treating patients who were "so out of touch with daily life as to preclude any possibility of their living outside." Influenced by the psychoanalytic turn and inspired by the challenge of bringing psychoanalysis to a large public hospital, he was optimistic about the possibility of a "psychic treatment that would attempt to reach the cause of their difficulties, and thereby effect relief from the abnormal mental state" and that might be more effective than the palliative hydrotherapy and occupational therapy routinely practiced in hospitals like Saint Elizabeths.[74] In an effort to excavate their unconscious conflicts, Karpman began engaging his patients in the recording and analysis of their dreams, asking them to complete psychological questionnaires, and soliciting their autobiographical writing.

Among the few American psychiatrists to write about homosexuality in the 1930s and 1940s, Karpman initially hewed closely to the Freudian framework that assumed a state of universal bisexuality. He identified homosexuality as a neurotic symptom of, and solution to, an unconscious conflict that arrested a person's psychosexual development at an immature stage. Like many American psychoanalysts, Karpman considered himself "an eclectic who is not committed to any particular point of view." While he accepted "a good deal of Freud's basic tenets," he was not a slavish disciple to Freudianism in toto. Yet he "invariably came back to the Freudian approach," he wrote, for its "helpful clinical demonstrations of effective psychotherapy and cure."[75]

Karpman began to boast of his ability to "cure" homosexuals in the 1940s. "I am sure I am not the only one who has been successful in curing homosexuality and perversions," he wrote in 1946, tempering his brag with a nod to humility.[76] But over the course of less than a decade of working with queer and gender-nonconforming patients, Karpman's belief in the feasibility of cure, or perhaps his faith in the wisdom or ethics of it, seemed to fade. In his 1954 book, *The Sexual Offender and His Offenses*, and against the grain of the psychoanalytic consensus of the time, Karpman character-ized homosexuality as "often too deeply rooted to be eradicated." He de-voted a chapter of that book to "the normal pervert": one who "despite the handicap imposed by an unorthodox and socially unacceptable sexual orientation, does manage to lead an otherwise normal life according to general standards of ordinary behavior."[77] The formulation of the "normal pervert" would have struck most at the time as oxymoronic. But Karpman insisted, contrary to most mid-century American psychoanalysts, that not all homosexuals were mentally disordered. He made that claim even at the expense of circumscribing the authoritative ambit of his own profession. About a lesbian under his care whose difficulties he judged to be "mainly those of social maladjustment and emotional frustration resulting from her homosexuality," Karpman concluded that "psychiatry cannot solve her problem."[78] "It must be admitted that the majority of homosexuals are be-yond psychoanalysis," he confessed. "Perhaps the best way to treat them is to leave them alone."[79]

Through his work with queer patients, Karpman also became more aware of the hostile social and political conditions, external to whatever psychic conflicts and unconscious processes he believed them to be wres-tling with, that made their lives difficult and sometimes unlivable. Karpman criticized what he termed the "wholesale persecution of homosexuals" in the years after the Second World War, a coordinated crackdown that cre-ated a culture of terror for queer people in Washington, DC, and beyond.[80] As a psychiatrist and resident of the District of Columbia, Karpman was aware of the purges of gay men and lesbians from federal jobs following a Senate investigation into the employment of "sex perverts" in 1950 and the increased policing of gay life in city parks, cruising areas, and bars in what the U.S. Park Police termed the "Pervert Elimination Campaign" in the late 1940s and early 1950s. Karpman and Saint Elizabeths superintendent Win-fred Overholser offered expert testimony in congressional debates in 1948 on the sexual psychopath law known as the Miller Law, in which congres-sional representatives made it clear that gay men were the law's primary target. He was drawn into those debates as an "expert"; he also heard about the laws and their terrorizing effects from his queer patients.

Karpman's psychoanalytic position on homosexuality gave way, under the influence of his work with patients and the pressures of the historical moment, to an explicitly political one, even when that position undermined his own authority as a psychiatrist. As efforts to police and prosecute homo-sexuality ramped up after the Second World War, Karpman's own concerns shifted from the psychoanalytic to the social and political, as evidenced in his writing and in his case notes about patients. About a lesbian under his care, Karpman observed that she was "beset by fears—as all homosexuals are at this time."[81] He wrote publicly about his own apprehensions as well. Karpman became a vocal critic of the government purges in Washington, DC, which he characterized as a "witch hunt" driven by "hysterical prejudice and mob psychology."[82] He condemned what he called an "all-out campaign against homosexuality" in Washington, DC, describing it as "a campaign characterized in great measure by extortion, blackmail, and a wholesale violation of civil rights."[83] "The idea of declaring all homosexuals *persona non grata* in all Government agencies is predicated on prejudice and prejudice only," Karpman wrote in 1952.[84] To the charge that gay people's vulnerability to blackmail made them security threats, he argued that "the easiest way to prevent the blackmailing of homosexuals is to recognize homosexuality as a fact and to remove the unreasonable laws which discriminate against it."[85] Karpman was among the few in this period to argue publicly for the decriminalization of homosexuality, stating before Congress in 1948, "I believe we ought to follow the experiences of Europe," where "they do not punish for the commission of [homosexual] acts unless they are a violation of the public sense of decency."[86] At a time when American Civil Liberties Union (ACLU) lawyers considered it too risky to meet with the Mattachine Society, Karpman accepted invitations to speak at its meetings and welcomed an honorary membership in the organization. "People are entitled to their own form of sex life," he proclaimed, and "we must not brand as psychogenic people different from us merely because they are different."[87] "What is to be the ultimate place of the homosexual in society?" he asked in a memorandum that never found its way to publication. In the next stunning sentence, he proposed that psychiatrists pause, step back from their curative agenda, and shift course: "Psychiatry should take time out from discussing homosexuality as an individual 'disease,'" Karpman wrote, "and offer a constructive plan for dealing with it as a social problem."[88]

Karpman's clinical engagement with questions of race and with Black patients, too, came to influence his understanding of homosexuality. Race and racism were not incidental interests for him. In addition to his clinical work with people diagnosed with various forms of sexual and gender difference and his prolific writing on sexuality and criminality, Karpman was interested in bringing psychoanalytic inquiry to problems of racial inequality. With a faculty affiliation in the psychiatry department at historically Black Howard University and a commitment to training and mentoring Black psychiatrists, Karpman considered himself a "specialist in minorities." He maintained a long friendship and correspondence with the writer Richard

Wright in the hope of collaborating with him on a book on the "psychology of race relations" that he described as a "scientific parallel" to Wright's novel *Native Son*.[89] Perhaps it is not surprising, then, that Karpman called on racial analogies to understand his queer patients—a practice that would become central to homophile arguments for gay rights and to an emerging sexual liberalism. He drew as well on his own experience as a Jew who had experienced antisemitism. Puzzling over the case of one gay patient's insistence on his own normalcy, for instance, he mused, "How can we expect any other answer? One might almost as well ask a Negro if he considers it normal to be black, or a Hebrew if he considers it normal to be a Jew." "The case of the homosexual is not exactly in point," he conceded," "but his emotional reaction is the same, for to him it is as natural for him to be a homosexual as it is to be one of a particular color or of a particular race of people."[90] He came to understand discrimination against homosexuals as "no different from social discrimination against Negroes and Jews."[91]

For people in psychiatric treatment, too, the psychiatric encounter could be a site of unexpected political vision and voice, in some cases anticipating insights and arguments that would not circulate in activist discourse until years later. A number of patients ventured utopian visions, some untethered to realistic possibility but no less remarkable for their unreason. Walter Webster, a twenty-nine-year-old man who had been discharged from the army for homosexuality and hospitalized at Saint Elizabeths in the late 1930s, declared his hope "for getting a bill through Congress to provide for a sanctuary for homosexuals" as well as a plan to "hire an army of homosexuals to overthrow the government."[92] Others formulated political critiques in more conventional terms. "The difficulties of the homosexual are largely man-made, society-made," a naval officer institutionalized at Saint Elizabeths declared in 1942. "They consist of having to fight an unfair fight against the stacked cards of social pressure, convention, orthodox Christian religion and Judaism, the obsolete law, blackmail, and social disapproval."[93] Joseph Frazier, a gay man committed indefinitely to Saint Elizabeths under the Miller Law in the mid-1950s, recognized that "no amount of psychiatric help to me is going to change the attitude of society."[94] Terry Willis, in analysis with Karpman in the late 1940s, realized that his "feelings of guilt and inferiority in regard to homosexuality [were] nothing more than the results of society's intolerant attitude toward homosexuality."[95] Benjamin Rogers conceded that the chances of the homosexual "being neurotic or immature are greater than those of the heterosexual," but he attributed that to "society's current attitude" rather than "anything inherent in homosexuality." "Everything is done to encourage the heterosexual struggling toward maturity," he wrote, "everything to smooth his path."[96] Rogers judged the homosexual to be "the most implacably persecuted of all minorities in America," one who lives life as "a pariah, outside the law."[97]

Some of Karpman's patients pondered other worlds and times less hostile to queerness, in which they imagined that life might be lived more freely. For many, that horizon of queer freedom lay beyond the borders of the United States. One man "heard that the homosexual has it kinder abroad" and fantasized about moving to "the Orient, Egypt, Paris, Vienna, India."[98] Others took heart in learning about the acceptance of homosexuality in earlier times and places. "Oh! How I wish I, and other such unfortunate victims as myself, victims who are stigmatized with an abnormality which we cannot help and for which society has no sympathy, were living in those days of Rome and Greece," one man wrote to Karpman.[99]

Another of Karpman's patients, Helen Pell, offers a stunning example of how people could make use of the psychiatric encounter, and especially Karpman's unusual solicitation to write, to articulate a prescient and intersectional political critique. A Black woman in her forties, Pell had worked at the hospital as a psychiatric nurse, with ambitions of becoming a supervisor who might be able to "break up segregation and the old stereotype regime at St. Elizabeths."[100] The circumstances of her hospitalization at Saint Elizabeths are not entirely clear; Pell wrote that what she called her "sickness" had "been like a rolling snowball that was tossed down a hill. As it rolls along it gathers more snow. My sickness grew along with me," she explained, "until it became like a mass of tangled wires."[101] In a narrative she wrote for Karpman, an apologetic and often shame-filled account of a life lived at odds with prevailing sexual norms titled "How I Got Sick and Why," Pell expressed regret and embarrassment for what she called her "queer ways." But she ultimately located the cause of her "sickness" beyond herself, and instead in the structural oppressions of sexuality, gender, and race. Pell speculated that she was sick "partly because . . . I did not stay in my own group and with my own race, partly because I set out to do something no other Negro woman had done." "I had set my goal too high in life," Pell wrote, and "had too many obligations for this one body." Here, she anticipated the arguments of psychiatrists in the 1960s who would attribute "psychopathogenic effects" to what they characterized paternalistically as "goal-striving behavior" in Black Americans.[102] Pell lamented that she was "weak and feeble and [did] not have the guts or power to speak up for my own rights," a self-criticism contradicted by her own powerful writing. But in a stunningly direct and searing conclusion, Pell pushed her critique beyond what she took to be her own failings and attributed her mental illness to the fact that "I am of the minority race of people."[103] In that unadorned line, Pell combined an indictment of the material injuries of racism, in particular the limits placed by racism and sexism on her own ambition, with an acknowledgment that those structural forces (rather than individual, psychic ones) could make one sick. Her comment can also be read as a critique of the long-standing racialization of mental illness, a tradition in which Saint Elizabeths Hospital was directly implicated.[104]

In the early 1950s, around the same time that Pell was putting Karpman's therapeutic writing assignments to the purpose of political theorization and critique, gay men committed to Mendocino State Hospital as sex offenders under California's Sexual Psychopath Act were exploiting an experiment in therapeutic psychodrama to forge and articulate their own critiques of normalizing psychiatric treatment. Trumpeted as an "effective means of treating sexual deviates" by the hospital's clinical director, Walter Bromberg, the theatrical exercises were initially scripted by psychiatrists as pedagogical dramas to "help young people . . . from falling into homosexuality." But as directed, staged, and performed by men incarcerated as sex offenders, the therapeutic performances became platforms to dramatize "the struggle for social acceptance of homosexuality," providing an opportunity for these men to articulate publicly the "disinclination to be cured of homosexuality."[105] In one dramatic exercise, patients staged a "legislative session" in which they assumed the roles of senators "considering a pending bill on sex offenders." Incarcerated patients used the performative opportunities of psychodrama to lampoon hospital administrators and doctors as "inefficient and confused."[106] In therapeutic theatrical sessions, gay patients who "called each other 'she'" and "demonstrated 'swish' openly" defied demands for gender as well as sexual normativity. During the psychodrama sessions, Bromberg and Franklin reported, gay participants "were vivacious with each other, living out their own special community life to the exclusion of other members of the group. It was obvious that the homosexuals were testing the social value of homosexuality within the group," the psychiatrists noted, "for the 'benefit' . . . of the therapist and staff." Thus, rather than promoting individual cure, the therapeutic modality of psychodrama consolidated the group identity of institutionalized gay men who, in the process, developed a critique of psychiatry's normalizing project and forged a new relationship with one another. Gay patient-inmates "talked sneeringly of the heterosexual deviates, were prideful of their assumed superior status and gained leadership in the plays because of their intellectual and artistic facility."[107] The most striking development in the behavior and attitude of the patients, Bromberg and Franklin observed, "was a feeling of solidarity, a 'we' feeling in the group" that emerged and strengthened over the course of the therapeutic theatrical experiment.[108]

Queer life and positive queer identity were made in community, historians have told us. George Chauncey and others urge against the tendency to see queer life in the past as isolated and solitary and have documented vibrant queer urban cultures in mid-twentieth-century cities.[109] Some Saint Elizabeths patients had been active participants in those cultures, and in the writing assignments they produced for Karpman, the social world rather than the psychic one sometimes flickers into view. Leslie Fuller described cruising in Washington, DC's Lafayette Park and frequenting the city's many gay clubs and cafeterias. At the Rival Club and E-Club in Baltimore, Fuller first saw floor shows that featured female and male impersonators, inspiring him to "see if I could be convincing dressed as a woman."[110] Leigh Stafford, a divorced woman troubled by her bisexuality who underwent analysis with Karpman in the 1940s, frequented New York City's 181 Club and recalled lesbians in tuxedos singing the opening number of the night, "Follow the Girls." Stafford chronicled her tumultuous relationship with a woman named Dorothy and their friendship with a gay man, describing her annoyance when Dorothy and the man "compar[ed] their Homeric emotional notes."[111] Of Dorothy's bohemian "village lesbian friends," Stafford recalled disdainfully, they "all smelled of dirt."[112] Raymond Shea marveled at the fairies in Los Angeles's 808 Club, who would "flirt with sailors, marines, and civilians."[113]

Most forms of psychotherapeutic treatment, by contrast, were profoundly atomizing and individuating in both intention and effect. Some people confessed to psychiatrists their deep loneliness, which was compounded by a feeling of gender and sexual difference that made them wonder if they were the only one like themselves, alone in the world. When walking around Los Angeles, Shea longed to meet "another boy with the same desire to live the life of a girl" so that they might live together. "We'd be less lonely and less ashamed of ourselves," Shea imagined; "then one acquaintance would lead to another and soon we would be in a circle of people like ourselves." "I was always looking for a person such as myself," Shea wrote, "but I never even caught a glimpse of such a person."[114] Eugene Lee, a young Black man who had spent time in a monastery before being institutionalized at Saint Elizabeths in the early 1940s, wrote to Karpman that he "wish[ed] he knew of some person who is homosexual himself" so that he would "have a chance of mutual companionship and understanding."[115] "I need gay friends," a thirty-seven-year-old Black gay man who was also blind wrote to psychotherapist Albert Ellis in 1966. He asked Ellis for "any suggestions that you have that will help me to find another lonely gay person who sits at home a lot."[116]

But while for some patients the psychiatric encounter could compound a sense of loneliness and singularity, it introduced others to a wider queer world—conceptually, through reading and learning of others with the same diagnosis, and sometimes literally, by providing an opportunity to meet other queer people. For some, an encounter with psychiatric thinking and practice led them to learn that their numbers were so legion that they constituted a "type" of person. For those who were institutionalized, the communal nature of hospital life cut against the individuating effects of psychiatric treatment. Some hospitals organized social and recreational activities, such as movie nights, concerts, excursions into town, group athletics, and dances, and those projects in rehabilitation and normalization could be remade into sites of queer connection. Benjamin Miller formed a social group at the hospital's weekly dances with other patients at Saint Elizabeths whom he identified as fellow "homosexual neurotics." "Our conversation was much like you might hear at a fag joint downtown," he wrote.[117] He and his friends sometimes dished about "handsome attendants or better looking patients." One night they discussed "the trials and tribulations and the high cost paid all around in many ways for being homosexually inclined."[118] Miller and his friends also participated in the time-honored practice, familiar to anyone who has ever been to a gay bar, of removed and disdainful judgment. At one dance, he reported, he and his friends didn't dance at all, "just observed . . . while my friend and I talked and criticized the others."[119] Miller recognized the value of queer community in the hospital: "I show a natural preference for associating with people whom I think understand me and my homosexual ways and language," he wrote, "even though no mention or thoughts of sexual activities have occurred."[120] Marina Harris "danced with many young men" at a Saint Elizabeths dance, but she most enjoyed "sitting and talking to Pauline. That was the only reason I went to that dance," she wrote, "so I could see Pauline again."[121] For some patients, hospitalization could provide the first opportunity to meet other queer people. "Whitey," a teenage lesbian, met other lesbians and gay men for the first time at the state mental hospital where she was committed by her parents: "That's where I actually learned the facts of life," she recalled.[122] Historian Gustavus Stadler observes that to live in a mental hospital in this period "was to dwell in an environment suffused in talk about sex's relationship to mental health and, in particular, about nonconformist sexual practices like homosexuality." That made it the only place, Stadler notes, in which "such discussion wasn't viewed with suspicion, as obscene or even, particularly in the postwar era, seditious."[123]

The psychiatric hospital figures in queer history and cultural memory, across generations, as a terrifying, violent, and profoundly stigmatizing site, and with good reason. That reputation stretches back to the late nineteenth century, when both mental asylums and homosexual identity were still in formation. When nineteen-year-old Alice Mitchell murdered her lover Freda Ward in Memphis in 1891, she was found incurably insane and was committed to the Western Hospital for the Insane in Bolivar, Tennessee, where she died in 1898. Psychiatrists took Mitchell's unfeminine behavior, her masculine interests, and her plan to marry Freda all as symptoms of her mental illness.[124] Joseph Israel Lobdell, who was assigned as female at birth, lived a transient life as a man for many decades, spending years trapping and hunting in upstate New York, northern Minnesota, and Pennsylvania. Lobdell was arrested for vagrancy in 1876 and later for cross-dressing and was institutionalized in the Willard Insane Asylum in Ovid, New York, in 1880. Lobdell's diagnosis of insanity was based on his preference for men's clothing and his partnership with a woman, as well as his poverty and "inarticulate" religious proclamations.[125] At Willard, Lobdell became the patient of sexologist P. M. Wise, who characterized his case as one of "sexual perversion" and "a rare form of mental disease" in an article he published in 1883. In one of the earliest American medical writings that used the word "lesbian," Wise observed that Lobdell "considered herself a man in all that the name implies."[126] Lobdell spent the rest of his life involuntarily committed at Willard and died in 1890.

Those stories and more bolstered an understanding of the asylum as a place of crushing carceral power dedicated to extinguishing queer and trans life. Those fears were amplified in the mid-twentieth century, when psychiatrists consolidated their power and authority by claiming expertise regarding homosexuality and gender nonconformity. When, in the mid-1950s, Magora Kennedy's mother discovered that she was a lesbian, she threatened to send her to "Utica," the mental hospital in upstate New York.[127] Miriam Wolfson knew "four or five friends" from her gay circle in 1950s New York who were institutionalized by their parents.[128] Jason Serinus recalled that three of the ten members of his gay men's collective house in New York City had "survived incarceration in mental institutions because of their homosexuality, and were carrying deep wounds."[129] Historian Gary Atkins learned from oral history interviews with lesbians and gay men in Seattle that the Harborview Medical Center "loomed" in their imagination, and he included the story of fifteen-year-old Jackie Cachero, involuntarily committed in 1958 when she told her mother she liked girls.[130] When psychologist Evelyn Hooker asked her friend the writer Christopher Isherwood for his cooperation as a research subject in her studies, "he would often reply, 'Yes, if you will keep me out of Norwalk,'" an institution for the mentally ill in Los Angeles.[131]

Given this history and the long and well-earned association of the psychiatric hospital as a place of violence for queer people, it can be surprising to find evidence of the solidary and sometimes politicizing effects of institutional life. Indeed, the mental hospital could help create a queer counterpublic, a space in which people met other queer people, sometimes for the first time; reflected on their own subordination; developed critiques of dominant norms; and made private experiences newly legible as political.[132]

Those possibilities of institutional life made some queer people seek out the mental hospital or lean into life there rather than fighting it. "I felt safe there," Betty Berzon wrote of her commitment at a private mental hospital in the 1950s, where she felt "on vacation from the world."[133] For trans man Mark Rees, the psychiatric hospital "was something of a haven, a refuge from the world with all its sniggers and questions."[134] Rodney Frank felt that Saint Elizabeths was "an asylum from the outside world," which he was reluctant to leave.[135] When Benjamin Rogers was discharged from Saint Elizabeths, he panicked at the loss of "the protective walls" of the institution and returned by cab to check himself back in the next day.[136] Clearly, and surprisingly, and against the grain of our own expectations, institutions like Saint Elizabeths could be places where queer life was made and sustained rather than extinguished.

"If encounters are meetings," feminist and critical race scholar Sara Ahmed writes, "then they also involve surprise."[137] It is not surprising that the encounter of queer and gender-variant people with psychiatry often reinforced stigma and shame, given mid-century American psychiatrists' commitment to understanding gender and sexual difference as pathological forms of difference and treatable mental disorders. More unexpectedly, queer and trans people used encounters with psychiatry to acknowledge and weigh the psychic costs of that stigma, to address questions of the self, and sometimes to articulate radical new political visions and imagine new ways of being.

At the same time, beyond the clinic and the asylum, gay men and lesbians were beginning to innovate new political arguments and forge new strategies to attack the authority of psychiatry and critique the stigmatizing effects of diagnosis. That would turn out to be a challenging proposition, one that they took to require distancing healthy gayness from the asylum and the clinic and the stigmatized subjects associated with those spaces. In the process, activists both narrowed the lens of gay political vision and delivered the early movement's first major victory.

## CHAPTER FIVE

# The Queer Politics of Health

In January 1964, the New York Academy of Medicine, an organization founded in 1847 to elevate the medical profession and promote public health, took up the question of the medical status of homosexuality (scheduled on their agenda between discussions of perinatal mortality and rat control) and appointed a subcommittee to study it.[1] A few months later, the academy issued a formal report urging that homosexuality be recognized as an illness, one that would respond to preventive measures and could, in many cases, be cured.

Echoing the arguments of psychiatrists and psychoanalysts who had been making that case for over two decades, the report's tone of marked defensiveness signaled an important shift. "Homosexuality is indeed an illness," the academy stated, "the contrary conviction and protestations of the confirmed homosexual notwithstanding."[2] The academy's interest in homosexuality had been sparked by what it believed to be its implication in other areas of their concern and investigation—the increasingly widespread availability of "salacious literature" and the rising incidence of venereal disease in New York City—but was made more urgent by the academy's observation of "a growing aggressiveness on the part of homosexuals in trying to promote their way of life."[3] Not only do they want to be "accepted," the authors of the report pronounced. "They would have it believed that homosexuality is . . . a desirable, noble, preferable way of life."[4] The headline of the *New York Times* article reporting on the academy's statement read, "Homosexuals Proud of Deviancy."[5]

In the 1950s and 1960s, as psychiatry grew in power and prestige, gay men and lesbians began to conceive of themselves in radically new ways. Contrary to the claims of medical professionals that homosexuality was a treatable mental disorder, gay activists insisted that it was a benign manifestation of human difference, an unfairly oppressed minority identity to be defended, and a way of life to be accepted and even celebrated. Psychiatric authority and affirmative gay identity thus embarked on a collision course that would culminate in one of the first and most celebrated gay political victories in 1973, when, under pressure from activists and supportive psychiatrists, the American Psychiatric Association removed homosexuality from its reference for classifying mental disorders, the *Diagnostic and Statistical Manual of Mental Disorders* (*DSM*). That battle with psychiatry would shape gay politics in profound and indelible ways, as activists worked to associate homosexuality with health and normalcy and to disavow a stigmatized past.

## "Normal Homosexuals"

Ammunition for that battle had been forged decades earlier. In 1953, as psychiatrists honed and popularized their evaluations of homosexuality as a mental disorder, psychologist Evelyn Hooker applied for a grant from the newly established National Institute of Mental Health (NIMH) for a study of what she termed "normal homosexuals." Echoing Benjamin Karpman's reference to the "normal pervert," Hooker's framing of her research subjects as normal was audacious in its implicit critique of the psychiatric and psychological consensus. When she told the chair of her department at the University of California at Los Angeles (UCLA) of her plan, she recalled that he "rose from his chair" and asked, "What do you think you are doing? There is no such person."[6] After sending an agent across the country to meet with Hooker in Los Angeles (Hooker suspected that the purpose of the on-site visit was to confirm that she was not a lesbian), the NIMH awarded her a six-month grant and renewed her funding through 1961, when the agency granted her its Research Career Award. That funding launched and supported Hooker's groundbreaking research, which would come to provide empirical support for gay activists' assault on the psychiatric pathologization of homosexuality.

Years later, Hooker would explain her interest in research on gay men by recalling her own experience of marginalization, discrimination, and social stigma and her witness to it in others. The sixth of nine children, Evelyn Gentry was born in 1907 in a sod house in North Platte, Nebraska. The family then moved to eastern Colorado, where they lived in a two-room tarpaper shack and her father worked as a tenant farmer. Having grown up "dirt poor," Hooker later observed that "the fact that I should end up studying an oppressed, a deprived people comes from my own experiences, in part, of being stigmatized."[7] After attending the University of Colorado on scholarship, she hoped to pursue a PhD in psychology at Yale to study with the psychologist Robert Yerkes, but the department chair at Colorado refused to recommend a woman to his alma mater. Hooker earned her PhD in experimental psychology from Johns Hopkins University in 1932, one of very few women to do so. Two years later, Hooker's early career was interrupted when she contracted tuberculosis and spent two years in sanitariums. While on a fellowship at the Institute for Psychotherapy in Berlin in 1937–38, she witnessed the violence of Kristallnacht and boarded with a Jewish family who were later killed in Nazi concentration camps. After a brief trip to the Soviet Union in 1938, she was fired from her academic post at Whittier College as a suspected subversive. When seeking a position at UCLA, Hooker was told by the chair of the Department of Psychology that there were already three women in the department, all "cordially disliked" by their male colleagues, and she was offered a teaching job as research associate in UCLA's extension division rather than on the tenure-track faculty.[8]

As influential as anything in shaping Hooker's research agenda, by her own account, were her close friendships with gay men. Those friends included the writer Christopher Isherwood, who rented a guesthouse in Hooker's backyard in the early 1950s; Isherwood's lover, the artist Don Bachardy; and the poet W. H. Auden. Sam From, a young gay man whom Hooker met in 1945 when he was a student in one of her night classes, took Hooker and her first husband, Donn Caldwell, on tours of gay bars and drag shows in Los Angeles. (Years later, Hooker would boast that she had "been in every gay bar in the whole of L.A." regretting only that she had never gained access to a gay bathhouse.)[9] After a weekend trip to San Francisco and a night out that ended at the city's famous drag club Finocchio's, From told Hooker, "We have let you see us as we are, and now it is your scientific duty to make a study of people like us."[10]

By "people like us," Hooker explained, her friend meant gay men who "don't need psychiatrists"—those who were "not insane" and were "not any of those things they say we are."[11] Hooker initially resisted the idea, fearing that she could not be objective about people who were her friends. She was encouraged, though, by her UCLA colleague and office-mate psychologist Bruno Klopfer, who insisted, "'Evelyn, you must do it [because] we don't know anything—all we know about are the sick ones.'"[12] From helped connect Hooker with research subjects from among his friends and members of Los Angeles homophile organizations like the Mattachine Society and ONE, Inc. Hooker was originally interested in the life histories of gay men selected as "normal," identified as such for having never sought psychiatric help and showing "no gross signs of psychological disturbance." She set out to study the developmental paths that led these "normal" men to identify as gay, with a particular interest in how they reconciled homosexuality with masculine gender identity.[13] After several rounds of interviews and a battery of psychological tests, however, Hooker found it impossible to diagnose "homosexual trends in individual personality." From there, she speculated that "the essential problem is our insistence on thinking of homosexuality as a clinical entity," a problem she sought to resolve through a novel experiment.[14]

Hooker assembled a group of thirty gay men and a control group of thirty heterosexual men, matched for age and IQ scores, and gave them a series of projective psychological tests that psychologists at the time used to detect homosexuality. Among them was the Rorschach inkblot test. Developed in 1921 by Swiss psychiatrist Hermann Rorschach and inspired by his observation that people diagnosed with schizophrenia often interpreted visual images in unusual ways, the Rorschach test was used to detect underlying thought patterns in order to identify mental illness more broadly. Psychiatrists believed that the Rorschach test could reliably reveal homosexuality and was purportedly especially useful in those who tried to conceal it. During the Second World War, Rorschach testing was used to screen recruits and service members for homosexuality along with alcoholism and other disorders.[15] Two naval officers reported that homosexual subjects' interpretation of the Rorschach inkblots tended "toward the abnormal" and that they were inclined to project "unreal and modified human figures," speculating that their "inability to project ordinary human beings" reflected their difficulty "in identifying with normal persons." They also observed what they took to be gay subjects' "confusion and evasiveness with respect to the identification of the gender" of images and their "preoccupation" with phallic symbolism that led them to see "snakes, poles, towers" in the inkblots.[16]

In the 1950s, Hooker noted, "Every clinical psychologist worth his soul would tell you that . . . he could tell whether a person was gay or not" based on their responses to projective psychological tests.[17] But few clinicians had either the opportunity or the interest in examining gay subjects "who neither came for psychological help nor were found in mental hospitals, disciplinary barracks in the Armed Services, or in prison populations."[18] Hooker set out to determine whether, when blinded to their sexual identities, psychiatrists and psychologists could distinguish between gay test subjects and the straight control group by analyzing their responses to the Rorschach test as well as the Thematic Apperception Test (TAT) and the Make-a-Picture-Story Test (MAPS), all of which were projective psychological tests that were used widely at the time. Submitting the subjects' responses to three expert analysts, including her office-mate Bruno Klopfer, who was a specialist in Rorschach testing, Hooker asked them to rank each subject on a 5-point scale of psychological adjustment ranging from "1, superior, to 5, maladjusted; with 3 representing average adjustment."[19]

To their surprise, the judges found no significant differences in adjustment between the homosexual and heterosexual groups (to gay activists' delight, the gay test subjects scored slightly higher on the adjustment scales than the straight control group). Most importantly, the experts were unable to distinguish the Rorschach protocols of homosexual subjects from those of the matched heterosexual group.

From those results, and with notable restraint given the boldness of her claim, Hooker stated that "homosexuality may be a deviation in sexual pattern which is within the normal range psychologically."[20] She presented her findings at the annual meeting of the American Psychological Association in Chicago in 1956, to an overflow and electrified audience and a reception that Hooker characterized as "very mixed," with some attendees thrilled to have scientific evidence to support what they had believed to be true and others defensive in the face of the threat Hooker's work posed to the legitimacy of scientific claims about homosexuality.[21] Hooker's study, judged to be one of the most important works of psychological research of the decade, was published in 1957.[22] In later years she moved to assert more definitively that homosexuality was not a form of mental illness, and indeed was not a clinical entity at all but rather was a "way of life" characterized by diversity and creativity and worth studying "as a collective phenomenon" rather than psychologically.[23] Hooker committed herself to that work, turning from psychological experiments to ethnographic studies of gay community life.[24]

## Homophile Activists and Psychiatric Authority

When Hooker's findings were published, as homophile activist and *ONE* magazine business manager W. Dorr Legg recalled, "It was as if a new order had come about."[25] As transformative as Hooker's work was, Legg's memory glosses over a long and ambivalent relationship between homophile activists and psychiatric authority. From the 1950s and through the mid-1960s, members of Mattachine, ONE, Inc., and the Daughters of Bilitis (DOB) were inclined to defer to psychiatrists and even to engage politely with their claims that homosexuality was a form of mental illness. Eager to cultivate a reputation for reason and open-mindedness, homophile activists courted psychiatrists and other professionals as allies, inviting them to speak at their meetings and conferences and publish in their journals. "The doctors have a variety of theories, and some solid work behind them," Jim Kepner wrote in 1955 (under the pseudonym Lyn Pedersen), urging readers of *ONE* magazine to "not write off too hurriedly their still plausible thesis that homosexuals are mentally ill . . . and sometimes curable."[26] In 1959,

ONE, Inc., dedicated its Midwinter Institute, an annual forum organized to bring together experts and members of the gay community to discuss "scientific, philosophical, legal, and social questions pertaining to homosexuality," to the topic of "Mental Health and Homosexuality." "Although the question of whether mental health for the homosexual can be possible was never resolved," one participant observed, it was "beneficial" to discuss "possible relationships between the mental health of the individual and the community and the homosexual."[27]

Homophile activists' closest and ultimately most vexing relationship was with the maverick clinical psychologist Albert Ellis. A psychoanalytically trained psychologist-turned-behavioralist who considered homosexuality a maladaptive "learned reaction" that could be "unlearned," Ellis boasted of his success in "curing" many of the gay men and lesbians he treated in his private practice.[28] While those commitments would seem to make him an unlikely ally of homophile activists, Ellis was better known to them for having written a generally approving (if qualified) foreword to the groundbreaking 1951 book *The Homosexual in America* by Donald Webster Cory (the pseudonym of Edward Sagarin), a work that provided the ideological scaffolding for the homophile movement by documenting widespread discrimination against gay men and proposing that homosexuals be understood as an oppressed minority group. Homophile activists were also drawn to Ellis as a popular writer and unabashed sexual liberal who spoke out publicly for the decriminalization of homosexuality at a time when few were willing to do so.

Members of the Mattachine Society and ONE, Inc., regularly invited Ellis to speak at their conferences and publish in their journals and newsletters. Ellis's article "Are Homosexuals Necessarily Neurotic?" was published as the cover story of *ONE* magazine in April 1955.[29] All "exclusive" homosexuals were undeniably neurotic, Ellis asserted, describing homosexuality (to the gay readership of *ONE*) as an immature and compulsive fixation and a "fetishistic sickness" and characterizing homosexuals as sex perverts who should "run, not walk, to the nearest psychotherapist."[30] Some homophile activists in those early years broached criticisms of Ellis (with some pushing back to ask if his argument called into question the mental health of "exclusive" heterosexuals), but they were respectful and restrained in their engagement. Declining to take issue with the substance of Ellis's claims, one reader from Indianapolis expressed the fear that *ONE* "may be publishing some material . . . that discourages homosexuals or leaves them depressed."[31] Another reader judged Ellis's "main point" about the neurotic basis of exclusive homosexuality to be "sound" but felt that his use of "the invidious term 'pervert'" was "misleading when applied to a person with such a neurosis."[32]

Over the next decade, Ellis continued to be a regular speaker at homophile meetings and conferences. In 1957, he spoke again at ONE's Midwinter Institute, where he advised gay men to "refrain from flaunting their homosexual tendencies in public"; avoid their tendency toward "self-pity"; police "their own ranks" in order to "discourage exploitative, rash, and patently illegal behavior by other homosexuals"; and finally, "keep up with recent scientific and clinical findings regarding homosexuality and be able to accept facts that controvert their own pro-homosexual prejudices."[33] Over time, as Ellis became more aggressive in his assertions that homosexuals were not simply neurotic but rather dangerously psychotic, gay activists began to distance themselves from him and challenge him more forcefully.[34] In 1965, Randy Wicker went so far as to revoke Ellis's honorary membership in the Mattachine Society, telling him that his arguments undermined "the fight we are waging for equal treatment in government work, educational rights, etc."[35] (Apparently stung by the rejection, Ellis replied to Wicker that "when word gets around" about Mattachine's actions, "the heterosexual world will . . . be even more convinced of how nutty and defensive the homosexual movement in America is.")[36]

The Daughters of Bilitis (DOB), the first organization for lesbians, founded in San Francisco in 1955 as a "secret society" and social alternative to lesbian bars, also initially treated psychiatric experts with deference.[37] In 1961, DOB research director Florence Jaffy (under the pseudonym Florence Conrad), wrote approvingly of a radio broadcast of a panel consisting of Edmund Bergler and two other psychiatrists, all of whom agreed that the treatment of homosexuality was both possible and desirable. Jaffy took the psychiatrists at their word when they claimed that they were simply trying to help homosexuals. "When these three psychiatrists plead to homosexuals that they are not criminal but only ill—and curable," she wrote, "listeners will feel that the case of enlightenment is being served" and "their message will seem helpful and optimistic."[38] In her review of Irving Bieber's influential 1962 study of homosexuality, Jaffy offered only the most restrained critique of his pathologizing conclusions, proposing that "the usefulness of the work would have been considerably enhanced" had Bieber defined "psychopathology" when describing homosexuality, as it was a word that to the "ordinary citizen" might "reinforce crude prejudices."[39]

Deference to psychiatric authority was enshrined in the DOB's mission statement, which was drafted in 1955 and printed on the inside cover of their periodical the *Ladder* until 1970. The statement opened by declaring the group's commitment to the "education of the variant" and the DOB's dedication to enlightening her about "the psychological, physiological, and sociological aspects" of homosexuality in order to "enable her to understand herself and make her adjustment to society." The mandate to gendered respectability and normative femininity was written into the DOB's mission as well, pledging the organization to work toward "the integration of the homosexual into society . . . by advocating a mode of behavior and dress acceptable to society."[40]

DOB members also pledged themselves to participate in "research projects by duly authorized and responsible psychologists, sociologists, and other such experts directed towards further knowledge of the homosexual."[41] In the early 1960s, the DOB began to receive requests from researchers eager to interview its members and include them as subjects in their research. (By the end of the decade, DOB member Kay Lahusen noted the growth of what she called "a new market: desire for information on homosexuality.")[42] In 1963, Jaffy announced the organization's formal collaboration with University of Washington–based psychologist Ralph Gundlach and urged DOB members to respond to his initial questionnaire and later to participate in hour-long interviews with his team of clinical psychologists. "This can be a significant step towards D.O.B.'s official objective of 'promoting further knowledge of the homosexual,'" Jaffy wrote. "When the time comes, please help!!"[43]

Not all DOB members were sold on this agenda, however. Some questioned the organization's relationship with Gundlach and the value of his research. One worried in particular about Gundlach's interest in causation and his assumption of pathological etiology, as communicated pointedly, if grammatically oddly, in the title of his article in the *Ladder*, "Why Is a Lesbian?," in which he expressed his curiosity about lesbians' "family relations in childhood," their relationships to siblings, and their "adult patterns of living."[44] That respondent was especially suspicious of Gundlach's bias "in favor of environment's being the generally predisposing factor toward homosexuality," which suggested to her his belief that "homosexuality is undesirable and if we can find out enough about its cause we can cut back on it or cure it."[45] Over time, some DOB members began to question the organization's stance toward research and researchers more generally and to pose bold critiques of psychiatric authority. In 1964, one contributor to the *Ladder* criticized her DOB peers "who have an inflated respect for the psychiatric profession and who take masochistic pleasure in inviting psychiatrists to their meetings to tell them that homosexuals are 'sick, sick, sick.'"[46]

A turning point came a year later, in March 1965, when Barbara Gittings, then editor of the DOB's journal the *Ladder*, defied the DOB's respectful and accommodationist stance toward psychiatrists by publishing an article by activist Frank Kameny with the provocative title, "Does Research into Homosexuality Matter?" In his sweeping critique of psychiatric research on homosexuality, Kameny invoked the authority of his own scientific training as well as anger at the discrimination he had experienced. An astronomer and Second World War veteran, Kameny had been fired from his position with the United States Army Map Service in 1957 and barred from government employment when a background investigation turned up a record of his past arrest on a charge of "lewd conduct" (a charge often used for people caught up in police raids on gay bars or in sweeps of cruising areas. Kameny had been arrested in a San Francisco public restroom). Kameny appealed his dismissal before the U.S. District Court for the District of Columbia, and although he consulted with Benjamin Karpman at Saint Elizabeths, who provided a statement that Kameny "entered the lavatory for legitimate purposes," remaining "somewhat longer than was absolutely necessary" out of scientific curiosity and not sexual intent, his appeal was overturned.[47] Kameny's request for a hearing before the U.S. Supreme Court, the first gay rights legal brief ever brought to the Court, was rejected. He went on to devote his life to gay activism, founding the Mattachine Society of Washington, DC, in 1961. Setting a bold agenda for the organization, Kameny pressed for full citizenship for gay men and lesbians and an end to discrimination in federal employment, the U.S. military, and criminal law.

Crucial to progress on those political fronts and essential to gaining civil rights for gay men and lesbians, Kameny argued, was countering psychiatry's determination of homosexuality as a mental disorder. He believed that the claim to gay health was a grounding political move, necessary for gay people's political intelligibility and for their claims to rights. "The entire homophile movement is going to stand or fall upon the question of whether homosexuality is a sickness," Kameny insisted, "and upon our taking a firm stand on it."[48] "We cannot declare our equality and ask for acceptance . . . from a position of sickness," he emphasized. "Our entire position . . . falls to the ground unless we are prepared to couple our requests . . . with an affirmative, definitive assertion of health."[49] To that end, Kameny framed a resolution—bold for its time and approved and adopted by the Mattachine Society of Washington, DC, in 1965—that "in the absence of valid evidence to the contrary, homosexuality is not a sickness, disturbance, or pathology in any sense, but is merely a preference, orientation, or propensity, on par with, and not different in kind from, heterosexuality."[50]

Kameny staked his case for those claims in his 1965 article in the *Ladder*. Rather than being a "passive battlefield across which conflicting 'authorities' fight their intellectual battles," he argued, gay men and lesbians must "play an active role" in the determination of their fate.[51] He focused his critique in particular on research into the etiology of homosexuality—the "why" question so central to the psychiatric and psychoanalytic project, one that contained within it an assumption of pathological origins. Following the example of homophile advocate Edward Sagarin and echoing Benjamin Karpman, Kameny invoked racial and ethnic analogies, observing that "the Negro is not engrossed in questions about the origins of his skin color, nor the Jew in questions about the possibility of his conversion to Christianity." Questions of causality, Kameny argued, likewise "ought not to be burning ones for the homophile movement." "It is time for us to move away from the comfortingly detached respectability of research," Kameny proposed, "into the often less pleasant rough-and-tumble of political and social activism."[52]

At the core of Kameny's argument was his charge that psychiatric and psychoanalytic claims were based on "bad science," tainted by what he characterized as an "abysmally poor sampling technique."[53] Psychiatrists began their research with the assumption that homosexuality was a disease, he observed, and so it was not surprising that their conclusions supported that view. Noting that psychiatrists based their assumptions on their observations of people who were in psychiatric treatment, Kameny argued that such a sample was unrepresentative of homosexuals as a whole. "Obviously, all persons coming to a psychiatrist's office are going to have problems[,] . . . are going to be disturbed or maladjusted or pathological, in some sense," Kameny wrote, "or they wouldn't be there. To characterize ALL homosexuals as sick, on the basis of such a sampling . . . is clearly invalid, and is bad science."[54]

Among lesbian activists, too, the question of how and whether to participate in research and how to think about psychiatric assessments of homosexuality grew increasingly divisive. Florence Jaffy pushed for "dialogue" and collaboration with scientific experts, since "they, not we, carry weight with the majority" on the question of homosexuality. "It is totally unrealistic to assume that we can make opinion on our own," she wrote, "in flat contradiction to those who deal in psychological matters professionally."[55] Jaffy worried that "shouting, as Franklin Kameny would have us do, that 'no, no, we're not sick'—would make us sound like a bunch of lunatics—as we sometimes do sound, I fear."[56] But Barbara Gittings, Jaffy's most vocal critic in the DOB, teamed up with Kameny to push for a more direct assault on psychiatric assessments of homosexuality. In 1964, and speaking on behalf of the DOB, Gittings denounced the New York Academy of Medicine statement in an editorial in the *Ladder*, writing that "the shoddy work behind this report is a discredit to a professional group in a scientific field."[57] Uncomfortable with Gittings's growing militancy on the question of psychiatry, the DOB fired her from her position as editor of the *Ladder* in 1966.

## Showdown

Through the late 1960s, gay and lesbian activists continued to debate about how and whether to engage with psychiatrists. In 1968, New York Mattachine activist Dick Leitsch chided Frank Kameny for "becoming too defensive, almost paranoid about research into homosexuality." "Let them study," Leitsch wrote to Kameny, reasoning that "we need to know all we can about ourselves and our world." In response to Leitch's comment that "there is no denying that children are often directed toward homosexuality because of mother-son and father-son relationships," Kameny scribbled in the letter's margin: "Yes, I can deny."[58]

But in the space of only about five years, gay activists went from debating the value of research into the etiology of homosexuality, inviting psychiatrists to speak at their meetings and conferences, and awarding them honorary memberships in homophile organizations to condemning them as "mind-pigs," castigating their promises of treatment and cure as "genocide," and engaging them in direct and sometimes physical confrontation.[59] Gay activists were inspired by the Black Panther Party's critiques of the racialized practices of medicine and by their fiery rhetoric.[60] They drew inspiration as well from the growing antipsychiatry movement and its characterization of psychiatry as an instrument of oppression and social control.[61] Gay activist Ronald Lee referenced psychiatrist and leading antipsychiatry theorist Thomas Szasz directly and appreciated Szasz's identification of the homosexual as "the model psychiatric scapegoat."[62] Beginning in the late 1960s, gay activists joined a larger effort to pull back the curtain to expose psychiatric diagnosis as an act of power rather than a statement of scientific fact, and one with damaging consequences for those who were diagnosed as homosexual.

Both the people involved in these events at the time and historians chronicling them years later struggle to explain the relatively rapid shift from gay activists' polite engagement with psychiatric authority through the mid-1960s to the direct assault that would ramp up just a few years later. Psychiatrist William Bennett, who came out as gay during this time of tumult, recalled that the turn from a world that assumed homosexuality was a mental disorder to one in which that assumption was widely questioned felt like "tectonic plates shifting."[63] Martin Duberman attributed the change to the rise of a new generation of gay men and lesbians, "many of whom had not been brought into the notion that they were 'sick.'"[64] Edmund White credited the Stonewall Rebellion of June 1969 with generating a dramatic epistemic rupture. "Up until that moment we had all thought that homosexuality was a medical term," he recalled. "Suddenly we saw that we could be a minority group—with rights, a culture, an agenda."[65] "Soon enough Freudian psychology went up in flames and became no more powerful or present than the smell of ashes in a cold fireplace the morning after."[66] Certainly the movements against the Vietnam War and for racial justice and women's rights had a powerful effect on gay activists, many of whom were participants in those movements and drew directly on their strategies and rhetoric. Duberman recognized the work of activists who managed to wrest authority from experts and claim it for themselves, which resonated with claims made by disability rights activists around the same time: "Once gay people began to think of themselves as experts on their own lives," he wrote, "the modern gay/lesbian political movement flowered—and the misrule of the psychiatric homophobes drew to a close."[67]

As gay and lesbian activists worked to delegitimize the psychiatric assessment of homosexuality, they took aim at the American Psychiatric Association (APA) and focused on the demand that the APA remove homosexuality from their *Diagnostic and Statistical Manual of Mental Disorders* (*DSM*). Known as the psychiatric "bible," the *DSM* provided the nationally accepted nomenclature and taxonomy of mental disease, one used by courts, social agencies, insurance companies, and policymakers as well as by clinicians; it also functioned as an account of psychiatric knowledge and an assertion of psychiatric jurisdiction and power. In its first edition in 1952, the *DSM* identified homosexuality as a "Sexual Deviation" under the larger category of "Personality Disorders" and alongside "transvestism, pedophilia, fetishism, and sexual sadism (including rape, sexual assault, mutilation)."[68] In 1968 in the second edition, known as *DSM-II* (and the *DSM*'s first major revision), homosexuality was again listed as one of ten sexual deviations, a category reserved "for individuals whose sexual interests are directed primarily towards objects rather than people of the opposite sex, toward sexual acts not usually associated with coitus, or toward coitus performed under bizarre circumstances as in necrophilia, pedophilia, sexual sadism, and fetishism."[69]

Beginning in 1970, gay activists turned the APA's annual meetings into a national stage on which to wage their battle against psychiatric diagnosis and pathologization and garner publicity for their new assertion of healthy and happy gay identity. Gay liberationist Gary Alinder described the experience of "invading" the APA's annual meeting in 1970, held that year in San Francisco, as "walking into the enemy's inner sanctum."[70] Among the sessions on the program that year was "Transsexualism vs. Homosexuality: Distinct Entities?," featuring Irving Bieber among the panelists. "When we heard that Bieber and company were coming," Alinder recalled, "we knew that we had to be there."[71] A panel titled "Penile Plethysmograph Responses to Aversive Therapy of Homosexuality" also drew the ire of activists, who were appalled at the cruelty of aversive treatment.[72] In conference sessions, exhibit halls, and hotel hallways, gay men and lesbians traded the deferential engagement of the previous decade for confrontational tactics, disrupting panels, heckling speakers, and seizing the podium. "We've listened to you long enough; you listen to us," a gay liberationist in drag yelled at one session. "We're fed up with being told we're sick. . . . We're gay and we're proud."[73]

Gay activists again disrupted the APA meeting the following year, in Washington, DC. Members of the newly formed Gay Activists Alliance (GAA) obtained phony credentials to enter the conference and attended wearing business suits; some members of the newly formed Gay Liberation Front (GLF) arrived in drag.[74] Storming a session on aversion therapy, Kameny grabbed the microphone and damned psychiatry as the "enemy incarnate." "Psychiatry has waged a relentless war of extermination against us," Kameny shouted; "You may take this as a declaration of war against you.'"[75] In a thwarted attempt to avoid the disruption of the previous year, the APA program chair had taken the unprecedented step of offering the protesters their own place on the conference program, so for the first time gay activists addressed psychiatrists from the stage as well as from the audience. On a panel titled "Lifestyles of Non-Patient Homosexuals," they insisted that psychiatrists recognize gay men and lesbians "as human beings, not as patients."[76] "Yes, we are sick," Gittings told psychiatrists; "we are sick of your manipulation and exploitation of us. We stand here before you to make you aware that we are equal human beings and not your guinea pigs."[77]

The next year, at the 1972 APA meeting in Dallas, Texas, gay activists staged a dramatic rebuke to psychiatric authority with a panel titled "Psychiatry: Friend or Foe to Homosexuals—a Dialogue." In a stunning act of political theater organized by Gittings and Kameny, the panel featured John Fryer, an untenured clinical psychiatrist at Temple University who was also gay. Gittings persuaded Fryer to speak on the panel, but out of reasonable fear for his job security, Fryer insisted on concealing his identity. Donning a distorted rubber mask and an oversized tuxedo and wig and speaking into a device that altered his voice, Fryer appeared as "Dr. H. Anonymous" and delivered a riveting account of the discrimination that he had faced as a gay psychiatrist: he had been dismissed from a residency and lost a job because he was gay. To a shocked audience of psychiatrists, and at a time when homosexuality disqualified candidates for psychiatric and psychoanalytic training, Fryer also revealed that more than two hundred members of the APA were also gay, referring to themselves as the GAYPA and meeting secretly at bars and hotel rooms during the annual meetings.[78]

Gay activists had cultivated new allies among psychiatrists critical of the psychoanalytic line on homosexuality. In 1972, psychiatrist Robert Spitzer encountered GAA activists when they disrupted the annual meeting of the Association for the Advancement of Behavior Therapy in New York City. Intrigued by their arguments that psychiatric claims about homosexuality were baseless, Spitzer invited them to present their case to the APA's Committee on Nomenclature (on which he was a member), which was charged with the task of deciding which mental disorders would be listed in the *DSM*. The GAA chose gay psychologist Charles Silverstein to present their argument to the committee. Silverstein decided "not . . . to play the role of gay activist with the Nomenclature Committee," knowing that "they'd be expecting that," and instead opened his presentation with an erudite account of the history of psychiatry and diagnostic labeling.[79] "Homosexuality," he asserted, "is not a diagnostic label"; instead, he countered, it was "a social and religious label, a pejorative label slipped in for religious and moral reasons." Silverstein went on to attack psychiatric arguments about the pathology of homosexuality by critiquing psychiatrists' scientific method. "The 'old' research with which you are familiar is the subjective psychoanalytic theory," Silverstein told the committee. But since psychoanalysts had all been taught the "so-called etiology of homosexuality" before they met their first patients, "selective perception takes over from there." "How can a treatment be evaluated without the comparison with appropriate control groups?" he asked. What about "experimenter bias and placebo effects?" He followed with evidence, some from disciplines beyond psychiatry, that called into question the understanding of homosexuality as a pathological condition, including Hooker's 1957 study as well as newer work by psychologist George Weinberg and psychological and ethnographic research by psychologist Frank Beach and anthropologist Clellen S. Ford, which documented same-sex sexual behavior in different human societies around the world and across animal species.[80] "Our position here is simple," Silverstein concluded. "Unless [psychiatrists] can establish the veracity of their theories through the established techniques of scientific research, their theories remain creative, but unsubstantiated."[81] Psychiatrist Robert Jean Campbell, a member of the APA Assembly who was gay and closeted at the time, recalled that Silverstein and the GAA "had a lot of data that I had never seen. I don't know where they got it, but I was really overwhelmed by the data."[82]

The data mattered; so did the timing. Gay activists were far from alone in the late 1960s and early 1970s in their assault on psychiatric authority. Their critique landed as part of a larger and broader challenge to the APA's conservatism in those years. A varied collection of radical thinkers and activists grouped under the designation of "antipsychiatry" lambasted psychiatrists for pursuing a project of social control and the enforcement of conformity under the guises of science and care.[83] At the same annual APA meetings where gay activists zapped panels on aversion therapy, antiwar activists introduced resolutions against the Vietnam War and the invasion of Cambodia. Feminists charged that psychiatrists perpetuated the "myth of male superiority" and in 1970 demanded that "reparations" be paid to women who had suffered mistreatment by their "piggish" therapists.[84] This broader context of critique and radical ferment and the turn of some psychiatrists from the individual psyche to the social world created fertile ground for gay activists' challenges.[85]

Gay activists also benefited from alliances forged with dissident psychiatrists. Perhaps the most important and consequential defection from the psychiatric orthodoxy on homosexuality was that of Judd Marmor. A widely respected mainstream psychoanalyst, Marmor had trained at the New York Psychoanalytic Institute in the late 1930s, where he "first encountered the formulations of organized psychoanalytic theory concerning homosexuality."[86] Moving to Los Angeles in 1946, he set up a private practice and began a prolific research and publishing career. In the late 1940s and 1950s, along with most of his colleagues, Marmor treated gay patients with the aim of changing their sexual orientation. "We all used to think in those days that psychoanalysis could cure everything," he recalled, "from chilblains to homosexuality."[87] When he learned of Hooker's claim in 1956 that homosexuality was not a mental illness, he confessed that he "wasn't prepared to go all the way" because "I still had a feeling that it was a developmental deviation."[88] But by the 1960s, moved in part by his own lack of success in effecting sexual conversion in his gay patients, Marmor began to publicly question the psychiatric doxa about homosexuality as a treatable mental disorder. Homosexuality was better understood as a benign variant of sexual behavior, Marmor came to argue, one with psychosocial and possibly also genetic and biological roots. In 1965, Marmor published *Sexual Inversion: The Multiple Roots of Homosexuality*, including contributions from a wide range of fields, including history, zoology, genetics, endocrinology, sociology, and anthropology as well as psychology and psychiatry. Marmor included an essay by Evelyn Hooker, with whom he would come to work closely on the National Institute of Mental Health Task Force on Homosexuality, established in 1967.[89] In his introduction, Marmor echoed gay activist arguments that psychoanalytic thinking relied on bad sampling, pointing out that the assumption that homosexuality was an illness was based on a "skewed sample because psychoanalysts saw only disturbed homosexuals in their offices."[90] At the APA's annual meeting in 1972, Marmor appeared on a panel alongside Kameny and Gittings, throwing his lot in publicly on the side of gay activists before an audience of his psychiatric colleagues. And in 1973, he delivered a paper at the annual meeting in which he stated his conviction that "there is now an incontrovertible body of evidence that there are homosexual individuals who, except for their variant object choice, are happy with their lives and have made a constructive and realistic adaptation to being members of a minority group in our society." "It is our task to be healers," Marmor asserted, "not watchdogs of our social mores."[91] While serving as vice president of the APA that year, Marmor was a powerful voice for change and a critical ally for gay activists.

It also helped gay activists' cause that they made their case to the APA at the same moment that some psychiatrists were challenging the dominance of psychoanalysts in the profession and calling for greater specificity in the definition of mental disorders and a more scientistic orientation in psychiatry more generally. Both *DSM-I* and *DSM-II* bore the imprint of psychoanalytic ideas that were in ascendence in the 1950s and 1960s, replacing the somatic emphasis of early psychiatry's search for organic causes of mental illness with psychodynamic concepts drawn from Freudian psychoanalysis that emphasized underlying psychological conflicts. The fortuitous timing of gay activists' assault on psychiatric authority, initiated at a moment of internal battle within the APA concerning the definition of mental disorders and Spitzer's determination to move psychiatry away from psychoanalysis to more empirical ground, helps explain their remarkable and rapid success—a victory that came in the very early days of the gay rights movement and would be followed by many setbacks and defeats. Spitzer may have been genuinely sympathetic to the arguments of gay activists; it is also clear that he made strategic use of them to gain power in a struggle internal to psychiatry and in an effort to dethrone psychoanalysis and move the discipline to purportedly firmer medical and scientific grounding, to forge definitions of mental disorders that might better hold up to empirical scrutiny, and to support the sweeping revision he would promote for the third edition of the *DSM*.[92] Spitzer was, by his own account, "becoming disenchanted with psychoanalysis" and growing more interested in behavior therapy and other forms of nonanalytic psychotherapy.[93] He claimed to have been inspired by gay activists' critique to ask broader questions about what constituted a mental disorder, questions he recognized that psychiatry had failed to answer with any specificity. When considering the claims made by gay activists, Spitzer wrote, "I was confronted with the absence of any accepted definition of mental disorder." Convinced that "no precise definition of disorder . . . was possible or even useful," Spitzer came to believe that "the consequences of a condition, and not its etiology" should be central in determining whether the condition should be considered a "disorder." Evidence of distress or impairment would come to dominate definitions of mental disorders in the *DSM-III*, replacing the psychoanalytic concepts of psychosis, neurosis, and perversion.[94] Breaking with psychoanalytic explanations, Spitzer wrote that "it seemed irrelevant . . . whether or not a condition is the result of childhood conflicts and interpsychic anxieties." Instead, he proposed that "either subjective distress or generalized impairment in social effectiveness" be the criteria for judging a condition to be a disorder.[95]

The final showdown came in May 1973, when the APA convened in Honolulu for their annual meeting. There, Spitzer organized a panel that posed the direct question, "Should Homosexuality Be in the APA Nomenclature?" A raucous and divided audience of over a thousand people came to hear psychiatrists Judd Marmor, Richard Green, and Robert Stoller, joined by gay activist Ron Gold, argue for the removal of homosexuality from the *DSM* and Irving Bieber and Charles Socarides defend its continued inclusion. Stoller began by arguing that homosexuality failed to fill the criteria of a "true diagnosis." "Since that is true for most of the rest of the 'diagnoses' of psychiatry," Stoller proposed, psychiatrists should "scrap the system . . . and start afresh."[96] Gold was more pointed in his critique, accusing psychiatrists of being "willing accomplices" in the discrimination perpetrated on gay people by a hostile society.

At the 1973 meeting, after several years of protest and with Spitzer's sanction, the Committee on Nomenclature recommended that the APA remove "homosexuality per se" from the *DSM*. That recommendation wended its way through the APA's councils and committees and was approved at each stage. Later that year, on December 15, 1973, the organization's Board of Trustees voted 13–0 (with 2 abstentions) to remove it. Psychiatrists opposed to the decision, led by Socarides and Bieber, demanded a referendum of the entire APA membership in an attempt to overturn it and obtained enough signatures on their proposal to force a popular vote. The APA sent a ballot to its 10,000 members in 1974, and to the surprise of the psychiatric establishment, the motion carried the vote of the majority (if far from an overwhelming one), with 58 percent of APA members voting to delete homosexuality from the *DSM*, 38 percent voting to keep it, and 4 percent abstaining.

## "Non-Patient, Non-Prisoner Homosexuals"

With no small sarcasm, Frank Kameny would name December 15, 1973, as the date on which "we were cured *en masse* by the psychiatrists."[97] The decision was broadcast by newspapers across the country in headlines such as "Twenty Million Homosexuals Gain Instant Cure" and "Doctors Rule Homosexuality Not Abnormal."[98] The APA's resolution to remove homosexuality from the *DSM*, however, was a less definitive victory than was celebrated by gay activists at the time or has been described later by historians. The APA stopped short of declaring homosexuality a "normal variant of human sexuality," as activists had hoped they would. In fact, to the contrary, Spitzer stated explicitly that while "homosexual activist groups will no doubt claim that psychiatry has at last recognized that homosexuality is as 'normal' as heterosexuality," "they will be wrong."[99] And while homosexuality was removed from the *DSM* in 1973, it was quietly replaced with a new diagnostic category, initially designated "Sexual Orientation Disturbance," a classification identifying "individuals whose sexual interests are directed primarily toward people of the same sex and who are either disturbed by, in conflict with, or wish to change their sexual orientation."[100] Spitzer presented this new disorder as a compromise between what he characterized as "two extreme viewpoints," in the hope that it might appease the hardline psychoanalysts adamantly opposed to removing homosexuality from the *DSM*.[101] His motivation, he acknowledged, was at least in part "political": "I knew that there was no way that homosexuality was going to be removed entirely from *DSM-II*, but if you had a category where you could say, 'Okay, for the homosexual who's dissatisfied, you can still treat it and that's the disorder—sexual orientation disturbance.'"[102] By including the new category, Spitzer wrote, the APA "acknowledges that at least in some cases, an appropriate therapeutic activity is to help the individual develop a normative sexual arousal pattern and not merely to become more comfortable with his or her homosexuality."[103] Spitzer and others represented their commitment to "sexual orientation disturbance" as essential in holding out hope for unhappy homosexuals and supporting the psychiatrists who treated them; they also surely acted out of an interest in preserving their own client base and income stream.

Four years later, in 1977, when members of an APA advisory committee sat down to hammer out the details of revisions to the section of the *DSM-III* on Psychosexual Disorders, the inclusion of the new diagnostic category sparked an acrimonious debate. That debate began over the most basic question, that of the new category's name. As chair of the APA task force responsible for overseeing the revisions and as the architect of the revisionist *DSM-III*, Spitzer first suggested the term "homodysphilia" "in an effort to improve upon the lack of specificity in the term Sexual Orientation Disturbance," but his colleagues pushed back.[104] ("What the fuck is Homodysphilia?" psychiatrist Richard Green wrote to a comember of the Psychosexual Disorders Advisory Committee, which was responsible for drafting the revision).[105] Judd Marmor proposed in protest that they add the "equally meaningless" diagnostic classification "heterodysphilia" as a "balancing term."[106] Spitzer offered another awkward neologism, "dyshomophilia," and then "Homosexual Conflict Disorder," both also roundly rejected by his colleagues. The committee finally settled, in "exhaustion rather than agreement," on "Ego-dystonic Homosexuality," the official designation that would be entered into the third major revision of the *DSM* (known as *DSM-III*) in 1980.[107] "Ego-dystonic homosexuality" remained in the *DSM* until it was quietly removed in 1986 and replaced with the more neutral term, "sexual disorder not otherwise specified." The pathologized status of homosexuality, however, continued to linger in a symptom listed under this new category, "persistent and marked distress about one's sexual orientation," which remained until 2013, forty years after the formal declassification of homosexuality, when it was finally deleted in revisions that would be published in the *DSM-V*.

Terminology aside, many psychiatrists, including some members of the committee tasked with revising the *DSM*, disagreed more fundamentally with the decision to include the new category at all. Judd Marmor believed the introduction of "homodysphilia" into the *DSM*, or any of its substitutes that singled out anxiety about same-sex orientation for a special diagnostic category, to be "a highly regressive step," one that "is really letting the old diagnostic category in under another guise."[108] "The only reason we treat individuals who feel distressed by their homosexual impulses as though they are a separate diagnostic category," Marmor wrote to Spitzer in September 1977, "is because we have not yet fully accepted the idea that homosexual impulses per se do not necessarily constitute psychopathology."[109] Spitzer conceded the point, acknowledging to gay psychiatrist Richard Pillard in 1977 that "for many of us, the issue as to whether or not . . . homosexuality is *in some cases* pathological is still not resolved."[110] The truth of that observation was borne out in a survey of psychiatrists in 1977, fielded four years after the removal of homosexuality from the *DSM*, in which 69 percent of the respondents said they believed that homosexuality was "usually a pathological adaptation."[111]

While gay activists were troubled by the inclusion of the new diagnostic category, few expended much energy to publicly oppose it or allowed it to undermine their claim to a larger victory. On December 15, 1973, the day the

APA's decision to remove homosexuality from the *DSM* was announced, Kameny sent a celebratory note to supporters who had helped fund his trip to Honolulu to attend the APA conference that year. He acknowledged that while the revised nomenclature asserted that "a Homosexual wishing to change to heterosexuality *IS* sick," the decision to remove homosexuality nonetheless represented "the happy and successful conclusion of a more-than-ten-year effort on my part."[112] Members of the newly formed Gay, Lesbian, and Bisexual Caucus of the APA were also eager to celebrate the victory of the declassification of homosexuality, deciding that the inclusion of the new category "was not worth spending effort to combat."[113] Barbara Gittings recalled "some worried talk" about the new diagnostic category and a proposal for "an equivalent category of 'Ego-Dystonic Heterosexuality' to show plainly that homosexuality in and of itself isn't still being looked at askance." She and other activists feared, though, that any such proposal "would likely trigger another referendum call by Dr. Socarides and his gang," and they decided that "we ought not do anything that would allow that shut door to be re-opened."[114] While "none of us liked the diagnosis of ego-dystonic homosexuality," gay psychiatrist Robert Cabaj recalled, "we suspected it was rarely used in clinical treatment anyway. Maybe if we didn't draw attention to it, nobody else would either, so maybe we should just let it be." Debate over the new category, he confessed, "left us drained, and for a while we indeed gave up."[115] Kameny was more flippant in his assessment, telling Gittings, "I don't have any problem with 'Ego-Dystonic Homosexuality,'" since "anyone who's gay and doesn't want to be has to be crazy!"[116]

Kameny's gay-pride quip aside, his disinterest in contesting the new diagnostic category of ego-dystonic homosexuality aligned with his broader investment in distinguishing healthy gay men and lesbians from those who were mentally ill or distressed by their sexuality. The effort to differentiate healthy gays from sick ones was at the core of Kameny's main argument against psychiatric assessments of homosexuality: that they were based on faulty sampling methods, generalizing from people in psychiatric treatment to make overarching and false assessments of homosexuals as a group. That strategy kept Kameny and others from stopping short of arguing that homosexuals were not, by default of their sexual choices, sick, arguing instead that *most* were not. That claim, and that core distinction, would become foundational to the gay challenge to psychiatric thinking and practice.

Kameny's emphasis on representative sampling, and his rhetorical distinction between gay people worthy of recognition and rights and those who might appropriately be pathologized or criminalized echoed a stance taken earlier by homophile activists and their allies and continued a longer pattern of cleaving and disavowal. In 1951, Edward Sagarin (writing under the pseudonym Donald Webster Cory) argued for differentiating between the "anti-social and the socially useful homosexual," with the latter deserving of social tolerance and civil rights.[117] "All minorities suffer because of the few undesirables in their midst," one lesbian wrote in 1957.[118] "If Dr. Bergler actually believes the statements he makes against homosexuals per se," a lesbian DOB member wrote to the *Ladder* the same year, "he must have studied only emotionally immature and mentally disturbed homosexuals. Perhaps he should meet some cheerful, constructive, and stable members of the sexual minority."[119] Eager to find evidence to bolster that claim of healthy lesbianism and counter research based on studies of "badly maladjusted women who have sought psychiatric help or from women in prison," the DOB sent a questionnaire to subscribers of the *Ladder* in 1958.[120] Their survey of what they characterized as a "quite different type of group from that usually studied by doctors and criminologists" found that such "normal" lesbians reported higher-than-average levels of education, income, professional status, and home ownership—in the words of the survey's author, they were lesbians who live "a relatively stable, responsible mode of life by certain conventional . . . standards." Respondents also reported "fairly conventional" family backgrounds, with most reared in two-parent households by a mother and father. The data, they were pleased to report, also "presents a picture considerably different from the stereotype of homosexuals as heavy drinkers." Finally, and importantly, the DOB found that a "large majority" of those surveyed "have not had, and do not want, psychotherapy."[121]

Those distinctions and disaggregations were evident as well in the work of Evelyn Hooker. Hooker characterized her own research subjects as "non-patient, non-prisoner" homosexuals, a depiction that would be repeated with admiration and approval by historians describing her work and one that worked, too, to differentiate rights- and tolerance-deserving homosexuals from the sick and criminalized minority.[122] "I didn't want anyone who had extended therapy or arrest records," Hooker emphasized, explicitly distinguishing her research subjects from criminalized populations and from people who sought (or were coerced into) psychiatric treatment.[123] Proposing to study gay men "who lead relatively stable, occupationally successful lives," Hooker also made gainful employment a criterion for research subjects she characterized as "responsible, reliable, productive, well-functioning."[124] Along with their lack of psychopathology and criminal history and their record of employment, Hooker emphasized that many such normal gay men were involved in long-term relationships that were

not organized around masculine and feminine roles, and so gender normativity too was part of what Hooker claimed, and consequently reinforced,
as "normal" homosexuality.

Hooker's critique of the concept of the clinical entity "homosexuality"
effectively refuted psychiatrists' wholesale pathologization, but she also believed that there were some "forms" of homosexuality that were "very destructive."[125] That assessment was reflected in the 1969 report of the NIMH
Task Force on Homosexuality, which Hooker chaired. Calling for the decriminalization of "private homosexual acts" and an end to discrimination in
employment, Hooker's report was hailed as a model of liberal reform (and
was shelved by President Richard Nixon when it was first released. It was
later leaked to the gay press and was first published in *Homophile Studies*, a
quarterly journal sponsored by the homophile organization ONE, Inc.). But
Hooker believed that "one of the most crucial questions" for the task force to
address was "the means of distinguishing between those homosexuals who
are dangerous to society and those who are not."[126] The final report confirmed the "wide diversity" among homosexuals, some of whom "function
well in everyday life" and others who are "severely maladjusted or disturbed
in their functioning." The latter were identified as those "whose total life is
dominated by homosexual impulses."[127] The report also reinforced the association between homosexuality and pedophilia, distinguishing the homosexual who engages in sex "only with another consenting adult in private"
from the one "whose sexual behavior is with children and adolescents or
who otherwise violates public decency."[128] To the dismay of many of her gay
admirers, Hooker also endorsed "prevention of the development of a homosexual orientation in a child or adolescent" as one of the "most important
goals" supported in the final report of the NIMH's Task Force on Homosexuality.[129] When pressed by gay men and lesbians at a public talk about her support for "prevention," Hooker made clear that she hoped to "prevent what
everybody in this room knows as well as I know, that there are some forms
of homosexuality which are very destructive." She insisted that "we have an
obligation as a society to bring up children in such a way that they will not
have to endure" the "agony" of vulnerability to arrest or violent assault.[130]

Hooker and the DOB were hardly alone in yoking healthy homosexuality to a range of broader cultural norms and values. The title of the panel
organized by gay activists in 1971 at the meeting of the APA, "Lifestyles of
Non-Patient Homosexuals," spoke powerfully to the desire to distinguish
healthy gays from sick ones. As Barbara Gittings insisted,

> We are really just like any other people in society. We get up in the morn-
> ing and go to work or school, we watch the boob tube or go to movies,

we go on picnics and we hike, we have hobbies or go in for sports, we shop at the super market and do our housework and all the other humdrum things that make up American life today. And sometimes we make love. We don't spend all our time in bed any more than other people do, however.[131]

At the 1972 meeting of the APA, Gittings and Kameny distributed a manifesto titled "Gay, Proud, and Healthy," a slogan they proposed, along with "Gay Is Good," as the official "theme" of the gay rights movement. "Gay, Proud, and Healthy" was also the title they chose for their exhibit—the first time gay activists were allowed to have exhibit space at the conference— which they used to make the visual case for health through photographs of "loving couples."

Sometimes gay claims to health were posed in temporal terms, as part of a forward-looking gay modernity. Activists worked to redraw the definitions

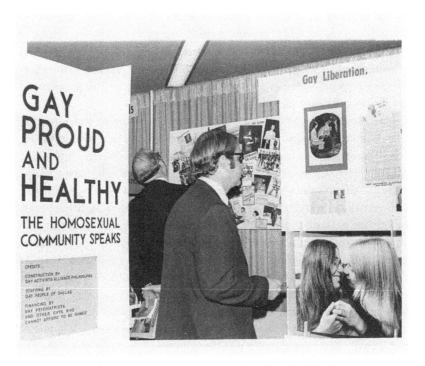

FIGURE 5.1. Psychiatrists looking at "Gay Proud and Healthy" display, American Psychiatric Association meeting in Dallas, Texas, May 1–4, 1972, Barbara Gittings and Kay Tobin Lahusen Gay History Papers and Photographs, Manuscripts and Archives Division, New York Public Library, New York, NY (photograph by Kay Tobin).

of the modern gay and lesbian as opposed to the anachronistic homosexual, aligning modern gayness with the linked values of gender normativity, pride, and happiness and the latter with mental instability and a retrograde and melancholic attachment to the past. In this formulation, "self-hating" or "masochistic" people in psychiatric treatment were atavistic holdovers of an antiquated gay past, unable or unwilling to join the bandwagon of gay happiness, health, and pride.

The norm most readily tied to health, although perhaps less recognizable as a norm than monogamy, home ownership, or gender normativity, was *happiness*. "Happy" plus "healthy" was probably the most common discursive pairing in gay politics in this period, naming the prescribed affect of properly politicized and modern gay men and lesbians and the obligatory response to psychiatrists' claims that gay lives were defined by misery. "Happiness" appeared so often in gay activist responses to psychiatry that it effectively operated as a mandate. Countering psychoanalytic representations of the homosexual as neurotically depressed and constitutionally melancholic or of homosexuality as way of life incommensurate with happiness, activists insisted on gay happiness. As sociologist Deborah Gould notes, social movements provide language for people's affective states as well as "a pedagogy of sorts regarding what and how to feel and what to do in light of those feelings."[132] Happiness occupied a central place in the affective pedagogy promoted by gay activists, tutoring queer people in new ways to feel about themselves and their sexuality.

Like the claim to health, the claim to happiness can be understood as a revolutionary act against the grain of every cultural narrative of the inevitable *unhappiness* of homosexuals. Psychiatrists in particular emphasized unhappiness to the point of despair as a defining feature of homosexual life. Indeed, unhappiness was the primary symptom by which "ego-dystonic homosexuality" was diagnosed. But while the insistence on gay happiness might have been a canny response to dominant assumptions of its impossibility, the mandate to happiness for people with a history of oppression, exclusion, and attributions of mental illness followed a perverse logic. As historian Abram J. Lewis has observed, activists' insistence on gay psychic fortitude put them in the position of having to argue that, "as a group, homosexuals were uniquely impervious to their own oppression."[133] And as critical theorist Sara Ahmed proposes, happiness, like health, is a quality that is easily naturalized into a transparent good but that is often used to reinscribe social norms and "make certain forms of personhood valuable." Ahmed asks "whether queer happiness involves an increasing proximity to social forms that are already attributed to happiness-causes (the family, marriage, class mobility, whiteness), which of course suggests that promoting queer happiness might involve promoting social forms in which other queers will not be able to participate."[134] By extension, of course, claims to gay happiness as the condition of recognition required for gay rights rendered other forms of queer affective subjectivity and personhood less valuable, less worthy, and less authentically gay.

The critical engagement of gay and lesbian activists with psychiatric authority, then, mobilized a set of prescriptions and hierarchies of worth, setting in motion a process of disaffiliation, disidentification, and disavowal that narrowed the lens and shrunk the reach of gay politics. For Kameny, distinguishing "most" gay men and lesbians from the mentally ill and the criminalized was a strategic move that was essential to the political progress of gay men and lesbians. "Whatever definitions of sickness one may use," he wrote, "sick people are NOT EQUAL to well people in any practical, meaningful sense."[135] Kameny seemed to comprehend the exclusionary effects of an antisickness position when he wrote that "properly or improperly, people ARE prejudiced against the mentally ill. Rightly or wrongly, employers will NOT hire them. Morally or immorally, the mentally ill are NOT judged as individuals, but are made pariahs. If we allow the label of sickness to stand," Kameny wrote, "we will then have *two* battles to fight—that to combat prejudice against homosexuals per se, and that to combat prejudice against the mentally ill—and we will be pariahs and outcasts twice over. One such battle is quite enough."[136] Here, Kameny defended his decision to organize around a single axis of oppression as pragmatic.[137] His words also suggest an awareness of the stigmatizing dynamics that sociologist Erving Goffman described during moments of "mixed encounter," as underlined by disability studies scholars, when an "affirmation of one's own health depends on the constant recognition, and indeed the creation, of the spoiled health of others."[138]

It is clear what was gained by such claims. Kameny and others did not underestimate the extent to which the understanding of homosexuals as mentally ill sanctioned a web of stigmatizing cultural attitudes and criminalizing laws and policies, from sexual psychopath laws to the denial of parental rights and the exclusion of immigrants.[139] At the same time, that project required distancing queer people from a long history of injury and illness by disavowing traumatic pasts and disentangling "gay" from the most stigmatized, minoritized, and criminalized subjects. In a painful irony, it is likely that those subjects, largely disavowed by gay activists, bore the brunt of the most invasive and violent psychiatric modalities, such as electroshock, lobotomy, and aversive treatment, those the gay activists most loudly decried. Activists' turn away from queer people with criminalized and psychiatric histories would make it difficult for them to recognize the expansion of psychiatric control and authority into prisons and jails and the use of behavior modification to control people, especially women, gay men, and gender-nonconforming people, as issues of concern to them. Their political strategy kept them from seeing what historian Emily Thuma characterizes as a "fusion of the 'therapeutic state' and the carceral state" and kept them from recognizing the most marginalized queer people as members of the group on whose behalf they were fighting.[140]

Gay activists sheared off the psychiatrized and criminalized from the rights-deserving and healthy; they also worked to sever ties between homosexuality and gender nonconformity in their effort to break free from psychiatric diagnosis. As Joanne Meyerowitz, Jennifer Terry, Jules Gill-Peterson, and others have shown, contemporary understandings of sex, gender, and sexuality as ontologically distinct categories did not take shape until the mid-twentieth century.[141] Gender variance had been central to nineteenth- and early twentieth-century ideas about homosexuality, as sexologists theorized same-sex desire through the concept of gender inversion, understood as a constitutional reversal or mixture of gender traits.[142] Those ideas continued to echo decades later in the writing of psychoanalysts, who often understood transvestism and transsexuality as symptoms of a more overarching homosexuality.

In the 1950s and 1960s, those connections between sexuality and gender began to loosen, prised apart by gay and gender-variant people as well as by psychiatrists, psychologists, and other physicians. Both gay and cross-gender-identified people in this period began to engage in what Meyerowitz terms a "social practice of taxonomy," a project of distinguishing different sexual and gender minorities that was driven in part by the respectability politics of both queer and trans people, who "sometimes attempted to lift their own group's social standing by foisting the stigma of transgression onto others."[143]

The new visibility of transsexuality in the 1950s and 1960s prompted some gay people to differentiate themselves from transsexuals. Gay people with aspirations to civil and social recognition in those decades also engaged in the policing of gender nonconformity among those whom they considered their own. Historian Craig Loftin documents the growing anxiety and resentment on the part of white gay men in the 1950s and 1960s with "swishes and swishiness," a style of gay male effeminacy with roots in early twentieth-century working-class and African American sexual cultures. For homophile leaders, Loftin writes, swishes "represented a degrading stereotype, an irritating throwback to an outdated model of homosexual identity."[144] Others read effeminacy as evidence of neurosis or another mental disorder. Blanche Baker, a psychologist who consulted with homophile groups and was a regular columnist in *ONE* magazine, diagnosed the effeminacy of the "swish" as a "neurotic retaliation."[145] Of the association of the "male homosexual" with the "'fairy' and the female impersonator, the transvestist at the drag," Edward Sagarin (under the pseudonym Donald Webster Cory) wrote, "this effeminacy is psychologically induced." The effeminate gay man was found "only in a small proportion of homosexuals," Cory insisted, and he was *persona non grata* among the more virile."[146] In defense against the charge that gay men often "make a public display of themselves," "swishing and screaming" and "placing themselves on exhibition like museum pieces or circus freaks," Cory countered that "most of us make no display at all of our tendencies. Will you punish the many for the few?"[147]

Lesbians engaged in their own complex navigation and policing of gender conformity in this period. DOB rules dictated that if a woman wore pants to a meeting, they had to be "women's slacks" (though violation of that rule, it seems, was common and tolerated).[148] With embarrassment and regret, Gittings recalled an incident in which a person she described as having lived "pretty much as a transvestite most of her life," passing socially as a man and wearing men's clothes, was "persuaded" by Gittings and other DOB members "to don female garb, [and] to deck herself out in as 'feminine' a manner as she could" to attend an early DOB national convention, even though women's clothes "were totally alien to her."[149] Hostility to trans women ramped up in some lesbian feminist circles in the 1970s. In 1972, new separatist leaders of the San Francisco chapter of the DOB that had elected trans woman and lesbian folksinger Beth Elliott to the position of vice president the year before ousted her for not "really" being a woman and voted to bar transsexual women from the DOB. In 1973, Elliott was forced off the stage at the West Coast Lesbian Conference and condemned by keynoter Robin Morgan as an infiltrator, a "male transvestite," and a "rapist."[150]

The campaign to remove homosexuality from the *DSM* raised the stakes for gay activists and supportive psychiatrists eager to emphasize the distinction between transsexuality and homosexuality. Writing to Dick Leitsch about "the question of gender-change" in 1968, Kameny insisted that "transsexuality is not our problem, and I don't believe in mixing causes, as you well know."[151] In a speech in 1973, gay activist Ron Gold countered popular associations of homosexuality with transsexuality, stating that he knew of "very few gay men who are 'frightened' of their genitals." Gold attributed the effeminacy of some gay men to the residual and emasculating effects of stigma, suggesting that gender variance would and should wither away with the declassification of homosexuality as a mental disorder.[152] A few years after the removal of homosexuality from the *DSM*, Kameny wrote

to Robert Spitzer in 1977 to weigh in on the debate about the new inclusion of "ego-dystonic homosexuality" in the *DSM-III*. Kameny condemned
psychiatrists' tendency to "confuse Homosexuality with both gender role
and gender identity" and warned Spitzer against perpetuating "a common
conceptual confusion" of gender and sexual identity to which he believed
psychiatrists were particularly prone.[153]

One skirmish in the larger battle between gay activists and psychiatrists
made clear how gay and lesbian activists could argue for the recognition
of their own health at the expense of trans people. Aversion therapy, using
painful shocks or nausea-inducing drugs in an effort to alter "maladaptive"
behaviors, was particularly abhorrent to gay activists, and practitioners
and advocates of aversive modalities were among their prime targets. The
Nebraska company Farrall Instruments, the main manufacturer of aversion
therapy equipment, regularly sponsored a booth at the annual meeting of
the APA, where they exhibited aversive conditioning shock units like the
"Office Shocker," advertised as "ideal for the desk of the private practitioner"; the "Personal Shocker," which could be carried in a shirt pocket;
selections of their extensive library of 35mm slides of nude men and women
designed to elicit arousal; and penile plethysmograph technology, used to
measure penile circumference in order to assess erotic response to visual
stimuli.[154] While gay activists denounced psychiatrists and psychologists
who practiced aversive conditioning, charging them with carrying out torture under the guise of therapy, Barbara Gittings went after Farrall Instruments itself. After the APA's decision to remove homosexuality from the
*DSM* in 1973, Gittings lobbied Farrall to remove "homosexuality" from the
list of "disorders" their instruments could be used to "treat" and to delete
any reference in their promotional materials to their success in "converting
homosexuals to heterosexual activity."[155] Gittings sent Farrall her recommended edits and deletions on copies of their own advertisements, crossing
out references to homosexuality in green ink.[156] But Gittings did not object
to Farrall's continued inclusion of "transsexuality" as a disorder treatable by
aversive conditioning. Going carefully through the bibliography that Farrall
featured in its advertisement for their Visually Keyed Shocker device, Gittings crossed out two articles that mentioned homosexuality but marked
"OK" next to the references to studies of the use of aversion therapy for
"transvestism."[157] With her edits, Gittings asserted a distinction between
gay and trans people rather than a relationship of kinship or linked fate.
Indeed, many gay activists felt that their own fate depended on severing
associations with trans people.

As gay and lesbian activists struggled for recognition as healthy, rights-
deserving citizens in these years, some trans people who desired access to

medical transition gained in their own quest for recognition as people most appropriately "treated" with surgery and hormones rather than with psychotherapy to "adjust" to their sex assigned at birth. Harry Benjamin had proposed a diagnostic category of the "true transsexual," as distinguished from the transvestite and the homosexual, in his 1966 book, *The Transsexual Phenomenon*, and he offered an affirmative treatment pathway that led to an upsurge in the number of people requesting hormone therapies and gender-confirming surgeries.[158] The 1960s and early 1970s witnessed the rise of transsexual medicine and the opening of gender identity clinics at several major universities, even as access to medical transition remained limited in the extreme and by design. The gender clinic at Johns Hopkins University limited its evaluations to two people per month.[159] Gender-affirming surgery was restricted to those who could afford the expense, constrained by rigid medical gatekeeping that demanded convincing heteronormative gender presentation and a posttransition heterosexual orientation, required a commitment to living a "stealth" life, and was guided by an overarching suspicion of fraudulence and mendacity.[160] Access to medical gender transition was limited as well by medical professionals preoccupied with the possibility that their patients would regret their transition and seek legal recourse.[161]

Part of the price of legal recognition and access to trans medical care was the classification of the desire for gender transition as a mental disorder.[162] Access to medical transition in the United States, from its beginning in the 1960s, required a psychiatrist's certification of "true transsexuality," so even as proponents of medical transition appeared to prevail over the opposition of psychoanalysts who viewed trans people as "borderline psychotics" and victims of "paranoid schizophrenic psychosis" and gender-affirming surgery as "a surgical acting out of psychosis," psychiatrists continued to assert authority over trans lives and embodiment and undercut people's claim to knowledge and authority over their own bodies and identities.[163] As the director of a counseling service wrote to Lou Sullivan in 1979, when he applied to Stanford University's Gender Dysphoria Program, "There is no way of telling if you are a transsexual unless you are tested and evaluated by a psychiatrist/psychologist."[164] (Sullivan was denied entry into the program because he did not hide his intention to live as a gay man.) The inclusion of Gender Identity Disorder (GID) in the revised version of the *DSM* in 1980 known as *DSM-III* (the first edition of the manual to omit homosexuality from its pages), confirmed and consolidated psychiatric authority over transgender health care. The *DSM-III* added a cluster of new diagnostic categories in a section on Psychosexual Disorders under the heading of Gender Identity Disorder, identified as "an incongruence between anatomic sex and gender identity."[165] The *DSM-III* defined the new diagnosis of "Transsexualism" as a disorder characterized by "a persistent sense of discomfort and inappropriateness about one's anatomical sex and a persistent wish to be rid of one's genitals and to live as a member of the other sex."[166] This was joined by Gender Identity Disorder of Childhood, defined as "a profound disturbance of the normal sense of maleness and femaleness," and "Atypical Gender Identity Disorder," a "residual category" covering disorders in gender identity "not classifiable as a specific Gender Identity Disorder."[167] The *DSM-III* cordoned off the new types of Gender Identity Disorder from the older diagnostic category of transvestism. Listed in the first two editions of the *DSM* under a subgroup of sexual deviations and alongside homosexuality, transvestism remained in the *DSM-III* but was now classified under the "Paraphilias," the essential feature of which was the requirement "that unusual or bizarre imagery or acts are necessary for sexual excitement."[168]

While the *DSM-III* confirmed the distinction between cross-gender identification and homosexuality by including the former and omitting the latter, psychiatrists continued to pull the two into association. Some called on the same psychoanalytic arguments used to explain the etiology of homosexuality to account for transsexuality, including "excessively close mother-son relationships" and detached and rejecting fathers.[169] Some continued to diagnose transsexuals as "basically homosexual."[170] Some subsumed homosexuality, along with transsexuality, transvestism, exhibitionism, and voyeurism, under the larger "core problem" of "the establishment of the solid gender identity."[171] And some understood the relationship between cross-gender identity in childhood and homosexuality in adulthood in temporal and developmental terms, arguing that early gender nonconformity portended and predicted homosexuality. In 1987, psychiatrist Richard Green published results from his fifteen-year study comparing "conventionally masculine" with "feminine" boys he treated in his clinic, which showed that the latter group disproportionately identified as gay in adulthood.[172] Childhood gender nonconformity, Green and others found, was strongly correlated with both adult homosexuality and transsexuality.[173] Intervening in those devalued outcomes through behavior modification was the explicit goal of childhood gender-identity clinics in the 1960s and 1970s.

Some scholars and activists have argued that the new inclusion of gender identity disorders in the *DSM* was an effort on the part of psychiatrists to fill the void created by the removal of the diagnosis of homosexuality in 1973 and that they were pathologizing gender identity as a proxy for homosexuality. Psychiatrists could justify continuing to treat homosexuality as a mental disorder, those critics propose, through recourse to the diagnostic category of GID. In her essay "How to Bring Your Kids Up Gay," queer theorist Eve Kosofsky Sedgwick rightly discerns the anxiety about adult gay futures evident in the post-*DSM-III* psychiatric studies of effeminacy in boys, as well as the "conceptual need of the gay movement to interrupt a long tradition of viewing gender and sexuality as continuous and collapsible categories," rendering the effeminate boy the "haunting abject of gay thought itself." "This is how it happens," Sedgwick concludes, "that the *de*pathologization of an atypical sexual object-choice can be yoked to the *new* pathologization of an atypical gender identification."[174]

While homosexuality and gender variance were indeed historically entangled and the coincidence of the removal of homosexuality and inclusion of GID worked to consolidate their categorical and ontological distinction, however, the new diagnosis of GID did not simply replace the older diagnosis of homosexuality in the *DSM* and was not evidence simply of the durability of psychiatric homophobia. Psychiatrists who remained steadfast in their belief that homosexuality was a mental disorder and committed to continuing to treat gay patients could make use of the diagnosis of "ego-dystonic homosexuality," at least until it was removed from the *DSM* in 1986, and after that with the diagnosis of "sexual disorder not otherwise specified." Psychiatrists Robert Stoller and Richard Green, both of whom served on the *DSM-III* subcommittee that recommended including GID as a new diagnostic category, had been among the most prominent psychiatrists to support the APA's decision to remove homosexuality from the *DSM*; they were also leaders in the growing field of research on gender identity in children and adults. Psychologist John Money, who is responsible for coining the term *gender role*, likewise supported deleting homosexuality and its surrogates from the *DSM-III*, arguing that including "ego-dystonic homosexuality" was "simply to readmit homosexuality into psychiatric nosology through the back door."[175] Rather than searching for a new proxy to replace homosexuality, it is more likely the case that psychiatrists who advocated for the additions of these new diagnostic categories were interested in elevating the status of their own work on gender.[176]

The effort of gay activists to disaggregate healthy homosexuality from gender nonconformity, which some deemed retrograde or neurotic, and the subsequent declassification of homosexuality as a mental illness and insertion of GID in the *DSM* offers an important example of the narrowing and normalizing effects of the gay embrace of a politics of health. The vexing challenges of diagnosis and the question of how to respond politically did not end with gay activism, however. Trans people were divided about the inclusion of GID in the *DSM*, as well as about the use of the medical model to explain and describe gender variance more broadly. Some welcomed the formal classification of GID in the *DSM*, hoping that it might pave the way for greater access to gender-affirming medical care and the possibility of insurance coverage (even if that possibility rarely if ever panned out in these years). "Transsexuals need the medical profession's support since physicians heretofore have been the only advocates for them in society," Sarah Seton wrote in 1991; "this is why the *DSM-III-R* diagnosis 302.5 ('Transsexualism') is politically as well as medically necessary for their credibility."[177] In 1997, the editors of the magazine *Transgender Tapestry* wrote that "the TG [transgender] community has been torn by the question of whether the American Psychiatric Association's diagnosis of transsexualism as a form of 'Gender Identity Disorder' (GID) harms or benefits transsexuals" and published essays on opposing sides of "The GID Controversy."[178] Margaret Deirdre O'Hartigan wrote in support of the new diagnostic category, underlining its necessity for trans-identified people who wished to access gender-affirming health care. "Provision of healthcare is dependent upon a need for treatment," she wrote, "and where there is no pathology, there is no need."[179] O'Hartigan went on to criticize opponents of GID for contributing to the stigma of disability more broadly. "Rather than condemning such stigmatization," O'Hartigan observed, "GID opponents reinforce it by attacking the diagnosis rather than the prejudice itself." Aware of the claims of disability rights activists and promoting an analysis sensitive to questions of multiple marginalization, O'Hartigan also pushed trans people to recognize the "class privilege" that she discerned in the anti-GID campaign, arguing that it threatened to harm less privileged members of the trans community.[180]

Opposing the inclusion of GID, trans activist Riki Ann Wilchins argued that "you cannot wage a progressive national struggle by bricking yourself deeper and deeper into the confines of a mental category." Drawing directly from the history of the gay rights struggle, Wilchins echoed arguments that Frank Kameny had made about homosexuality nearly three decades earlier. "The reality is that we are not mentally ill," she wrote. "And most of us bridle at the implication. I will not be told that I am mentally ill. I will not be told that I am disabled. And I will not live within the confines of a mental diagnosis which is a lie." Wilchins resisted calls to embrace the inclusion of a diagnostic category of GID that suggested "that we are somehow bizarre, freakish, or embarrassing simply because we need, want, or deeply desire to change our bodies, lives, and identities in ways of which [the culture] disapproves."[181] The stigma faced by trans people, Florence Ashley wrote, "is frequently predicated on the belief that being trans is a mental illness and, more specifically, a delusion."[182] Wilchins and other activists were particularly concerned about the possibility of abuse of the diagnostic category of Gender Identity Disorder of Childhood, which Wilchins recognized, rightly, as "a cocked and loaded gun" that invited and licensed psychiatric intervention into the lives of trans children.[183]

The debate about how to preserve trans people's access to gender-affirming health care while minimizing the stigma of psychiatric diagnosis and the licensing of psychiatric authority over trans lives continues to this day. Activism on the part of trans people and their allies resulted in the removal of GID from the fifth edition of the *DSM* in 2013 and its replacement with the purportedly less pathologizing "Gender Dysphoria." Like the APA's intentions concerning "ego-dystonic homosexuality," the change to Gender Dysphoria aimed to foreground distress and impaired functioning as the clinical problems indicating disorder, rather than cross-gender identity in and of itself. The APA defines gender dysphoria as "the distress that may accompany the incongruence between one's experienced or expressed gender and one's assigned gender."[184] The persistence of the diagnostic category and debates about it testify to the enduring power of psychiatry over sexual and gender difference, the enduring stigma of mental illness, and ongoing queer and trans engagements and entanglements with psychiatric authority.

# The Queer Afterlives
# of Psychiatric Power

The success of the campaign to remove homosexuality from the American Psychiatric Association's compendium of mental disorders in 1973 has been understood to mark the end of an era: the end of psychiatric authority over homosexuality and the formal delegitimization of psychiatric claims that homosexuality was a pathological condition. There's a case to be made for organizing the story of the queer encounter with psychiatric power around a *before* and a distinct *after*. The APA's decision knocked away one of the most important props supporting larger structures of discrimination and exclusion. The same year it removed homosexuality from the *DSM*, the APA issued a position statement condemning antigay discrimination in employment, housing, and public accommodations and supporting broad civil rights for gay men and lesbians.[1] The granting of those rights and protections remains only partial, and the decades-long fight for them has been punctuated by defeats, setbacks, and reversals. But the emancipation of homosexuality from its status as a mental disorder helped secure the conditions of possibility for lesbian and gay rights to workplace protection, custody of their children, the right to marry, and more.

And yet, psychiatric authority and queer experience, historically co-constituted and tightly imbricated as they were, were not easily disentangled. Psychiatric power, thinking, and logics continued to reverberate in queer and trans lives long after 1973, in uneven, sometimes surprising, and consequential ways.

## Psychotherapy "For Gays—by Gays"

Looking to the future from the heady vantage point of 1972, gay activist Louis Landerson declared that the success of the gay liberation movement would be measured "by the decrease in numbers of homosexuals seeking professional help."[2] Gay activists who were invested in that metric, though, would have been sorely disappointed. Studies undertaken in the 1970s, 1980s, and 1990s showed that gay men and lesbians turned to psychotherapy at "considerably higher" rates than their heterosexual counterparts.[3] A national survey of nearly two thousand lesbians undertaken in 1984–85 showed that 73 percent were currently in therapy or had previously sought the services of a mental health professional, in striking contrast to 13.4 percent of their nonlesbian peers.[4] Walt Odets, a gay psychologist who began working in the San Francisco Bay Area in the early 1980s, estimated that gay men entered into psychotherapy at about three times the rate of heterosexual men, "and for good reason." Among those reasons, Odets noted, were "the complexity of growing up gay in a heterosexist society," the trauma of the HIV/AIDS epidemic, and "ongoing marginalization in adult life."[5]

Queer people successfully fought their formal pathologization at the hands of psychiatry and psychology. But the bad feelings that gay liberationists had tried to mandate out of existence, countering psychiatry's assertion of gay misery with an insistence on gay happiness, eventually had to be acknowledged and accommodated. The recognition of the toll exacted on mental health by conditions of discrimination, exclusion, and stigma led many queer people to explore the possibility of psychotherapy outside the confines of mainstream psychiatry and stripped of psychiatry's longstanding hostility to queerness and commitment to conversion.

Some of those efforts long predated the successful drive in the early 1970s to remove homosexuality from the *DSM*. In 1954, Los Angeles homophile activist Chuck Rowland drew up plans for what he called the Walt Whitman Guidance Center, a community center he envisioned would offer "help for gays—by gays," including counseling, employment assistance, legal referrals, and recommendations for care with psychiatrists who were not dedicated to "curing" gay people. Though Rowland's ambitious plan for a physical center never came to fruition, the Los Angeles homophile organization ONE, Inc., arranged with psychologist Blanche Baker to connect gay men with peer counselors. By 1960, homophile activist Dorr Legg estimated, counselors affiliated with ONE, Inc., had responded to over seven thousand requests for help from queer and trans people.[6]

In the early 1970s, in the midst of lobbying and protesting the APA and after the APA's removal of homosexuality from the *DSM*, gay men and lesbians began to build the infrastructure to support their aspirations. In founding and staffing their own mental health clinics and counseling centers, they drew inspiration from other radical social movements, like the Black Panther Party, the disability rights movement, and feminist health advocates, who criticized mainstream medicine and envisioned access to health care as a liberatory goal.[7] In 1970, psychiatrist Richard Pillard helped found Boston's Homophile Community Health Center, which was staffed by nurse-therapists, social workers, and psychologists and offered counseling services to "the first flush of post-Stonewall's openly gay men and lesbians," who "couldn't—or didn't want to—pass for straight."[8] In 1971, psychologist Charles Silverstein, social worker Bernice Goodman (one of New York's few openly lesbian therapists at the time), and several others founded Identity House as a "counter-therapy environment for gays and lesbians" and a walk-in peer counseling center, which was first housed in a church basement and later in Silverstein's apartment on New York City's Upper West Side.[9] Psychotherapist Ralph Blair opened the Homosexual Counseling Center in New York City in 1971, prompted by his awareness of "the need for counseling which does not oppress troubled clients with myths of sickness and sin but allows them to become more fully-functioning persons on their own terms."[10] Gay and lesbian counseling centers were established in cities far from the coasts as well. In 1971 Minneapolis activists founded Gay House on the principle of "Gay help for Gay people."[11]

Gay and lesbian health centers bore the imprint of the revolutionary ethos of their activist roots. "Gay liberation has blown apart the traditional mind-set of mental health professionals," wrote Cindy Hanson and John Preston, founders and directors of Gay House and its affiliated mental health group in Minneapolis in 1972. "Drastic reevaluations of philosophies of treatment, and even the concept of there being such a thing as treatment, have taken place."[12] One lesbian therapist in 1975 who described herself as "extremely sensitive to issues of imposed value in judgments of 'pathology'" characterized her therapeutic method as "anarchy."[13] Gay and lesbian mental health centers were among the early innovators of the practice of peer counseling, which was offered by trained nonprofessionals who guided and mentored their peers. "Peer counseling is a very special understanding and emotional support a (gay) person can offer another," one participant wrote in 1975, "not by virtue of being 'professionally' trained, but by being humanly aware."[14] Some clinics worked to democratize psychotherapy by offering a sliding scale or refusing to charge for their services and instead welcoming donations.

What would become known as gay-affirmative mental health services offered a place for gay men and lesbians to go for help without having to worry that their therapist would locate the root of their problems in their sexuality or act as an agent of the surveilling state. As gay men and lesbians rejected the assumptions of mainstream psychiatry, Seattle-based counselor and gay activist Charna Klein noted, "the need grew for a gay mental health delivery system based on the premise that gays have legitimate mental health needs and that gayness itself is not a sickness."[15] "Homosexuals who come seeking psycho-therapy are pretty much like anybody else who seeks psycho-therapy," Ronald Lee wrote in 1972. "They come with problems of depression, of anxiety, of drug abuse, chronic inter-personal difficulties, of problems in self-esteem, and in some cases with mental illness."[16] At the same time, gay and lesbian mental health advocates and practitioners developed an analysis of what gay activists in Los Angeles named "oppression sickness," moving away from blanket proclamations of gay health and happiness to acknowledge the trauma of oppression and its effects on mental health.[17] One gay psychologist urged psychotherapists to be aware that many of the problems facing gay men and lesbians seeking psychotherapy "are a function of social, legal, and political circumstances, rather than a reflection of intrapsychic problems."[18] If a "high percentage" of gay men and lesbians have symptoms of neurosis, gay activists came to argue, "we're made neurotic by a hostile society."[19] Psychiatrist Judd Marmor asked "whether it is at all possible for a person to have a pattern of behavior that is as strongly condemned by his culture as homosexuality is by ours, and not end up with basic feelings of insecurity, inadequacy, and self-rejection."[20] "We found that our problems are not individual illnesses," a group of gay men who formed a consciousness-raising group found, "but are generated by our oppression as a class of people."[21]

The post-*DSM* moment made it possible for activists to acknowledge the human reality of psychic distress suffered by some gay men, lesbians, and trans people and to forge new analyses of it. Organizing around queer mental health also opened up the possibility of a new political imaginary, one that was fragile, sometimes quixotic, and far from universally taken up, and was less invested in disassociating gay men and lesbians from other minoritized queer and trans subjects who might undermine their claims to health, and more intersectional and expansive in its vision of a queer "we."

Those politics were embraced in the mission and operation of the Eromin Center. Founded in Philadelphia in 1973 by members of the city's Gay Activists Alliance, who crafted a name that was an acronym for "erotic minorities," the Eromin Center offered mental health services "for members of sexual minority groups (male and female homosexuals, transvestites, transsexuals, and other minorities)."[22] The activists who established the center "wanted a name which would not only apply to gays" but instead to "the spectrum of people concerning any sexual conflicts" and hoped to "expand the current civil rights efforts beyond the single issue of homosexuality."[23] Accordingly, Eromin's intake questionnaire asked clients to "label your present sexual orientation," instructing them to "circle all that you feel apply" among a capacious list of choices: "heterosexual, homosexual, transvestite, transsexual, pedophile, sadist, gay, necrophile, masochist, exhibitionist, voyeur, asexual, autosexual, male, female, human, bisexual, ambisexual, lesbian, feminist, uncertain, other _____."[24] Eromin counseling staff committed themselves to having "no a priori value judgments or assumptions" about the pathology of any kind of sexual inclination, behavior, or identity.[25] Eromin counselors understood their clients' problems as "due not only to [their] own personality organization, but also to the realities of oppression and to the incorporation of society's homophobia, etc."[26] In striking contrast to gay activists who worked to dissociate themselves from any stigmatized association that might have called their health into question, Eromin staff members dedicated themselves to "sexual minority people who are particularly vulnerable," aligning themselves with the gender variant (including "transsexuals and heterosexual transvestites"), the criminalized, "youth prostitutes," "alcoholic gays," and "disabled gays."[27] In 1980, the Eromin Center initiated a program to sponsor gay and trans-identified Cuban youth who had arrived in the United States as part of the Mariel boatlift. Eromin also created a group home in Philadelphia that housed LGBT young people, mostly youths of color.[28] Eromin's expansive vision extended to its own composition. In 1979, Eromin Center workers committed themselves to reserving a minimum of one-third of the board member positions for "third-world people."[29]

The APA's decision in 1973 to remove homosexuality from the *DSM*, then, did not mark the end of queer engagements with mental health—far from it. For some, and for a time, it opened up the possibility of a less exclusionary, more coalitional and intersectional political vision; a broader recognition of queer and trans kinship and linked fate; and a deeper and more honest engagement with the psychic costs of stigma and marginalization. The infrastructure of community health care, new ways of conceiving queer collectivity, and new tools to fight the conjoining of gayness with sickness that were developed in the 1970s would serve queer people with the onset of the AIDS epidemic in the early 1980s and its painful and stigmatizing remedicalization of gayness less than ten years after the declassification of homosexuality as a mental illness.[30]

Still, the effects of psychiatry's pathologization of queerness lived on, and they live on still. In 1991, when Martin Duberman published *Cures: A Gay Man's Odyssey*, some read his memoir about turning to psychiatrists to "cure" himself of his homosexuality in the 1950s through the 1970s as the historical account it was meant to be. "It's taking me on a remembrance of things past, déjà vu," psychologist John Money wrote to Duberman.[31]

Some younger readers registered their distance from the time Duberman wrote about in their lack of understanding and sympathy. Duberman was devastated when members of Princeton University's gay student group asked him, "Why didn't you just leave therapy?" and "Why didn't you decide to just feel better about yourself?"[32] Some reviews of the book were quick to locate Duberman's suffering in a dark but comfortably *past* past, one of "psychiatric indignities that seem scarcely credible these days."[33] But many of Duberman's readers read *Cures* not as a work of history, but rather as a guide to navigating their own present-day struggles with psychiatry's stigmatizing stamp. A twenty-four-year-old reader told Duberman that his account "was almost identical to feelings and thoughts that I have had myself."[34] A forty-year-old Black man incarcerated in Louisiana's state prison at Angola told Duberman that his experiences "were either identical to some I've had or brought on memories of others related to them."[35] For Duberman as well, the "self-loathing" effect of pathologization "was deeply imprinted, and it remains." "There are things you don't get over," he reminds us.[36]

## Conversion Therapy and Time Warps

Queer people worked to bend psychiatric thinking and practice toward their interests, to frame mental distress in politicized rather than pathologized terms, and to reckon with the ongoing legacies of life in the shadow of diagnosis. Likewise, psychiatry and psychiatrists continued to wrestle with their relationship to queerness and gender nonconformity. Psychiatric claims that homosexuality was a symptom of mental disorder persisted, even in the absence of official sanction by the psychiatric profession and despite mainstream psychiatrists' outright disavowal.

The APA's decision in 1973 to remove homosexuality from the *DSM* was momentous. But it was not a magic wand. That decision was supported by a relatively slim majority (58 percent) of the APA's ten thousand voting members. Many psychiatrists, and according to some surveys *most* of them, continued to conceive of homosexuality as a pathological deviation from normal human behavior and to treat queer patients with the aim of conversion and cure. When APA members were surveyed in 1977, four years after their organization's resolution to declassify homosexuality as a mental disorder, 69 percent agreed with the statement that "homosexuality is usually a pathological adaptation, as opposed to a normal variation." Only 18 percent disagreed (13 percent were uncertain).

And 70 percent believed that the problems of gay men and lesbians "have more to do with their own inner conflicts than with stigmatization by society at large."[37]

Some of the most prominent and vocal opponents of the APA's decision to declassify homosexuality as a mental disorder continued to promote their ideas, a few joining forces with religious organizations and ministries that practiced what they called "reparative" therapy and trumpeted the heterosexual conversion of "ex-gay" members. Historians and other scholars typically locate the rise of ex-gay ministries and the resurgence of interest in sexual conversion in the "culture wars" of the 1980s and 1990s and the emergence of evangelical Christians as political actors. But the religious ex-gay movement spoke in the language of science as well as religion, bolstered by a close association with psychiatrists and psychologists whose research and writing lent it legitimacy.[38] In 1992, Charles Socarides joined psychologist Joseph Nicolosi and psychiatrist Benjamin Kaufman to found the National Association for Research and Therapy of Homosexuality (NARTH). Operating as the "science-oriented wing" of the ex-gay movement, NARTH promoted itself as a secular and scientific organization, arguing that the APA had stifled scientific inquiry into the malleability of homosexuality by bowing to political pressure from gay activists.[39] NARTH extolled conversion therapy as a scientifically supported method and trained hundreds of therapists who continued to treat gay patients with the intention of curing them.

Despite NARTH's insistence on its own scientific standing, psychiatrists committed to the idea that homosexuality was pathological were increasingly marginalized by psychiatric, psychoanalytic, and psychological professional organizations. But in 2001, nearly thirty years after the APA's historic decision, a prominent figure at the very center of mainstream psychiatry lent his authority and prestige to the idea that gay people could be converted to straight. Robert Spitzer had been lauded (and, by critics, condemned) as the "architect" of the removal of homosexuality from the *DSM* in 1973. But in 1999, Spitzer's encounter with ex-gay protesters at the annual meeting of the APA in Washington, DC, piqued his curiosity about their claims. "I started to talk to one of those guys," he recalled, "and he tried to tell me about how he had changed." Confessing that he was "always looking for trouble or something to challenge the orthodoxy," and perhaps trying to regain the attention he had attracted decades earlier, Spitzer set out to test the hypothesis "that some individuals whose sexual orientation is predominantly homosexual can, with therapy, become predominantly heterosexual."[40] In 2001, he presented his findings at the annual meeting of the APA in New Orleans, explaining that, following some kind of "reparative" therapy ranging from talk therapy to Bible study and prayer, many of the two hundred gay men and lesbians he had studied were able to change from a "predominantly homosexual orientation to a predominantly heterosexual orientation."[41] Spitzer leaked the study to the media in advance, and the results were reported in every newspaper across the country and featured on talk shows in what one critic called a "media frenzy."[42] Those findings were all the more "explosive," journalists noted, given Spitzer's role in the APA's decision decades earlier. "What translated in the culture," journalist Gabriel Arana wrote, was that "the father of the 1973 revolution in the classification and treatment of homosexuality, who could not be seen as just another biased ex-gay crusader with an agenda, had validated ex-gay therapy."[43]

Ignoring his colleagues' criticism, Spitzer published the results of his study in the journal *Archives of Sexual Behavior* in 2003.[44] His article was accompanied by twenty-five responses solicited from psychiatrists, psychologists, social workers, and sexologists. Most were critical, and some harshly so. Psychiatrist Lawrence Hartmann condemned Spitzer's study as "too flawed to publish" and "likely to do harm."[45] Other critics denounced the study as tainted by biased sampling and criticized Spitzer's willingness to take his subjects at their word. By his own admission, Spitzer had worked directly with NARTH and the Exodus ministry to recruit his research subjects. In fact, 43 percent of the two hundred participants in Spitzer's study were recruited through ex-gay religious ministries and 23 percent were recruited directly from NARTH. Another 19 percent were mental health professionals or directors of ex-gay ministries. The vast majority of Spitzer's participants (93 percent) reported that religion was "extremely" or "very" important in their lives, but he failed to acknowledge that many of his subjects may have been drawn to conversion therapy or motivated to exaggerate its effects by the stigma, shame, and guilt imposed on them by families and churches. Many of Spitzer's critics were troubled by his reliance on the self-reporting of his subjects, who, given their commitment to the agenda of promoting gay conversion, had compelling motivations to overestimate the extent and permanence of their change. Some of Spitzer's critics anticipated "widespread suffering for homosexual minorities" that would result from the publication of his study.[46] "We fear the repercussions of this study," the multiple authors of one response wrote, "including an increase in suffering, prejudice, and discrimination."[47]

Spitzer's study was disputed by a nearly united critical front among his professional colleagues, but the publication of his findings put the idea of queer pathology and the possibility of conversion back into the world with renewed legitimacy. Ex-gay movement leaders gleefully referenced Spitzer's study as objective and scientific evidence that conversion therapy worked, and the study was widely cited as proof that gay men and lesbians could change their sexual orientation to heterosexual.

In the years that followed, a series of scandals, exposés, and controversies chipped away at the legitimacy that the ex-gay movement had been able to garner. In 2008, John Smid, the former director of the ex-gay Christian ministry Love in Action, apologized for harm the program had done; in 2014, he married a man. Two of the five founders of Exodus International, Michael Bussee and Gary Cooper, quit the group, divorced their wives, and married each other. Other prominent "ex-gay" leaders recanted and came out as gay or were outed by others. Some "reparative" therapists were accused of sexually assaulting their clients. In 2010, NARTH board member George Rekers was exposed for traveling abroad with a male sex worker. Exodus International collapsed in 2013, and its president apologized for the "pain and hurt" the organization had caused.[48] Worried that his 2001 study would "tarnish his legacy," Spitzer issued a formal apology in 2012 for "making unproven claims of the efficacy of reparative therapy."[49]

One might think that this string of humiliating defeats, scandals, recantations, and retractions would ring the death knell for the ex-gay movement and its agenda of normalization and conversion. And yet, claims about the psychopathology of queerness and transness live on, revivified through a recoupling of homosexuality with a pathologized understanding of transgender and redeployed by the American political right. NARTH founder Joseph Nicolosi helped forge that reconnection, theorizing that homosexuality is caused by a "gender deficit," which he characterized as insufficient masculinity in boys and insufficient femininity in girls.[50] NARTH has committed itself (under the organization's 2014 rebranding as the Alliance for Therapeutic Choice and Scientific Integrity) to "promoting a more complete truth, informed by Judeo-Christian values and natural law" about "the science of sexual orientation and biological sex," thus pulling queerness and transness back into pathologized association.[51] Where NARTH once amplified the voices of "ex-gays," the alliance now showcases people who regret their gender transitions. Weaponizing the *DSM* for its own ends, the Alliance states that "gender dysphoria" is a "mental health issue."[52] The group is committed to training and defending clinical and religious practitioners of gay conversion therapy and condemning gender-affirming medical care for trans people, especially children. It dedicates itself, too, to challenging state and municipal bans on conversion therapy.

While the alliance may be considered marginal, and it is indeed marginalized by professional psychiatrists, the ideas it promotes have entered the mainstream. Conversion therapy continues to be practiced, especially and routinely on trans children.[53] In the past several years, those ideas have gained new traction, and opposition to conversion therapy bans, gender-affirming health care for trans people, and recognition of the legitimacy of trans experience and identity are now mainstays of the Republican Party's agenda.[54] As I finish this book, their efforts are bearing legislative fruit.

∵

When I began work on this project, I sometimes wondered if psychiatric power was an antiquated form, and whether my interest in it, born of a particular generational experience, might seem antiquated too. Psychiatry's mid-century golden age is well and truly over, displaced and supplanted within psychiatry by biomedical models and psychopharmaceuticals, and beyond the psychiatric realm, by the rise of carceral power and the national security state (even as psychiatry has been and remains deeply implicated in those phenomena).[55] I did not anticipate the resurrection of psychiatry's claims about homosexuality as a mental disorder (albeit in the absence of support from most psychiatrists) or the resurgence of those ideas in mainstream political discourse.

Psychiatry launched modes of thinking and practice that made a deep and lasting impact on many people and crafted an adhesive connection among queerness, gender variance, and sickness. Those ideas have outlived their mid-century genesis, having survived the formal disavowal of psychiatry and psychiatrists, and they remain available for revitalization and appropriation. The extent to which the epithet "sick" or the more clinical characterization of "disordered" are still heard and understood in reference to queerness and transness shows this to be true. The association of queerness and sickness was not always thus, and presumably will not always be so. But as I conclude this book, fifty years after the APA's decision to declassify homosexuality as a mental disorder, we are still engaging with a set of meanings about same-sex desire and gender variance that were forged in the mid-twentieth century. In his 2002 afterword to the tenth anniversary edition of *Cures*, Duberman reminds us that "the past tends to leak into the future and is never entirely displaced."[56] The history I have charted in this book, tracing the ways in which psychiatry and modern queerness worked to constitute each other in the middle decades of the twentieth century, helps us understand why the associations of gender and sexual difference with pathology have been so enduring. That history also makes clear both the challenge and the urgency of undoing them.

# Acknowledgments

Writing acknowledgments is an act of giving thanks; it is also an exercise in taking account of the life of a project. This book has had a long life indeed, and my debts are many. I began mulling over these ideas during a year when I experienced a health crisis; I have finished the book in the midst of an enduring global pandemic. Those experiences have made me think a lot about questions of diagnosis and its effects that are at the heart of this book. They also made me especially attuned to and grateful for the supreme generosity of my friends and colleagues.

Historians are always beholden to archivists; that debt is multiplied several times over with this book, enabled as it was by one archivist's doggedness and dedication to preserving LGBTQ history. My first thanks, then, go to Jean-Nickolaus Tretter, founder and first archivist of the LGBTQ archive that bears his name at the University of Minnesota and acquirer of the collection that inspired this book and made it possible to write. Jean died just as I was finishing my final revisions, and I so regret that I wasn't able to show him what came from his tenacity and the collection that he worked so hard to preserve. I'm most grateful, too, to James Sheridan Kane, who recognized the importance of the documents he found at Saint Elizabeths Hospital and went above and beyond the call of duty to save them. I thank Jim and Jean for trusting me with these extraordinary materials.

Other librarians and archivists offered vital assistance. My thanks go to Tim Johnson, Kris Kiesling, and Lisa Vecoli, at the University of Minnesota Libraries; Velora Jernigan-Pedrick at the Saint Elizabeths Hospital archive; Loni Shibuyama at the ONE National Gay and Lesbian Archives; Tal Nadan at the New York Public Library; Bob Skiba at the William Way LGBT Community Center in Philadelphia; and Renata Vickrey at Central Connecticut State University's Special Collections. I also thank the librarians and archivists at Columbia University's Rare Books and Manuscripts Library; Cornell University's Human Sexuality collection; the Gerber/Hart Library and Archives; the GLBT Historical Society; the Historical Society of Pennsylvania; the LGBT Community Center National History Archive; the Library of Congress; Northeastern University's Archives and Special Collections; Smith College's Mortimer Rare Book Collection; Princeton University's Seeley G. Mudd Manuscript Library and Firestone Library; Temple University's Special Collections; the University of California, Los Angeles, Library Special Collections; the University of Pennsylvania's Kislak Center for Special Collections, Rare Books, and Manuscripts; and Yale University's Beinecke Library and Manuscripts and Archives.

I'm grateful for the help of a number of excellent research assistants over the years: Angela Carter, Stephen Dillon, Laura Luepke, Jessica Petocz, and Jayne Swift. My graduate students, past and present, have been a source of enormous inspiration. Thanks, too, to Tanya Matthews, who offered crucial help in navigating the institutional review board process.

My work on this book has been generously supported by the University of Minnesota, Princeton University, and Yale University. I gratefully acknowledge support as well from the American Council of Learned Societies, the Stanford Humanities Center, and the City University of New York's Advanced Research Collaborative. For my year at Stanford, my thanks to Caroline Winterer and my friends and fellow fellows, especially Elizabeth Anker, Melanie Arndt, Dorinne Kondo, Tanya Luhrmann, Benjamin Paloff, Uğur Peçe, Dylan Penningroth, Dan Rosenberg, and Matthew Sommer, who kept me company in a year of anxious but generative uncertainty about the project.

Tim Mennel at the University of Chicago Press has been an extraordinarily engaged editor. His incisive comments on an early draft of the manuscript emboldened me to restructure it, and I deeply appreciate his support. I will always be indebted to Doug Mitchell, for his interest in my early ideas for this book and for his support of the field of queer history. Thanks go, too, to Susannah Engstrom and Caterina MacLean, who helped shepherd the manuscript into production, and to Nicole Balant for her skillful copyediting. I also thank the two anonymous reviewers for the Press for their engaged and helpful feedback on the manuscript.

I thank Martin Duberman for facilitating my access to parts of his papers at the New York Public Library that were not yet processed and for his own remarkable work.

For help with oral history leads and tips, I thank Margot Canaday, Alix Genter, and Timothy Stewart-Winter. For sharing their stories with me, I thank William Bennett, Warren Goldfarb, Richard Pillard, Charles Silverstein, Miriam Wolfson, and others who asked to remain anonymous.

Some of the material that appears in this volume is derived from material originally published in various sources: *The Oxford Handbook of Disabil-*

*ity History*, ed. Michael Rembis, Catherine Kudlick, and Kim E. Nielsen, pp. 459–76, copyright 2018, Oxford University Press, reproduced with permission of the Licensor through PLSclear; *American Quarterly*, vol. 69, no. 2, June 2017, copyright 2017, The American Studies Association, published with permission by Johns Hopkins University Press; "Sex Panic, Psychiatry, and the Expansion of the Carceral State," in *The War on Sex*, ed. David M. Halperin and Trevor Hoppe, pp. 229–46, copyright 2017, Duke University Press, all rights reserved, republished by permission of the publisher; and "Sex Panic, Psychiatry, and the Expansion of the Carceral State," in *Intimate States: Gender, Sexuality, and Governance in Modern US History*, ed. Margot Canaday, Nancy F. Cott, and Robert O. Self, pp. 193–210, copyright 2021, University of Chicago Press.

I first tried out the ideas for this book at the University of Maryland's Queering the Archive/Archiving the Queer conference. There, Christina Hanhardt and Robert McRuer offered astute and encouraging comments that set me on my way. This book has benefited from the questions, insights, and critique posed by audiences at Brown University; Bryn Mawr College; Cornell University; Duke University; Haverford College; Humboldt-Universität zu Berlin; Louisiana State University; Northwestern University; Princeton University; Smith College; Stony Brook University; Trinity College; Tulane University; University of California, Berkeley; University of California, Irvine; University of California, Santa Cruz; University of Chicago; University of Illinois Urbana-Champaign; University of Kansas; University of Massachusetts, Amherst; University of Michigan; University of Minnesota; University of Oregon; University of Pennsylvania; University of Southern California; Williams College; and Yale University.

The kindness and generosity of friends and colleagues have kept me going over these years; many have been crucial interlocutors as well. For conversations, inspiration, support, and sustenance, I'm grateful to Betsy Armstrong, Karisa Butler-Wall, Susan Cahn, Margot Canaday, George Chauncey, Anne Cheng, Elizabeth Cohen, Pete Coviello, Rebecca Davis, Cornelia Hughes Dayton, Robin Dembroff, Jigna Desai, Steve Dillon, Jill Dolan, Finn Enke, Rod Ferguson, Joe Fischel, Paul Frymer, Jules Gill-Peterson, Katja Guenther, David Halperin, Marybeth Hamilton, Christina Hanhardt, Jeanne Walker Harvey, Lynn Hudson, Tera Hunter, Adria Imada, Janice Irvine, Jill Jarvis, Liza Johnson, Susan Lee Johnson, Benjy Kahan, Amy Kapczynski, Kathryn Kent, Caleb Knapp, Issa Kohler-Hausman, Tom Kohut, Greta LaFleur, Abram J. Lewis, Beth Lew-Williams, Heather Love, Rosina Lozano, Anna Lvovsky, Joanne Meyerowitz, Ali Miller, David Minto, Naomi Murakawa, Zein Murib, Kevin Murphy, Allison Page, Lisa Sun-Hee Park, David Pellow, Lizzie Reis, Jane Rhodes, Gayle Salamon, Nayan Shah,

Libby Sharrow, Siobhan Somerville, Hannah Srajer, Sarah Staszak, Cathe-rine Stock, Donna Tatro, Emily Thuma, Mara Toone, Stephen Vider, Keith Wailoo, Wendy Warren, Chris Waters, Spence Weinreich, Judith Weisen-feld, Barbara Welke, Katie White, Stacy Wolf, and Scott Wong.

I thank the members of my writing group, Margot Canaday, Jennifer Mit-telstadt, and Johanna Schoen, who managed to combine sometimes brac-ing critique with support and encouragement.

I'm especially indebted to the immense generosity of friends and col-leagues who took time away from their own work to read drafts of chapters: Katie Kent, Greta LaFleur, Lizzie Reis, Siobhan Somerville, Dara Strolo-vitch, Spence Weinreich, and Barbara Welke. Special thanks go to Janice Irvine, Joanne Meyerowitz, and Emily Thuma, who read drafts of the entire manuscript.

Kevin Murphy's provocations at this project's beginning and smart sug-gestions at its end have made this a much better book. Siobhan Somerville helped pull this project back into vision for me a dozen times or more over the years and helped restore my confidence in it at least as many times. Her sustaining friendship is one of the great gifts of my life. For Dara Strolovitch, who lived with this book from its wobbly beginnings, thank you hardly seems adequate to convey my gratitude. Her love and support brighten my life beyond measure.

# Archives

*Advocate* Records. ONE National Gay and Lesbian Archives, USC Libraries, University of Southern California, Los Angeles, CA

AGLP Records. Association of Gay and Lesbian Psychologists Records, 1973–1992, Division of Rare and Manuscript Collections, Cornell University, Ithaca, NY

Arvin Papers. Newton Arvin Papers, Mortimer Rare Book Collection, Smith College Library, Northampton, MA

Bertelson Papers. D. E. Bertelson Papers, GLBT Historical Society, San Francisco, CA

Berzon Papers. Betty Berzon Papers, ONE National Gay and Lesbian Archives, Los Angeles, CA

Bronstein Papers. Sidney Bronstein Papers, ONE National Gay and Lesbian Archives, USC Libraries, University of Southern California, Los Angeles, CA

Brown Center Records. Howard Brown Health Center Records, Gerber Hart Library, Chicago, IL

Canfield Papers. William J. Canfield Papers, Northeastern University Archives and Special Collections, Boston, MA

Cole Papers. Rob Cole Papers, ONE National Gay and Lesbian Archives, USC Libraries, University of Southern California, Los Angeles, CA

Duberman Papers. Martin Duberman Papers, Manuscripts and Archives Division, New York Public Library, New York, NY

Ellis Papers. Albert Ellis Papers, Rare Book and Manuscript Library, Columbia University, New York, NY

Eromin Records. Eromin Center Records, Special Collections Research Center, Temple University, Philadelphia, PA

Franzblau Papers. Rose Franzblau Papers, Rare Books and Manuscript Library, Columbia University, New York, NY

Fryer Papers. John Fryer Papers, Historical Society of Pennsylvania, Philadelphia, PA

GHP Papers. Gay Health Project Papers, GLBT Historical Society, San Francisco, CA

Gittings and Lahusen G/H. Barbara Gittings and Kay Tobin Lahusen Papers, Gerber / Hart Library and Archives, Chicago, IL

Gittings and Lahusen NYPL. Barbara Gittings and Kay Tobin Lahusen Gay History Papers and Photographs, Manuscripts and Archives Division, New York Public Library, New York, NY

Gittings and Lahusen ONE. Barbara Gittings and Kay Tobin Lahusen Papers, ONE National Gay and Lesbian Archives, USC Libraries, University of Southern California, Los Angeles, CA

Gittings and Lahusen Papers Wilcox. Barbara Gittings and Kay Tobin Lahusen Papers, John J. Wilcox, Jr., LGBT Archives, William Way LGBT Community Center, Philadelphia, PA

Gold Papers. Ron Gold Papers, LGBT Community Center Archive, New York, NY

Graves Papers. John C. Graves Papers, Northeastern University Archives and Special Collections, Boston, MA

Hadden Papers. Samuel Bernard Hadden Papers, University Archives and Records Center, University of Pennsylvania, Philadelphia, PA

Henry Foundation Papers. George W. Henry Foundation / Canon Clinton Jones Papers, Special Collections, Central Connecticut State University, New Britain, CT

Hooker Papers. Evelyn C. Hooker Papers, Department of Special Collections, Charles E. Young Research Library, University of California, Los Angeles, CA

Jackson Papers. Don Jackson Papers, Manuscripts and Archives Division, New York Public Library, New York, NY

Kameny Papers. Frank Kameny Papers, Library of Congress, Washington, DC

Karpman Papers. Benjamin Karpman Papers, Jean-Nickolaus Tretter Collection in Gay, Lesbian, Bisexual, and Transgender Studies, University of Minnesota, Minneapolis, MN

Kessler Papers. David Kessler Papers, GLBT Historical Society, San Francisco, CA

Langhorne Papers. Harry Langhorne Papers, Division of Rare and Manuscript Collections, Cornell University Library, Ithaca, NY

Lilienthal Papers. David E. Lilienthal Papers, Seely G. Mudd Library, Princeton University, Princeton, NJ

Long Papers. Jim Long Papers, ONE National Gay and Lesbian Archives, USC Libraries, University of Southern California, Los Angeles, CA

Lowinger Papers. Paul Lowinger Papers, Kislak Center for Special Collections, Rare Books and Manuscripts, University of Pennsylvania, Philadelphia, PA

Marmor Papers. Judd Marmor Papers, Department of Special Collections, Charles E. Young Research Library, University of California, Los Angeles, CA

Marmor Papers ONE. Judd Marmor Papers, ONE National Gay and Lesbian Archives, USC Libraries, University of Southern California, Los Angeles, CA

Mecca Papers. Tommi Avicolli Mecca Collection, John J. Wilcox, Jr., LGBT Archives, William Way LGBT Community Center, Philadelphia, PA

Moran Papers. Camille Moran Papers, GLBT Historical Society, San Francisco, CA

NGLTF Records. National Gay and Lesbian Task Force Records, Rare Books and Manuscripts, Cornell University, Ithaca, NY

Overholser Papers. Winfred Overholser Papers, Library of Congress, Washington, DC

Saint Elizabeths Records. Records of Saint Elizabeths Hospital, RG 418, National Archives and Records Administration, Washington, DC

Vincenz Papers. Lilli Vincenz Papers, Library of Congress, Washington, DC

Wright Papers. Richard Wright Papers, Beinecke Library, Yale University, New Haven, CT

Yoakem Papers. John R. Yoakem Papers, Jean-Nickolaus Tretter Collection in Gay, Lesbian, Bisexual, and Transgender Studies, University of Minnesota, Minneapolis, MN

# Notes

INTRODUCTION

1. See Edmund Bergler, *Homosexuality: Disease or Way of Life* (New York: Hill and Wang, 1957); Edmund Bergler, *One Thousand Homosexuals: Conspiracy of Silence, or Curing and Deglamorizing Homosexuals* (Patterson, NJ: Pageant Books, 1959); Irving Bieber, Harvey J. Dain, Paul R. Dince, Marvin G. Drellich, Henry G. Grand, Ralph H. Gundlach, Malvina W. Kremer, Alfred H. Rifkin, Cornelia B. Wilbur, and Toby B. Bieber, *Homosexuality: A Psychoanalytic Study of Male Homosexuals* (New York: Basic Books, 1962); Charles W. Socarides, *The Overt Homosexual* (New York: Grune and Stratton, 1968).

2. Following Michel Foucault's understanding of the clinic in *The Birth of the Clinic: An Archeology of Medical Perception* (*Naissance de la clinique: Une archéologie du regard médical* [Paris: Presses Universitaires de France, 1963]), Cindy Patton writes that the "'clinic' is as much a disposition and a relationship as a particular place and time" (Patton, "Clinic without the Clinic," in *Rebirth of the Clinic: Places and Agents in Contemporary Health Care*, ed. Cindy Patton [Minneapolis: University of Minnesota Press, 2010], 137). On psychiatric power, see Michel Foucault, *Psychiatric Power: Lectures at the Collège de France, 1973–1974*, trans. Graham Burchell (New York: Picador, 2008); Elizabeth Lunbeck, *The Psychiatric Persuasion: Knowledge, Gender, and Power in Modern America* (Princeton: Princeton University Press, 1994); Nikolas Rose, *Inventing Our Selves: Psychology, Power, and Personhood* (Cambridge: Cambridge University Press, 1996); Ellen Herman, *The Romance of American Psychology: Political Culture in the Age of Experts* (Berkeley: University of California Press, 1995).

3. Barbara Gittings, preface, in *American Psychiatry and Homosexuality: An Oral History*, ed. Jack Drescher and Joseph P. Merlino (New York: Harrington Park Press, 2007), xv.

4. Jonathan Ned Katz, *Gay American History: Lesbians and Gay Men in the U.S.A.* (New York: Thomas Y. Crowell, 1976; reprint, New York: Avon, 1977), 197.

5. Ronald Bayer, *Homosexuality and American Psychiatry: The Politics of Diagnosis* (Princeton: Princeton University Press, 1987).

6. Kenneth Lewes, *The Psychoanalytic Theory of Male Homosexuality* (New York: Simon and Schuster, 1988).

7. Martin Duberman, *Cures: A Gay Man's Odyssey* (New York: Dutton, 1991).

8. John D'Emilio, *Sexual Politics, Sexual Communities: The Making of a Homo-sexual Minority in the United States, 1940–1970* (Chicago: University of Chicago Press, 1983), 15.

9. For important exceptions and illuminating histories of medical and psychiatric conceptualizations of homosexuality, see Jennifer Terry, *An American Obsession: Science, Medicine, and Homosexuality in Modern Society* (Chicago: University of Chicago Press, 1999); Harry Oosterhuis, *Stepchildren of Invention: Krafft-Ebing, Psychiatry, and the Making of Sexual Identity* (Chicago: University of Chicago Press, 2000); Harry Minton, *Departing from Deviance: A History of Homosexual Rights and Emancipatory Science in America* (Chicago: University of Chicago Press, 2002); Bayer, *Homosexuality and American Psychiatry*; Lewes, *Psychoanalytic Theory of Male Homosexuality*.

10. George Chauncey, *Gay New York: Gender, Urban Culture, and the Making of the Gay World, 1890–1940* (New York: Basic Books, 1994), 26.

11. Martin Duberman, *Waiting to Land: A (Mostly) Political Memoir, 1985–2008* (New York: New Press, 2009), 44.

12. Margot Canaday, *The Straight State: Sexuality and Citizenship in Twentieth-Century America* (Princeton: Princeton University Press, 2009), 4.

13. See Aren Z. Aizura, Marquis Bey, Toby Beauchamp, Treva Ellison, Jules Gill-Peterson, and Eliza Steinbock, "Thinking with Trans Now," in "Left of Queer," ed. David L. Eng and Jasbir K. Puar, special issue, *Social Text* 38:4 (December 2020): 125–47; Jules Gill-Peterson, *Histories of the Transgender Child* (Minneapolis: University of Minnesota Press, 2018); Cameron Awkward-Rich, "'She of the Pants and No Voice': Jack Bee Garland's Disability Drag," *TSQ: Transgender Studies Quarterly* 7:1 (February 2020): 21; Marcia Ochoa, in "Trans*historicities: A Roundtable Discussion," *TSQ: Transgender Studies Quarterly* 5:4 (November 2018): 661.

14. Regina Kunzel, *Criminal Intimacy: Prison and the Uneven History of Modern American Sexuality* (Chicago: University of Chicago Press, 2008); Michel Foucault, *Discipline and Punish: The Birth of the Prison*, trans. Alan Sheridan (London: Penguin, 1975), 333. Saint Elizabeths is spelled without the possessive apostrophe, referring to the hospital's location on a land grant bearing that name.

15. The Benjamin Karpman Papers are housed in the Jean-Nickolaus Tretter Collection in Gay, Lesbian, Bisexual, and Transgender Studies, University of Minnesota (hereafter cited as Karpman Papers).

16. For histories of Saint Elizabeths Hospital, see Martin Summers, *Madness in the City of Magnificent Intentions: A History of Race and Mental Illness in the Nation's Capital* (New York: Oxford University Press, 2019); Matthew Gambino, "Mental Health and Ideals of Citizenship: Patient Care at St. Elizabeths Hospital in Washington, D.C., 1903–1962" (PhD dissertation, University of Illinois, 2010); Matthew Gambino, "'These Strangers within Our Gates': Race, Psychiatry, and Mental Illness among Black Americans at St. Elizabeths Hospital in Washington, D.C., 1900–1940," *History of Psychiatry* 19:4 (2008): 387–408; Sarah A. Leavitt, *St. Elizabeths in Washington, D.C.: Architecture of an Asylum* (Charleston, SC: History Press, 2019).

17. See Gambino, "Mental Health and Ideals of Citizenship," 74.

18. On the use of case files in historical analysis, see Franca Iacovetta and Wendy Mitchinson, *On the Case: Explorations in Social History* (Toronto: University of

Toronto Press, 1998); Linda Gordon, *Heroes of Their Own Lives: The Politics and Histories of Family Violence: Boston, 1880–1960* (New York: Viking, 1988); Birgit Lang, Joy Damousi, and Alison Lewis, *A History of the Case Study: Sexology, Psychoanalysis, Literature* (Manchester, UK: Manchester University Press, 2017); Warwick Anderson, "The Case of the Archive," *Critical Inquiry* 39:3 (2013): 532–47. Saidiya Hartman offers a powerful and lyrical reflection on the limits, violent erasures, and dehumanizing attributions of the case file in *Wayward Lives, Beautiful Experiments: Intimate Histories of Social Upheaval* (New York: Norton, 2020).

19. On the importance of the case study in psychiatry and psychoanalysis, see John Forrester, *Thinking in Cases* (Cambridge: Polity Press, 2017); Carol Berkenkotter, *Patient Tales: Case Histories and the Use of Narrative in Psychiatry* (Columbia: University of South Carolina Press, 2008).

20. Lauren Berlant, "On the Case," *Critical Inquiry* 33 (Summer 2007): 663.

21. Michel Foucault, "The Lives of Infamous Men," in *Essential Works of Foucault, 1954–1984*, vol. 3, *Power*, ed. James D. Faubion, trans. Robert Hurley (New York: New Press, 2000), 161.

22. Jennifer Terry, "Theorizing Deviant Historiography," *differences* 3:2 (1991): 59.

23. Karpman explains this method in Benjamin Karpman, "'Blitz' Psychotherapy," *Medical Annals of the District of Columbia* 11:8 (August 1942): 291–96, box 136, folder 2009, Richard Wright Papers, Beinecke Library, Yale University, New Haven, CT.

24. Karpman, *Case Studies in the Psychopathology of Crime*, vol. 3 (Washington, DC: Medical Science Press, 1948), xviii; KP42, Karpman Papers.

25. In a method that she calls "just reading," Sharon Marcus eschews the queer analytical practice of looking for what is excluded or searching for the hidden and marginal to find queer subtexts. Instead, Marcus looks to "what texts make manifest on their surface" (Sharon Marcus, *Between Women: Friendship, Desire, and Marriage in Victorian England* [Princeton: Princeton University Press, 2007], 2).

26. Cameron Awkward-Rich, *The Terrible We: Thinking with Trans Maladjustment* (Durham: Duke University Press, 2022), 8.

27. Gilbert M. Joseph, "Close Encounters: Toward a New Cultural History of U.S.– Latin American Relations," in *Close Encounters of Empire: Writing the Cultural History of U.S.–Latin American Relations* (Durham: Duke University Press, 1998), 8. See also Mary Louise Pratt, *Imperial Eyes: Travel Writing and Transculturation* (London: Routledge, 1992); Caitlin Janzen, Donna Jeffrey, and Kristin Smith, eds., *Unravelling Encounters: Ethics, Knowledge, and Resistance under Neoliberalism* (Toronto: Wilfrid Laurier University Press, 2015).

28. Sara Ahmed, *Strange Encounters: Embodied Others in Post-Coloniality* (London: Routledge, 2000), 8.

29. Simi Linton, *Claiming Disability: Knowledge and Identity* (New York: NYU Press, 1998), 114. For other examples of the use of analogy between disability and sexual orientation, see Tom Shakespeare, "Disability, Identity, and Difference," in *Exploring the Divide: Illness and Disability*, ed. Colin Barnes and Geof Mercer (Leeds, UK: Disability Press, 1996), 94–113. Susan K. Cahn puzzles through the consonances and dissonances between the identities of lesbian and disabled in "Come Out, Come

Out Whatever You've Got! Or, Still Crazy after All These Years," *Feminist Studies* 29:1 (Spring 2003): 7–18. Ellen Samuels discusses the analogizing of social identities, particularly queer and disability, in "My Body, My Closet: Invisible Disability and the Limits of Coming-Out Discourse," *GLQ: A Journal of Lesbian and Gay Studies* 9:1–2 (2003): 233–55. See also Anna Mollow, "'When *Black* Women Start Going on Prozac': Race, Gender, and Mental Illness in Meri Nana-Ama Danquah's 'Willow Weep for Me,'" *MELUS* 31:3 (Fall 2006): 67–99.

30. Emily Martin, *Bipolar Expeditions: Mania and Depression in American Culture* (Princeton: Princeton University Press, 2007), xix.

31. Nielsen, *A Disability History of the United States* (Boston: Beacon, 2012), 160. Other disability studies scholars have explored the associative links between queerness and disability. See Alison Kafer, *Feminist Queer Crip* (Bloomington: Indiana University Press, 2013); Cahn, "Come Out, Come Out Whatever You've Got!"; Robert McRuer, *Crip Theory: Cultural Signs of Queerness and Disability* (New York: NYU Press, 2006); Ellen Samuels, "My Body, My Closet"; Eli Clare, "Stolen Bodies, Reclaimed Bodies: Disability and Queerness," *Public Culture* 13:3 (2001): 359–66. For an insightful discussion of the ways in which the disavowal of "sickness" been foundational to the development of the field of trans studies, see Awkward-Rich, *The Terrible We*. See Awkward-Rich, too, on the coproduction of disability and gender in *The Terrible We*, esp. 31–59.

32. See Janet E. Halley, "'Like Race' Arguments," in *What's Left of Theory? New Work on the Politics of Literary Theory*, ed. Judith Butler, John Guillory, and Kendall Thomas (New York: Routledge, 2000), 40–74; Siobhan B. Somerville, "Queer *Loving*," *GLQ: A Journal of Lesbian and Gay Studies* 11:3 (2005): 335–70.

33. See Somerville, "Queer *Loving*." In her examination of the legal thinking of Pauli Murray, Serena Mayeri explores what analogy can reveal and make possible, even as she is critical of what it can obscure, in *Reasoning from Race: Feminism, Law, and the Civil Rights Revolution* (Cambridge, MA: Harvard University Press, 2011).

34. Robert McRuer and Anna Mollow, introduction, in *Sex and Disability*, ed. Robert McRuer and Anna Mollow (Durham: Duke University Press, 2012), 3. For engagements between queer studies and disability studies, see McRuer, *Crip Theory*; Carrie Sandahl, "Queering the Crip or Cripping the Queer: Intersections of Queer and Crip Identities in Solo Autobiographical Performance," *GLQ: A Journal of Lesbian and Gay Studies* 9:1–2 (2003): 25–56; Abby L. Wilkerson, "Normate Sex and Its Discontents," in McRuer and Mollow, *Sex and Disability*, 183–207.

35. Heather Love, *Feeling Backward: Loss and the Politics of Queer History* (Cambridge, MA: Harvard University Press, 2007). See also Awkward-Rich, *The Terrible We*.

36. Kadji Amin, *Disturbing Attachments: Genet, Modern Pederasty, and Queer History* (Durham: Duke University Press, 2017), 11.

37. George Chauncey, "The Trouble with Shame," in *Gay Shame*, ed. David Halperin and Valerie Traub (Chicago: University of Chicago Press, 2009), 280. Writing about the decades before the Second World War, Chauncy challenges what he terms "the myth of internalization," which "holds that gay men uncritically internalized the dominant culture's view of them as sick, perverted, and immoral" (Chauncey, *Gay New York*, 4).

38. Eli Clare, *Brilliant Imperfection: Grappling with Cure* (Durham: Duke University

Press, 2017), 26. See also Eunjung Kim, *Curative Violence: Rehabilitating Disability, Gender, and Sexuality in Modern Korea* (Durham: Duke University Press, 2017).

39. Sharon L. Snyder and David T. Mitchell, *Cultural Locations of Disability* (Chicago: University of Chicago Press, 2006), 12.

40. Barbara Gittings, preface, in *American Psychiatry and Homosexuality: An Oral History*, ed. Jack Dresher and Joseph P. Merlino (New York: Harrington Park Press, 2007), xvi.

41. Robert McRuer, "Shameful Sites: Locating Queerness and Disability," in *Gay Shame*, ed. David Halperin and Valerie Traub (Chicago: University of Chicago Press, 2009), 184.

42. See Jonathan M. Metzl and Anna Kirkland, eds., *Against Health: How Health Became the New Morality* (New York: NYU Press, 2010).

43. Nathan G. Hale Jr., *The Rise and Crisis of Psychoanalysis in the United States: Freud and the Americans, 1917–1985* (New York: Oxford University Press, 1995), 276.

44. See Lunbeck, *Psychiatric Persuasion*; Herman, *Romance of American Psychology*; Gerald N. Grob, *Mental Illness and American Society, 1875–1940* (Princeton: Princeton University Press, 1983); Grob, *Mad among Us: A History of the Care of America's Mentally Ill* (New York: Free Press, 1994); Michael E. Staub, *Madness Is Civilization: When the Diagnosis Was Social, 1948–1980* (Chicago: University of Chicago Press, 2011).

45. Lunbeck, *Psychiatric Persuasion*, 82.

46. See Canaday, *Straight State*; David K. Johnson, *The Lavender Scare: The Cold War Persecution of Gays and Lesbians in the Federal Government* (Chicago: University of Chicago Press, 2004); Elaine Tyler May, *Homeward Bound: American Families in the Cold War Era* (New York: Basic Books, 1988).

47. See Ellen Herman, *Romance of American Psychology*.

48. On sexual psychopath laws, see Estelle B. Freedman, "'Uncontrolled Desires': The Responses to the Sexual Psychopath, 1920–1960," *Journal of American History* 74:1 (June 1987): 83–106; George Chauncey, "The Postwar Sex Crime Panic," in *True Stories from the American Past*, ed. William Graebner (New York: McGraw-Hill 1993): 160–78; Simon Cole, "From the Sexual Psychopath Statute to 'Megan's Law': Psychiatric Knowledge in the Diagnosis, Treatment, and Adjudication of Sex Criminals in New Jersey, 1949–1999," *History of Medicine and Allied Sciences* 55:3 (2000): 292–314; El Chenier, *Strangers in Our Midst: Sexual Deviancy in Postwar Ontario* (Toronto: University of Toronto Press, 2008); Fred Fejes, "Murder, Perversion, and Moral Panic: The 1954 Media Campaign against Miami's Homosexuals and the Discourse of Civic Betterment," *Journal of the History of Sexuality* 9:3 (June 2000): 305–47.

49. See Cornelius F. Collins, "N.Y. Court Requests Psychiatric Service Clinic for Criminals Supplemental Memorandum," *Journal of Criminal Law and Criminology* 19:3 (November 1928): 337–43.

50. On the nexus of the carceral and therapeutic, see Emily Thuma, "Against the 'Prison/Psychiatric State': Anti-Violence Feminisms and the Politics of Confinement," *Feminist Formations* 26:2 (Summer 2014): 26–51; Liat Ben-Moshe, *Disability Incarcerated: Imprisonment and Disability in the United States and Canada* (New York: Palgrave

MacMillan, 2014); Jules Gill-Peterson, "A Trans History of Conversion Therapy," *Sad Brown Girl* (blog), Substack, April 22, 2021, https://sadbrowngirl.substack.com/p/a-trans-history-of-conversion-therapy.

51. Karpman, "The Problem of Homosexuality," box 16, Karpman Papers.

52. Lance Wahlert argues that the supposed liberation of queer people from the discourses of pathology and the effects of the clinic has been a failed exercise, in "The Painful Reunion: The Remedicalization of Homosexuality and the Rise of the Queer," *Bioethical Inquiry* 9:3 (July 2012): 261–75.

53. Roscoe W. Hall to Winfred Overholser, August 16, 1946, Annual Reports of Subordinate Units, box 4, Records of Saint Elizabeths Hospital, National Archives and Records Administration, RG 418, Washington, DC (hereafter cited as Saint Elizabeths Records).

54. Chauncey, *Gay New York*, 14–21.

55. Chauncey, *Gay New York*, 14–22. Siobhan Somerville finds that *queer* could also convey racialized meanings in the early twentieth century, "particularly in the context of mixed-race identities that exposed the instability of divisions between 'black' and 'white'" (Siobhan Somerville, "Queer," in *Keywords for American Cultural Studies*, ed. Bruce Burgett and Glenn Hendler [New York: NYU Press, 2014], 188). See also Sarah Haley, *No Mercy Here: Gender and the Making of Jim Crow Modernity* (Chapel Hill: University of North Carolina Press, 2016): 38–41.

56. Laura Doan, *Disturbing Practices: History, Sexuality, and Women's Experience of Modern War* (Chicago: University of Chicago Press, 2013), 51–52; quote from Eve Kosofsky Sedgwick, *Epistemology of the Closet* (Berkeley: University of California Press, 1990), 22.

57. John Oliven, *Sexual Hygiene and Pathology: A Manual for the Physician and the Professions* (Philadelphia: J. B. Lippincott & Co., 1965). See also Cristan Williams, "Transgender," *TSQ: Transgender Studies Quarterly* 1:1–2 (2014): 233; Susan Stryker, "Transgender History, Homonormativity, and Disciplinarity," *Radical History Review*, no. 100 (Winter 2008): 145–57; Joanne Meyerowitz, *How Sex Changed: A History of Transsexuality in the United States* (Cambridge, MA: Harvard University Press, 2004); David Valentine, *Imagining Transgender: An Ethnography of a Category* (Durham: Duke University Press, 2007); Paisley Currah, "Gender Pluralisms under the Transgender Umbrella," in *Transgender Rights*, ed. Paisley Currah, Richard M. Juang, and Shannon Price Minter (Minneapolis: University of Minnesota Press, 2006), 3–31; Marta V. Vicente, "Transgender: A Useful Category?: Or, How the Historical Study of 'Transsexual' and 'Transvestite' Can Help Us Rethink 'Transgender' as a Category," *TSQ: Transgender Studies Quarterly* 8:4 (November 2021): 426–42.

58. For useful discussions of choices regarding terminology in the history of sexuality and gender, see Emily Skidmore, "Troubling Terms: The Label Problem in Transgender History," *Notches* (blog), November 28, 2017, https://notchesblog.com/2017/11/28/troubling-terms-the-label-problem-in-transgender-history/; Scott Larson, "'Indescribable Being': Theological Performances of Genderlessness in the Society of the Publick Universal Friend, 1776–1819," *Early American Studies: An Interdisciplinary Journal* 12:3 (Fall 2014): 576–600.

59. Jules Gill-Peterson, "General Editor's Introduction," in "The Transsexual/Transvestite Issue," ed. Emmett Harsin Drager and Lucas Platero, special issue, *TSQ: Transgender Studies Quarterly* 8:4 (November 2021): 414.

60. Emmett Harsin Drager and Lucas Platero, "At the Margins of Time and Place: Transsexuals and the Transvestites in Trans Studies," *TSQ: Transgender Studies Quarterly* 8:4 (November 2021): 417.

61. Susan C. Lawrence writes that "the dead themselves have no right to privacy" because "they have ceased to be persons," in *Privacy and the Past: Research, Law, Archives, Ethics* (New Brunswick, NJ: Rutgers University Press, 2016), 14.

62. I am guided by other historians who have approached questions of historical ethics in thoughtful ways, especially Adria L. Imada, *An Archive of Skin, an Archive of Kin: Disability and Life-Making during Medical Incarceration* (Berkeley: University of California Press, 2022); Françoise N. Hamlin, "Historians and Ethics: Finding Anne Moody," *American Historical Review* 125:2 (April 2020): 487–97; Susan Burch, *Committed: Remembering Native Kinship in and beyond Institutions* (Chapel Hill: University of North Carolina Press, 2021). See also Thomas G. Couser, *Vulnerable Subjects: Ethics and Life Writing* (Ithaca, NY: Cornell University Press, 2004); Lawrence, *Privacy and the Past*; Brian Fay, "Historians and Ethics: A Short Introduction to the Theme Issue," *History and Theory* 43:4 (December 2004): 1–2.

## CHAPTER ONE

1. George W. Henry, "Psychogenic Factors in Overt Homosexuality," *American Journal of Psychiatry* 93:4 (January 1937): 905.

2. George W. Henry, *Sex Variants: A Study of Homosexual Patterns* (New York: Paul B. Hoeber, 1941). On Henry, see Jennifer Terry, *An American Obsession: Science, Medicine, and Homosexuality in Modern Society* (Chicago: University of Chicago Press, 1999), 178–267; Henry L. Minton, *Departing from Deviance: A History of Homosexual Rights and Emancipatory Science in America* (Chicago: University of Chicago Press, 2002), 33–57.

3. Alexis de Tocqueville, *Democracy in America*, vol. 2 (1840; repr., New York: Vintage, 1945), 432.

4. See David K. Johnson, *Lavender Scare: The Cold War Persecution of Gays and Lesbians in the Federal Government* (Chicago: University of Chicago Press, 2004); Elaine Tyler May, *Homeward Bound: American Families in the Cold War Era* (New York: Basic Books, 1988).

5. On "intimate governance," see Margot Canaday, Nancy F. Cott, and Robert O. Self, introduction, in *Intimate States: Gender, Sexuality, and Governance in Modern U.S. History*, ed. Margot Canaday, Nancy F. Cott, and Robert O. Self (Chicago: University of Chicago Press, 2021), 1.

6. Eve Kosofsky Sedgwick, "How to Bring Your Kids Up Gay," *Social Text*, no. 29 (1991): 23, 26. On the relationship between violence and cure, see Eli Clare, *Brilliant Imperfection: Grappling with Cure* (Durham: Duke University Press, 2017); Eunjung Kim, *Curative Violence: Rehabilitating Disability, Gender, and Sexuality in Modern Korea* (Durham: Duke University Press, 2017).

7. Nathan G. Hale Jr., *The Rise and Crisis of Psychoanalysis in the United States: Freud and the Americans, 1917-1985* (New York: Oxford University Press, 1995), 276.

8. See Terry, *American Obsession*; Benjamin Kahan, *The Book of Minor Perverts: Sexology, Etiology, and Emergences of Sexuality* (Chicago: University of Chicago Press, 2019); Siobhan B. Somerville, *Queering the Color Line: Race and the Invention of Homosexuality in American Culture* (Durham: Duke University Press, 2000); Vern L. Bullough, "Homosexuality and the Medical Model," *Journal of Homosexuality* 1:1 (1976): 99-110. The scholarly literature on sexology is robust. Key texts include Heike Bauer, *Sexology and Translation: Cultural and Scientific Encounters across the Modern World* (Philadelphia: Temple University Press, 2015); Janice Irvine, *Disorders of Desire: Sexuality and Gender in Modern American Sexology* (Philadelphia: Temple University Press, 2005).

9. Benjamin Kahan reminds us that etiology was a matter of considerable debate among sexologists. See Kahan, *Book of Minor Perverts*.

10. See Harry Oosterhuis, *Stepchildren of Nature: Krafft-Ebing, Psychiatry, and the Making of Sexual Identity* (Chicago: University of Chicago Press, 2000), 71.

11. See James D. Steakley, "Per scientiam ad justitiam: Magnus Hirschfeld and the Sexual Politics of Innate Homosexuality," in Vernon A. Rosario, ed., *Science and Homosexualities* (New York: Routledge, 1997), 133-54.

12. Richard von Krafft-Ebing, *Psychopathia Sexualis*, 7th ed., trans. Charles Gilbert Chaddock (Philadelphia: F. A. Davis Co. Publishers, 1893), 187, 227. Jay Prosser notes that "the reading of sexual inversion as about homosexuality is profoundly ironic" given its primary focus on gender ("Transsexuals and the Transsexologists: Inversion and the Emergence of Transsexual Subjectivity," in *Sexology in Culture: Labelling Bodies and Desires*, ed. Lucy Bland and Laura Doan [Cambridge: Polity Press, 1998], 117-18).

13. On the history of conceptions of human bisexuality, see Joanne Meyerowitz, *How Sex Changed: A History of Transsexuality in the United States* (Cambridge, MA: Harvard University Press, 2002), 23-29, 98-104; George Makari, *Revolution in Mind: The Creation of Psychoanalysis* (New York: Harper, 2008), 99.

14. See Oosterhuis, *Stepchildren of Nature*, 66-67; Chris Waters, "Havelock Ellis, Sigmund Freud, and the State: Discourses of Homosexual Identity in Interwar Britain," in *Sexology in Culture: Labelling Bodies and Desires*, ed. Bland and Doan, 165-79; Jeffrey Weeks, *Sexuality and Its Discontents: Meanings, Myths, and Modern Sexualities* (London: Routledge and Kegan Paul, 1985), 153-54.

15. See Kenneth Lewes, *The Psychoanalytic Theory of Male Homosexuality* (New York: Simon and Schuster, 1988), 35; Makari, *Revolution in Mind*, 99.

16. Sigmund Freud, *Three Essays on the Theory of Sexuality: The 1905 Edition*, trans. Ulrike Kistner, ed. Philippe Van Haute and Herman Westernk (London: Verso, 2017), 141-42; footnote added in 1915.

17. Freud, "The Psychogenesis of a Case of Female Homosexuality," *International Journal of Psycho-Analysis* 1:2 (January 1920): 129.

18. Freud, "Psychogenesis of a Case of Female Homosexuality," 148.

19. Freud, "A Letter from Freud," *American Journal of Psychiatry* 107:10 (April 1951): 786–87.

20. Lewes makes this important point in *Psychoanalytic Theory of Male Homosexuality*, 35.

21. Ellis, "A Note on the Treatment of Sexual Inversion," *Alienist and Neurologist* 17:3 (July 1896): 258. See Albert von Schrenck-Notzing, *Therapeutic Suggestion in Psychopathia Sexualis with Especial Reference to Contrary Sexual Instinct*, trans. Charles Gilbert Chaddock (Philadelphia: F. A. Davis, 1895).

22. Ellis, "Note on the Treatment of Sexual Inversion," 258.

23. Ellis, "Note on the Treatment of Sexual Inversion," 261.

24. Ellis, "Note on the Treatment of Sexual Inversion," 262.

25. Magnus Hirschfeld, "Adaption Treatment of Homosexuality (Adjustment Therapy)," *Homophile Studies: ONE Institute Quarterly* 5:2–4 (Fall 1962): 41–54; two chapters of his book, *De Homosexualität des Mannes und des Weibes* (Berlin: Louis Marcus Verlagsbuchhandlung, 1920), trans. Henry Gerber, 42–43.

26. Hirschfeld, "Adaptation Treatment of Homosexuality," 43.

27. Hirschfeld, "Adaptation Treatment of Homosexuality," 54.

28. Krafft-Ebing, *Psychopathia Sexualis*, 231. See Oosterhuis, *Stepchildren of Nature*, 157.

29. Wilhelm Stekel, "Is Homosexuality Curable?," trans. Bertrand S. Frohman, *Psychoanalytic Review* 17 (October 1930): 444.

30. Stekel, "Is Homosexuality Curable?," 443.

31. Stekel, "Is Homosexuality Curable?," 443.

32. James G. Kiernan, "Psychical Treatment of Congenital Sexual Inversion," *Review of Insanity and Nervous Disease* 4:4 (June 1894): 295, 293. On Kiernan, see Ivan Crozier, "James Kiernan and the Responsible Pervert," *International Journal of Law and Psychiatry* 25:4 (July–August 2002): 331–50. See also William J. Robinson, "My Views on Homosexuality," *American Journal of Urology* 10 (January–December 1914), 550–52.

33. Eli Zaretsky, *Secrets of the Soul: A Social and Cultural History of Psychoanalysis* (New York: Knopf, 2004), 277.

34. John C. Burnham, introduction, in *After Freud Left: A Century of Psychoanalysis in America*, ed. John Burnham (Chicago: University of Chicago Press, 2012), 16.

35. On the reception of Freud in America, see Hale, *The Rise and Crisis of Psychoanalysis*; Burnham, *After Freud Left*; Clarence Paul Oberndorf, *A History of Psychoanalysis in America* (New York: Grune & Stratton, 1953); Dagmar Herzog, *Cold War Freud: Psychoanalysis in an Age of Catastrophes* (Cambridge: Cambridge University Press, 2017); Nathan G. Hale Jr., *Freud and the Americans: The Beginning of Psychoanalysis in the United States, 1876–1971* (New York: Oxford University Press, 1971); Zaretsky, *Secrets of the Soul.*

36. Elisabeth Roudinesco, *Freud in His Time and Ours* (Cambridge, MA: Harvard University Press, 2016), 131. See also Hale, *Freud and the Americans*, 331–52.

37. Walter Bromberg, *Psychiatry between the Wars, 1918–1945: A Recollection* (Westport, CT: Greenwood Press, 1982), 147.

38. Sandor Rado, "A Critical Examination of the Concept of Bisexuality," in *Psychoanalysis of Behavior: The Collected Papers of Sandor Rado* (New York: Grune & Stratton, 1956): 139–50; originally published in *Psychosomatic Medicine* 2 (1940): 459–67. On Rado's rejection of Freud's concept of bisexuality, see Meyerowitz, *How Sex Changed*, 98–105; Ronald Bayer, *Homosexuality and American Psychiatry: The Politics of Diagnosis* (New York: Basic Books, 1981), 29–30; Matthew Tontonoz, "Sandor Rado, American Psychoanalysis, and the Question of Bisexuality," *History of Psychology* 20:3 (August 2017): 263–89.

39. Sandor Rado, *Psychoanalysis of Behavior: The Collected Papers of Sandor Rado* (New York: Grune & Stratton, 1956), 206.

40. Rado, *Psychoanalysis of Behavior*, 210. For an analysis of the arguments that Rado made for his rejection of bisexuality, see Tontonoz, "Sandor Rado, American Psychoanalysis."

41. Edmund Bergler, *One Thousand Homosexuals* (Patterson, NJ: Pageant Books, 1959), 244; Bergler, *Homosexuality: Disease or Way of Life?* (New York: Hill and Wang, 1956), 9, 28–29.

42. Bergler, *Homosexuality*, 9.

43. Bergler, *Homosexuality*, 8–9.

44. Bergler, *Homosexuality*, 188; Bergler, *One Thousand Homosexuals*, ix.

45. Irving Bieber, Harvey J. Dain, Paul R. Dince, Marvin G. Drellich, Henry G. Grand, Ralph H. Gundlach, Malvina W. Kremer, Alfred H. Rifkin, Cornelia B. Wilbur, and Toby S. Sieber, *Homosexuality: A Psychoanalytic Study of Male Homosexuals* (New York: Basic Books, 1962), 24, vii.

46. Phillip Wyle, *Generation of Vipers* (New York: Farrar & Rinehart, 1942). See also Edward Strecker, *Their Mother's Sons: The Psychiatrist Examines an American Problem* (Philadelphia: Lippincott, 1946); Ferdinand Lundberg and Marynia F. Farnham, *Modern Woman: The Lost Sex* (New York: Harper & Brothers, 1947).

47. For psychoanalytic studies of lesbians in this period, see Richard C. Robertiello, *Voyage from Lesbos: The Psychoanalysis of a Female Homosexual* (New York: Citadel Press, 1959); Cornelia B. Wilbur, "Clinical Aspects of Female Homosexuality," in *Sexual Inversion: The Multiple Roots of Homosexuality*, ed. Judd Marmor (New York: Basic Books, 1965), 268–81; Morris Wolfe Brody, "An Analysis of the Psychosexual Development of a Female: With Special Reference to Homosexuality," *Psychoanalytic Review* 30:1 (January 1943): 47–58; May E. Romm, "Sexuality and Homosexuality in Women," in *Sexual Inversion: The Multiple Roots of Homosexuality*, ed. Judd Marmor (New York: Basic Books, 1965), 282–301; Helene Deutsch, "Homosexuality in Women," *International Journal of Psychoanalysis* 14 (1933): 34–56; Donald Webster Cory (pseudonym of Edward Sagarin), *The Lesbian in America* (New York: Citadel Press, 1964); Frank S. Caprio, *Female Homosexuality: A Psychodynamic Study of Lesbianism* (New York: Citadel Press, 1954). On psychoanalysis and lesbianism, see Amanda Littauer, *Bad Girls: Young Women, Sex, and Rebellion before the Sixties* (Chapel Hill: University of North Carolina Press, 2015), 147–58.

48. Wilbur, "Clinical Aspects of Female Homosexuality," 276.

49. Emil A. Gutheil, "The Psychologic Background of Transsexualism and Transvestism," *American Journal of Psychotherapy* 8:2 (1954): 238. On psychoanalysts and transvestism, see Meyerowitz, *How Sex Changed*, 104–9.

50. David O. Cauldwell, "Psychopathia Transexualis," *Sexology* 16 (1949): 274–80.

51. Nikolas Golosow and Elliott L. Weitzman, "Psychosexual and Ego Regression in the Male Transsexual," *Journal of Nervous and Mental Disease* 149:4 (October 1969): 328.

52. Benjamin Karpman, "From the Emotional and Dream Life of a Transvestite, II," *Archives of Criminal Psychodynamics* 5:1 (Winter 1962): 61; Benjamin Karpman, "Dream Life in a Case of Transvestism, with Particular Attention to the Problem of Latent Homosexuality," *Journal of Nervous and Mental Disease* 106:3 (1947): 294.

53. Danica Deutsch, "A Case of Transvestism," *American Journal of Psychotherapy* 8 (1954): 242.

54. Albert Ellis, introduction to Cory, *Lesbian in America*, 12; Albert Ellis, introduction to Larry Maddock's "Femmepersonator," box 40, folder 13, Albert Ellis Papers, Rare Book and Manuscript Library, Columbia University, New York, NY (hereafter cited as Ellis Papers).

55. Herzog, *Cold War Freud*, 63.

56. Bergler, *One Thousand Homosexuals*, iv.

57. Steven Lee Myers, "Irving Bieber, 80, a Psychoanalyst Who Studied Homosexuality, Dies," *New York Times*, August 28, 1991.

58. "'Homosexuality,' A Report by the Committee of Public Health, New York Academy of Medicine," *Bulletin*, 1964, New York Academy of Medicine, New York, NY, 5.

59. Charles Socarides, "Homosexuality and Medicine" *JAMA* 212:7 (May 18, 1970): 1199; Jean M. White, "Center to Treat Homosexuals Urged," *Washington Post*, September 25, 1967, in Barbara Gittings and Kay Tobin Lahusen Papers, box 2, folder 5, ONE National Gay and Lesbian Archives, USC Libraries, University of Southern California, Los Angeles. Many psychiatrists and physicians understood homosexuality and alcoholism to be closely linked. See Michele Elaine Morales, "Persistent Pathologies: The Odd Coupling of Alcoholism and Homosexuality in the Discourse of Twentieth Century Science" (PhD dissertation, University of Michigan, Department of American Culture, 2006).

60. On the history of the development of the *DSM*, see Morton Kramer, "The History of the Efforts to Agree on an International Classification of Mental Disorders," *Diagnostic and Statistical Manual of Mental Disorders*, 2nd ed. (*DSM-II*) (Washington, DC: American Psychiatric Association, 1968); Herb Kutchins and Stuart Kirk, *Making Us Crazy: DSM: The Psychiatric Bible and the Creation of Mental Disorders* (New York: Free Press, 1997); Stuart Kirk and Herb Kutchins, *The Selling of DSM: The Rhetoric of Science in Psychiatry* (New York: A. de Gruter, 1992); Staub, *Madness Is Civilization*.

61. American Psychiatric Association, *Diagnostic and Statistical Manual of Mental Disorders* (Washington, DC: American Psychiatric Association, 1952), 38–39.

62. Herzog, *Cold War Freud*, 66.

63. See Lewes, *Psychoanalytic Theory of Male Homosexuality*; Susanna Drake, *Slandering the Jew: Sexuality and Difference in Early Christian Tests* (Philadelphia: University of Pennsylvania Press, 2013); Jeremy Webster, "The 'Lustful Buggering Jew': Anti-Semitism, Gender, and Sodomy in Restoration Political Satire," *Journal for Early Modern Cultural Studies* 6:1 (Spring–Summer 2006): 106–24.

64. Ernest Jones, *Free Associations: Memoirs of a Psychoanalyst* (1959; reprint, New Brunswick, NJ: Transaction Publishers, 1990), 201. See also Sander L. Gilman, *The Case of Sigmund Freud: Medicine and Identity at the Fin de Siècle* (Baltimore: Johns Hopkins University Press, 1994).

65. Kenneth Lewes, Elizabeth Young-Bruehl, Ralph Roughton, Maggie Magee, and Diana C. Miller, "Homosexuality and Psychoanalysis I: Historical Perspectives," *Journal of Gay & Lesbian Mental Health* 12:4 (2008): 239, 232, 302.

66. See Tontonoz, "Sandor Rado."

67. See Gerald N. Grob, *Mental Illness and American Society, 1875–1940* (Princeton: Princeton University Press, 1983), 235.

68. Ellen Herman, *The Romance of American Psychology: Political Culture in the Age of Experts* (Berkeley: University of California Press, 1995).

69. Alfred C. Kinsey, Wardell B. Pomeroy, and Clyde E. Martin, *Sexual Behavior in the Human Male* (Philadelphia: W. B. Saunders, 1948); Alfred C. Kinsey, Wardell B. Pomeroy, Clyde E. Martin, and Paul H. Gebhard, *Sexual Behavior in the Human Female* (Philadelphia: W. B. Saunders, 1953); William H. Masters and Virginia E. Johnson, *Human Sexual Response* (Toronto: Bantam Books, 1966); William H. Masters and Virginia E. Johnson, *Human Sexual Inadequacy* (Toronto: Bantam Books, 1970). On Kinsey's reception, see Miriam G. Reumann, *American Sexual Character: Sex, Gender, and National Identity in the Kinsey Reports* (Berkeley: University of California Press, 2005).

70. See Margot Canaday, *The Straight State: Sexuality and Citizenship in Twentieth-Century America* (Princeton: Princeton University Press, 2009).

71. Henry Gerber to Manual boyFrank, July 9, 1946, Manuel boyFrank Papers, Box 1, Folder 1:2, ONE National Gay and Lesbian Archives, Los Angeles, CA.

72. Jim Kepner, "Dr. Bieber's Enormous Carrot," *Tangents*, May–June 1968, 19.

73. Naoko Wake, *Private Practices: Harry Stack Sullivan, the Science of Homosexuality, and American Liberalism* (New Brunswick, NJ: Rutgers University Press, 2011), 166. On Sullivan's and other psychiatrists' participation in the policy to screen inductees for "fitness" for service, see Wake, *Private Practices*, 157–86; Allan Bérubé, *Coming Out under Fire: The History of Gay Men and Women in World War Two* (New York: Free Press, 1990), 8–28; Herman, *Romance of American Psychiatry*, 85–95.

74. See Bérubé, *Coming Out under Fire*, 147; Naoko Wake, "The Military, Psychiatry, and 'Unfit' Soldiers, 1939–1942," *Journal of the History of Medicine and Allied Sciences* 62:4 (October 2007): 461–94.

75. Bérubé, *Coming Out under Fire*, 147.

76. See George Chauncey, "The Postwar Sex Crime Panic," in *True Stories from the American Past*, ed. William Graebner (New York: McGraw-Hill 1993), 160–78;

Estelle B. Freedman, "'Uncontrolled Desires': The Responses to the Sexual Psycho-path, 1920–1960," *Journal of American History* 74:1 (June 1987): 83–106; Simon Cole, "From the Sexual Psychopath Statute to 'Megan's Law'"; El Chenier, *Strangers in Our Midst: Sexual Deviancy in Postwar Ontario* (Toronto: University of Toronto Press, 2008); Fred Fejes, "Murder, Perversion, and Moral Panic: The 1954 Media Campaign against Miami's Homosexuals and the Discourse of Civic Betterment," *Journal of the History of Sexuality* 9:3 (June 2000): 305–47; Philip Jenkins, *Moral Panic: Changing Concepts of the Child Molester in Modern America* (New Haven: Yale University Press, 1998).

77. See Morris Ploscowe, *Sex and the Law* (New York: Prentice-Hall, 1951), 216; Freedman, "Uncontrolled Desires."

78. "The Psychopathic Individual: A Symposium," *Mental Hygiene* 8 (1924): 175.

79. "The Psychopathic Individual," 175. See also Frederick J. Hacker and Marcel Frym, "The Sexual Psychopath Act in Practice: A Critical Discussion," *California Law Review* 43:5 (December 1955): 770.

80. Charles W. Cabeen and James C. Coleman, "The Selection of Sex Offender Patients for Group Psychotherapy," *International Journal of Group Psychotherapy* 12:1 (January 1962): 327.

81. Karpman wrote that "psychopaths exhibit a combination of hypersexuality with a strong homosexual component. Despite their intellectual capacity, they are unable to foresee the consequences of their acts since their primitive emotional organization presses for immediate release" (Benjamin Karpman, *The Individual Criminal: Studies in the Psychogenetics of Crime* [Washington, DC: Nervous and Mental Disease Publishing, 1935], 26); see also Benjamin Karpman, "The Sexual Psychopath," *Journal of Criminal Law & Criminology* 42 (1951–52): 185.

82. U.S. Congress, House, Committee on the District of Columbia, *Criminal Sexual Psychopaths*, 80th Cong., 2nd sess., 1948, 107.

83. U.S. Congress, House, Committee on the District of Columbia, *Criminal Sexual Psychopaths*, 115.

84. "2,000 Hear Experts on Sex Deviates at Star Forum Meeting," *ONE* 4:3 (1956): 12.

85. Karl M. Bowman and Bernice Engle, "A Psychiatric Evaluation of the Laws of Homosexuality," *American Journal of Psychiatry* 112:6 (February 1956): 577–83.

86. U.S. Congress, House, Committee on the District of Columbia, *Criminal Sexual Psychopaths*, 104.

87. U.S. Congress, House, Subcommittee on Health, Education, and Recreation, Committee on the District of Columbia, *Criminal Sexual Psychopaths*, February 20, 1948, 1; italics added.

88. U.S. Congress, Senate, *Providing for the Treatment of Sexual Psychopaths in the District of Columbia*, Senate, Committee on the District of Columbia, S. Rep. No. 1377, 80th Cong., 2nd sess., May 21, 1948, 1.

89. U.S. Congress, Senate, *Providing for the Treatment of Sexual Psychopaths in the District of Columbia*, 6.

90. U.S. Congress, House, Committee on the District of Columbia, *Criminal Sexual Psychopaths*, 103.

91. U.S. Congress, Senate, *Providing for the Treatment of Sexual Psychopaths in the District of Columbia*, 8. El Chenier makes a similar argument, tracing the genealogy of sexual psychopath laws in Canada to Progressive-Era laws that named the "defective delinquent" a "medicalized version of the habitual criminal" and suggests that "It is . . . useful to see criminal sexual psychopath legislation as one point on a century-long trajectory of psycho-medical thinking about criminality, sexual, and legal responsibility, and as part of a long tradition of social reform that took a dim view of punishment and repression" (Chenier, *Strangers in Our Midst*, 21, 40).

92. U.S. Congress, House, Committee on the District of Columbia, *Criminal Sexual Psychopaths*, 7.

93. U.S. Congress, House, Committee on the District of Columbia, *Criminal Sexual Psychopaths*, 97.

94. U.S. Congress, House, Committee on the District of Columbia, *Criminal Sexual Psychopaths*, 39–40. In the discussion of the bill in the Committee on the District of Columbia, O'Hara noted that the committee "endeavored in considering this subject, realizing the danger which might exist in a wave of hysteria of social workers or anything of that nature, that the right of the accused or the rights of an individual are safeguarded to the greatest extent that we could do so, even to the right of counsel, to insist upon counsel to appear before him in any and all of these cases" (H.R. 6071, 80th Cong., 2nd sess., March 31, 1948, 16–17).

95. Anna Lvovsky, *Vice Patrol: Cops, Courts, and the Struggle over Urban Gay Life before Stonewall* (Chicago: University of Chicago Press, 2021), 120. On psychiatrists' relationship to the courts, see Cornelius F. Collins, "N.Y. Court Requests Psychiatric Service Clinic for Criminals Supplemental Memorandum," *Journal of Criminal Law and Criminology* 19:3 (November 1928): 337–43; Manfred S. Guttmacher and Henry Weihoffen, *Psychiatry and the Law* (New York: Norton, 1952).

96. Guttmacher and Weihoffen, *Psychiatry and the Law*, vii.

97. Manfred S. Guttmacher, *Sex Offenses: The Problem, Causes, and Prevention* (New York: Norton, 1951), 142.

98. Hadden, "Homosexuality: An Experientially Determined and Treatable Condition," unpublished book ms., 1981, box 2, folder 41, Samuel Bernard Hadden Papers, University Archives and Records Center, University of Pennsylvania, Philadelphia, PA (hereafter cited as Hadden Papers).

99. Senate Committee of the Judiciary, *Revision of Immigration and Naturalization Laws*, S. Rep. 1137, 82nd Cong., 2nd sess., 1952, pt. 1.

100. Canaday interprets psychiatrists' disavowal of the concept of "psychopathic personality" as a sign of the crumbling of psychiatric consensus on homosexuality as a mental illness (Canaday, *Straight State*, 216). While a few may have questioned that idea in 1952, their more general complaint was with the diagnostic category of psychopathy.

101. In the major challenge to the law fifteen years later, in 1967, advocates for the defendant, Clive Michael Boutilier, asserted that Boutilier was unfairly excluded because homosexuality was not a mental disease and that he did not exhibit a "psy-

chopathic personality." But the Supreme Court concluded that "the Congress used the phrase 'psychopathic personality' not in the clinical sense, but to effectuate its purpose to exclude from entry all homosexuals and other sex perverts" (*Boutilier v. Immigration Service*, 387 U.S. 118 [1967], 122). On the McCarran-Walter Act and homosexuality, see Canaday, *Straight State*, 214–54; Siobhan B. Somerville, "Queer *Loving*," *GLQ: A Journal of Lesbian and Gay Studies* 11:3 (2005): 335–70; Marc Stein, *Sexual Injustice: Supreme Court Decisions from Griswold to Roe* (Chapel Hill: University of North Carolina Press, 2010). See also Eithne Luibhéid, "'Looking Like a Lesbian': The Organization of Sexual Monitoring at the United States–Mexican Border," *Journal of the History of Sexuality* 8:3 (January 1998): 477–506.

102. Lewes et al., "Homosexuality and Psychoanalysis I," 303.

### CHAPTER TWO

1. Irving Bieber, Harvey J. Dain, Paul R. Dince, Marvin G. Drellich, Henry G. Grand, Ralph H. Gundlach, Malvina W. Kremer, Alfred H. Rifkin, Cornelia B. Wilbur, and Toby S. Sieber, *Homosexuality: A Psychoanalytic Study of Male Homosexuals* (New York: Basic Books, 1962).

2. Robert Isay, *Becoming Gay: The Journey to Self-Acceptance* (New York: Pantheon, 1996), 19–20.

3. Albert Ellis, *Reason and Emotion in Psychotherapy* (New York: Lyle Stuart, 1962), 3. See also Ellis to Douglas Kennedy, Editor, *True*, February 26, 1966, box 125, folder 2, Albert Ellis Papers, Rare Book and Manuscript Collection, Columbia University, New York, NY (hereafter cited as Ellis Papers); Albert Ellis, *Homosexuality: Its Causes and Cure* (New York: Lyle Stuart, 1965), 94–98, 133.

4. Ellis, *Reason and Emotion in Psychotherapy*, 11.

5. Ellis, *Reason and Emotion in Psychotherapy*, 11.

6. Ellis, *Homosexuality*, 157.

7. Ellis, *Homosexuality*, 99. See also Samuel Hadden, "Trends in Treatment of Homosexuality and Sexual Deviants," October 10, 1955, box 2, folder 23, Samuel Bernard Hadden Papers, University Archives and Records Center, University of Pennsylvania, Philadelphia, PA (hereafter cited as Hadden Papers).

8. Ernest Bien, "Why Do Homosexuals Undergo Treatment?" *Medical Review of Reviews* 40:1 (January 1934): 7.

9. Irving Bieber, "Clinical Aspects of Male Homosexuality," in *Sexual Inversion: The Multiple Roots of Homosexuality*, ed. Judd Marmor (New York: Basic Books, 1965), 265.

10. KP31, responses to questions, 6, Benjamin Karpman Papers, Jean-Nickolaus Tretter Collection in Gay, Lesbian, Bisexual, and Transgender Studies, University of Minnesota, Minneapolis, MN (hereafter cited as Karpman Papers). Note: The Tretter Collection has assigned KP numbers to each case file. I have given them pseudonyms.

11. KP45, case history, Karpman Papers.

12. KP31, Karpman Papers.

13. Christine Jorgensen, *Christine Jorgensen: A Personal Autobiography* (New York: Paul S. Ericksson, 1967), 31, 63.

14. Jorgensen, *Personal Autobiography*, 101, 114, 115. On Jorgensen's self-representation, see Joanne Meyerowitz, *How Sex Changed: A History of Transsexuality in the United States* (Cambridge, MA: Harvard University Press, 2002), 51–97.

15. Robert Bogdan, ed., *On Being Different: The Autobiography of Jane Fry* (New York: Wiley and Sons, 1974), 126.

16. See Meyerowitz, *How Sex Changed*, 130–68. Jules Gill-Peterson notes that "for the first half of the century, trans people's embodied knowledge borrowed heavily from intersex discourses to negotiate this growing power of the doctor and the clinic" (Jules Gill-Peterson, *Histories of the Transgender Child* [Minneapolis: University of Minnesota Press, 2019], 16).

17. Elizabeth Mintz, "Overt Male Homosexuals in Combined Group and Individual Treatment," *Journal of Consulting Psychology* 30:3 (June 1966): 194.

18. Edmund Bergler, *Homosexuality: Disease or Way of Life* (New York: Hill and Wang, 1957), 21.

19. Edmund Bergler, *One Thousand Homosexuals: Conspiracy of Silence, or Curing and Deglamorizing Homosexuals* (Patterson, NJ: Pageant Books, 1959), 243.

20. Robert A. Harper, "Can Homosexuals Be Changed?" *Sexology* 26 (1959): 552.

21. KP9, Karpman Papers.

22. Samuel Hadden, "Attitudes toward and Approaches to the Problem of Homosexuality," paper delivered at the meeting of the Pennsylvania Psychiatric Society, Philadelphia, PA, October 26, 1956, box 2, folder 24, Hadden Papers.

23. Samuel Hadden, "Treatment of Male Homosexuals in Groups," paper delivered at AGPA [American Group Psychotherapy Association], January 29, 1965, box 2, folder 26, Hadden Papers. See also Carl Rogers, Howard Roback, Embry McKee, and Daniel Calhoun, "Group Psychotherapy with Homosexuals: A Review," *International Journal of Group Psychotherapy* 26:1 (January 1976): 3.

24. Samuel Hadden, "Trends in Treatment of Homosexuality and Sexual Deviants," October 10, 1955, box 2, folder 23, Hadden Papers.

25. Samuel Hadden, "Treatment of Male Homosexuals."

26. *Time* magazine, "Psychiatry: Homosexuals Can Be Cured," February 12, 1965, 44.

27. Samuel Hadden, "Treatment of Homosexuality," 812.

28. Samuel Hadden, "Male Homosexuality: Observations on Its Psychogenesis and on Its Treatment by Group Psychotherapy," paper delivered in London, 1964, box 2, folder 25, Hadden Papers.

29. Irving Bieber, "Clinical Aspects of Male Homosexuality," in *Sexual Inversion: The Multiple Roots of Homosexuality*, ed. Judd Marmor (New York: Basic Books, 1965), 266.

30. Alfred C. Kinsey, Wardell B. Pomeroy, and Clyde E. Martin, *Sexual Behavior in the Human Male* (Philadelphia: W. B. Saunders, 1948), 623.

31. Alfred C. Kinsey, Wardell B. Pomeroy, Clyde E. Martin, and Paul H. Gebhard, *Sexual Behavior in the Human Female* (Philadelphia: W. B. Saunders, 1953), 487.

32. Alfred Kinsey to Albert Ellis, January 25, 1952, box 118, folder 12, Ellis Papers.

33. Donald Webster Cory (pseudonym of Edward Sagarin), *The Homosexual in America: A Subjective Approach* (1951; reprint, New York: Castle Books, 1960), 91.

34. Kinsey et al., *Sexual Behavior in the Human Female*, 448.

35. Edmund Bergler, "The Myth of a New National Disease: Homosexuality and the Kinsey Report," *Psychiatric Quarterly* 22:1–4 (January 1948): 74. See also Miriam G. Reumann, *American Sexual Character: Sex, Gender, and National Identity in the Kinsey Reports* (Berkeley: University of California Press, 2005), 169; Jeffrey Escoffier, "Kinsey, Psychoanalysis, and the Theory of Sexuality," *Sexologies* 29 (April–June 2020): 35–42; Katie Sutton, "Kinsey and the Psychoanalysts: Cross-Disciplinary Knowledge Production in Post-War US Sex Research," *History of the Human Sciences* 34:1 (May 2020): 120–47; Jonathan Gathorne-Hardy, *Sex the Measure of All Things* (Bloomington: Indiana University Press, 1998), 326–27; Wardell Pomeroy, *Dr. Kinsey and the Institute for Sex Research* (New Haven: Yale University Press, 1972), 202; Paul H. Gebhard and Alan B. Johnson, *The Kinsey Data: Marginal Tabulations of the 1938–1963 Interviews Conducted by the Institute for Sex Research* (Philadelphia: W. B. Saunders Company, 1979), 28. On the conflict between psychoanalysts and Kinsey, see Kenneth Lewes, *The Psychoanalytic Theory of Male Homosexuality* (New York: Simon and Schuster, 1988), 122–40.

36. Bergler, *One Thousand Homosexuals*, 5.

37. Edmund Bergler, *Homosexuality: Disease or Way of Life* (New York: Hill and Wang, 1957), 16, 47.

38. Bergler, *Homosexuality*, 200.

39. Bergler, *One Thousand Homosexuals*, 162.

40. Bergler, *One Thousand Homosexuals*, 22.

41. Paul Moor, "The View from Irving Bieber's Couch: 'Heads I Win, Tails You Lose,'" *Journal of Gay and Lesbian Psychotherapy* 5:3–4 (2001): 28.

42. LASFR, August 28, 1964, box 91, folder 17, Ellis Papers.

43. KP 34, Karpman Papers.

44. Author's interview with Charles Silverstein, July 28, 2015, New York, NY.

45. Charles Silverstein, *For the Ferryman: A Personal History* (New York: Chelsea Station Editions, 2011), 80.

46. Ellis, *Homosexuality: Its Causes and Cure*, 239.

47. Bergler, *Homosexuality*, 9.

48. Robert J. Stoller, "Criteria for Psychiatric Diagnosis," in Robert J. Stoller, Judd Marmor, Irving Bieber, Ronald Gold, Charles W. Socarides, Richard Green, and Robert L. Spitzer, "A Symposium: Should Homosexuality Be in the APA Nomenclature?" *American Journal of Psychiatry* 130:11 (November 1973): 1207.

49. Samuel B. Hadden, "Newer Treatment Techniques for Homosexuality," *Archives of Environmental Health* 13:3 (September 1966): 286.

50. KP90, Karpman, memorandum, Karpman Papers.

51. KP90, Karpman Papers.

52. Author's interview with Warren Goldfarb, September 25, 2016, Cambridge, MA.

53. Betty Berzon, "Homosexuality Then and Now: A Gay Perspective," ms., n.d., box 4, folder 58, Betty Berzon Papers, ONE National Gay and Lesbian Archives, Los Angeles, CA.

54. Lionel Ovesey, Willard Gaylin, and Herbert Hendin, "Psychotherapy of Male Homosexuality: Psychodynamic Formulation," *Archives of General Psychiatry* 9:1 (July 1963): 23.

55. KP56, responses to questions, 1, Karpman Papers.

56. Karpman, *The Individual Criminal: Studies in the Psychogenetics of Crime* (Washington, DC: Nervous and Mental Disease Publishing Co., 1935), 107.

57. Cory, *Homosexual in America*, 5.

58. Cory, *Homosexual in America*, 6–7. Sagarin would come to reconsider and reverse these early views, aligning himself with the views of psychologist Albert Ellis and placing him at odds with the homophile and gay rights movements that he had done so much to inspire.

59. Karpman, February 10, 1932, KP9, Karpman Papers

60. KP92, "Comments on Survey," August 19, 1949, Karpman Papers.

61. KP45, case history, Karpman Papers.

62. KP82, Karpman Papers.

63. KP82, Karpman Papers.

64. KP33, Karpman Papers.

65. KP3, psychiatrist's memorandum, December 3, 1947, Karpman Papers.

66. KP3, Karpman Papers.

67. KP3, Karpman Papers.

68. Of psychiatrists earlier in the twentieth century, Naoko Wake finds that some "artfully separated what they argued in public from who they were in private" (*Private Practices: Harry Stack Sullivan, the Science of Homosexuality, and American Liberalism* [New Brunswick, NJ: Rutgers University Press, 2011], 3).

69. On the importance of the psychological concept of adjustment in the thinking of gay men and lesbians in the 1940s and 1950s, see Stephen Vider, *The Queerness of Home: Gender, Sexuality, and the Politics of Domesticity after World War II* (Chicago: University of Chicago Press, 2021), 43–47.

70. Justin Spring, *Secret Historian: The Life and Times of Samuel Steward, Professor, Tattoo Artist, and Sexual Renegade* (New York: Farrar, Straus and Giroux, 2010), 28.

71. R.P., "Case History," 18, Karpman Papers.

72. Jonathan Ned Katz, *Gay American History: Lesbians and Gay Men in the U.S.A.* (New York: Thomas Y. Crowell, 1976; reprint, New York: Avon, 1977), 201.

73. Quoted in Dan Wakefield, *New York in the Fifties* (New York: Houghton Mifflin Harcourt, 1992), 223, 224.

74. Charles Silverstein, *For the Ferryman: A Personal History* (New York: Chelsea Station Editions, 2011), 78.

75. KP27, Karpman to Marina Harris, May 16, 1942, Karpman Papers.

76. KP30, memorandum #1, February 21, 1944, Karpman Papers.

77. Benjamin Karpman, yearly report, July 1, 1948–June 30, 1949, annual reports of subordinate units, box 8, Records of Saint Elizabeths Hospital, National Archives and Records Administration, RG 418, Washington, DC (hereafter cited as Saint Elizabeths Records).

78. KP43, Karpman Papers.

79. KP 34, supplemental memorandum for Dr. Karpman, "Re Hal Richardson," March 14, 1936, Karpman Papers.

80. KP 43, memorandum for Dr. Karpman, December 3, 1935, Karpman Papers.

81. KP 43, Hal Richardson, case file, Karpman Papers.

82. KP43, "Observations of the Patient Hal Richardson by Mr. X," n.d., Karpman Papers.

83. On the work of the George W. Henry Foundation, see Henry Minton, *Departing from Deviance: A History of Homosexual Rights and Emancipatory Science in America* (Chicago: University of Chicago Press, 2002).

84. See Alfred A. Gross, *Strangers in Our Midst: Problems of the Homosexual in American Society* (Washington, DC: Public Affairs Press, 1962).

85. *17th Annual Report of the George W. Henry Foundation*, 1965, 10, box 3, folder 6 (hereafter cited as Henry Papers).

86. *The Nineteenth Annual Report on the State of the George W. Henry Foundation, Inc.*, 1967, box 3, folder 6, Henry Papers.

87. Alfred A. Gross, "Understanding the Homosexual," *NPPA Journal* 1:2 (1955): 146.

88. *The Fifteenth Annual Report of the George W. Henry Foundation, Inc.*, April 1963, "Homosexuality" (New York Academy of Medicine, New York, NY), 10.

89. *The Sixteenth Annual Report of the George W. Henry Foundation, Inc.*, April 1964, "Homosexuality" (New York Academy of Medicine, New York, NY), 3.

90. *4th Annual Report of the George W. Henry Foundation*, 1953, box 3, folder 16, Henry Papers.

91. Alfred Gross to Clinton R. Jones, March 24, 1965, box 1, folder 2, Henry Papers.

92. *The Nineteenth Annual Report on the State of the George W. Henry Foundation.*

93. Alfred A. Gross to Dear Mr. _____, August 10, 1969, box 1, folder 6, Henry Papers.

94. *Fifteenth Annual Report of the George W. Henry Foundation, Inc.*, "Homosexuality," 10.

95. *7th Annual Report of the George W. Henry Foundation*, 1955, box 3, folder 16, Henry Papers.

96. Gross, *Strangers in Our Midst*, 72.

97. George W. Henry, *The Sixteenth Annual Report of the George W. Henry Foundation, Inc.*, April 1964, 1, box 3, folder 16, Henry Papers. Henry Minton finds evidence that Alfred Gross ghost-wrote the annual reports of the foundation under George Henry's name, in *Departing from Deviance*.

98. *21st Annual Report of the George W. Henry Foundation*, 1971, box 3, folder 16, Henry Papers.

99. Alfred Gross to Harry Golden, December 14, 1967, box 1, folder 4, Henry Papers.

100. KP40, "Insulin Treatments," Karpman Papers. On patients' experience of electroshock therapy, see Heather Murray, *Asylum Ways of Seeing: Psychiatric Patients, American Thought and Culture* (Philadelphia: University of Pennsylvania Press, 2022), 57–59.

101. Paul Schilder, "Notes on the Psychology of Metrazol Treatment of Schizophrenia," *Journal of Nervous and Mental Disease* 89:2 (February 1939): 134.

102. See Gerald Grob, *Mental Illness and American Society, 1875–1940* (Princeton: Princeton University Press, 1983), 304; Grob, *Mad among Us: A History of the Care of America's Mentally Ill* (New York: Free Press, 1994), 180–81; Jonathan Sadowsky, *Electroconvulsive Therapy in America* (New York: Routledge, 2017); David J. Impastato, "The Story of the First Electroshock Treatment," *American Journal of Psychiatry* 116:12 (June 1960): 1112–14.

103. Winfred Overholser to Dr. Clarence O. Cheney, February 21, 1947, Saint Elizabeth Administrative Files, box 12, Saint Elizabeths Records. See also Sadowsky, *Electroconvulsive Therapy*, 4.

104. See A. A. Brill, "Homoeroticism and Paranoia," *American Journal of Psychiatry* 13 (1934): 957–74; George S. Sprague, "Varieties of Homosexual Manifestations," *American Journal of Psychiatry* 92 (1935): 143–45; James Page and John Warkentin, "Masculinity and Paranoia," *Journal of Abnormal and Social Psychology* 33 (1938): 527–31; Harry Stack Sullivan, "Peculiarity of Thought in Schizophrenia," in Harry Sullivan, *Schizophrenia as a Human Process* (New York: Norton, 1962), originally published in *American Journal of Psychiatry* 82 (1925): 21–86. Jules Gill-Peterson notes that "a typical misdiagnosis leading to conversion therapy" for trans children "was schizophrenia" (Gill-Peterson, "A Trans History of Conversion Therapy," *Sad Brown Girl* (blog), April 22, 2021, https://sadbrowngirl.substack.com/p/a-trans-history-of-conversion-therapy.

105. Newdigate M. Owensby, "Homosexuality and Lesbianism Treated with Metrazol," *Journal of Nervous and Mental Disease* 92:1 (1940): 65.

106. George N. Thompson, "Electroshock and Other Therapeutic Considerations in Sexual Psychopathy," *Journal of Nervous and Mental Diseases* 109 (June 1949): 549.

107. Russell H. Dinerstein and Bernard C. Glueck, "Sub-coma Insulin Therapy in the Treatment of Homosexual Panic States," *Journal of Social Therapy* 1 (1955): 182–86.

108. Dinerstein and Glueck, "Sub-Coma Insulin Therapy," 182.

109. Samuel Liebman, "Homosexuality, Transvestism, and Psychosis: Study of a Case Treated with Electroshock," *Journal of Nervous and Mental Disease* 99:6 (1944): 945.

110. Liebman, "Homosexuality, Transvestism, and Psychosis," 951.

111. Liebman, "Homosexuality, Transvestism, and Psychosis," 951–52.

112. Liebman, "Homosexuality, Transvestism, and Psychosis," 952.

113. Liebman, "Homosexuality, Transvestism, and Psychosis," 955.

114. Liebman, "Homosexuality, Transvestism, and Psychosis," 956.

115. Charles H. Jones and James G. Shanklin, "Transorbital Lobotomy: A Preliminary Report of Forty-One Cases," February 16, 1948, box 24, Administrative Files, Saint Elizabeths Records.

116. Quoted in Jack El-Hai, *The Lobotomist: A Maverick Medical Genius and His Tragic Quest to Rid the World of Mental Illness* (Hoboken, NJ: Wiley & Sons, 2005), 124; "Annual Report of St. Elizabeths Hospital," 1950, National Archives and Records Administration, Washington, DC, 3–4.

117. Walter Freeman and James W. Watts, *Psychosurgery in the Treatment of Mental Disorders and Intractable Pain*, 2nd ed. (Springfield, IL: Charles C. Thomas, 1950), x.

118. On Freeman and the use of lobotomy in the United States, see Mical Raz, *The Lobotomy Letters: The Making of American Psychosurgery* (Rochester, NY: University of Rochester Press, 2013); Jack Pressman, *Last Resort: Psychosurgery and the Limits of Medicine* (Cambridge: Cambridge University Press, 1998); El-Hai, *The Lobotomist*; Howard Dully and Charles Fleming, *My Lobotomy* (New York: Three Rivers Press, 2007).

119. Freeman and Watts, *Psychosurgery*, 517, xiii.

120. See Freeman and Watts, *Psychosurgery*, 347.

121. KP92, Case History, March 5, 1949, Karpman Papers.

122. Freeman and Watts, *Psychosurgery*, 347.

123. Don Jackson, "California Runs an Atascadero 'Dachau' for Queers," in box 1, folder 51, *Advocate* Records, ONE National Gay and Lesbian Archives, USC Libraries, University of Southern California, Los Angeles, CA (hereafter cited as *Advocate* Records).

124. Freeman and Watt, *Psychosurgery*, 132, 346; Freeman, "Sexual Behavior and Fertility after Frontal Lobotomy," *Biological Psychiatry* 6:1 (1969): 97–104.

125. Moses Zlotlow and Albert E. Paganini, "Autoerotic and Homoerotic Manifestations in Hospitalized Male Postlobotomy Patients," *Psychiatric Quarterly* 33:3 (1959): 491.

126. Ztotlow and Paganini, "Autoerotic and Homoerotic Manifestations," 493.

127. Ztotlow and Paganini, "Autoerotic and Homoerotic Manifestations," 492–93.

128. "Whitey," in Nancy Adair and Casey Adair, *Word Is Out: Stories of Some of Our Lives* (San Francisco: New Glide Publications, 1978), 8.

129. "Former Patient Tells What Life Is Like Inside Searcy State Mental Hospital," *Southern Courier*, August 5–6, 1967, 4.

130. Raz, *Lobotomy Letters*.

131. Raz, *Lobotomy Letters*, 44.

132. Joseph Wolpe, *The Practice of Behavior Therapy* (New York: Pergamon, 1970), vii.

133. N. V. Kantorovich, "An Attempt at Associative-Reflex Therapy in Alcoholism," *Psychological Abstracts* 4 (1930): 493.

134. Louis William Max, "Breaking Up a Homosexual Fixation by the Conditioned Reaction Technique: A Case Study," *Psychological Bulletin* 32:9 (November 1935): 734.

135. Kurt Freund, "Some Problems in the Treatment of Homosexuality," in *Behavior Therapy and the Neuroses*, ed. H. J. Eysenck (Oxford: Pergamon Press, 1960), 317.

136. See, for example, Otto Fenichel, "Psychology of Transvestism," *International Journal of Psycho-analysis* 11 (January 1, 1930): 211; Michael G. Gelder and Isaac M. Marks, "Aversion Treatment in Transvestism and Transsexualism," in *Transsexualism and Sex Reassignment*, ed. Richard Green and John Money (Baltimore: Johns Hopkins University Press, 1969), 383–413; J. C. Barker, "Behaviour Therapy for Transvestism: A Comparison of Pharmacological and Electrical Aversion Techniques," *British Journal of Psychiatry* 111 (1965): 268–76.

137. N. I. Lavin, J. G. Thorpe, J. C. Barker, C. B. Blakemore, and C. G. Conway, "Behavior Therapy in a Case of Transvestism," *Journal of Nervous and Mental Disease* 133:4 (1961): 346.

138. Lavin et al., "Behavior Therapy in a Case of Transvestism," 347.

139. "Specialists Offer Cure for Deviates," *Augusta Chronicle*, August 12, 1963, p. 16. The study by J. G. Thorpe, E. Schmidt, and D. Castell, "A Comparison of Positive and Negative (Aversive) Conditioning in the Treatment of Homosexuality" (*Behaviour Research and Therapy* 1 [October 1963]: 357–62), was covered in newspapers across the country.

140. Michael Serber, "Shame Aversion Therapy," *Journal of Behavior Therapy and Experimental Psychiatry* 1:3 (September 1970): 213.

141. David H. Barlow, E. Joyce Reynolds, and W. Stewart Agras, "Gender Identity Change in a Transsexual," *Archives of General Psychiatry* 28:4 (January 1973): 569.

142. Barlow, Reynolds, and Agras, "Gender Identity Change," 576.

143. See C. B. Blakemore, J. G. Thorpe, J. C. Barker, C. G. Conway, and N. Lavin, "The Application of Faradic Aversion Conditioning in a Case of Transvestism," *Behavioral Research Therapy* (1963): 29; R. J. McGuire and M. Vallance, "Aversion Therapy by Shock: A Simple Technique," *British Medical Journal* 1 (January 1964): 151.

144. M. P. Feldman, "Aversion Therapy for Sexual Deviations: A Critical Review," *Psychological Bulletin* 65:2 (1966), 75. See also Herbert Fensterheim, "Behavior Therapy of the Sexual Variations," *Journal of Sex & Marital Therapy* 1:1 (Fall 1974): 19; Tommy Dickinson, *"Curing Queers": Mental Nurses and Their Patients, 1935–74* (Manchester, UK: Manchester University Press, 2015), 160.

145. Lavin et al., "Behavior Therapy in a Case of Transvestism," 348.

146. Basil James, "Case of Homosexuality Treated by Aversion Therapy," in *Experiments in Behavior Therapy*, ed. H. J. Eysenck (London: Pergamon Press, 1964), 159–63;

reprinted from *British Medical Journal* 1:5280 (March 17, 1962): 768–70. See also J. C. Barker, "Behaviour Therapy for Transvestism: A Comparison of Pharmacological and Electrical Aversion Techniques," *British Journal of Psychiatry* 111 (1965): 270.

147. S. Rachman, "Aversion Therapy: Chemical or Electrical?" *Behavior Research and Therapy* 2:2–4 (1965): 290.

148. Quoted in Dickinson, *"Curing Queers,"* 160.

149. Rachman, "Aversion Therapy," 291.

150. Blakemore et al., "Application of Faradic Aversion Conditioning," 33.

151. Rachman, "Aversion Therapy," 297.

152. Wolpe, *Practice of Behavior Therapy,* 205; Saul Levin, Irwin S. Hirsch, Gerald Shugar, and Robert Kapache, "Treatment of Homosexuality and Heterosexual Anxiety with Avoidance Conditioning and Systematic Desensitization: Data and Case Report," *Psychotherapy: Theory, Research, and Practice* 5:3 (Fall 1968): 163.

153. Barry A. Tanner, "Shock Intensity and Fear of Shock in the Modification of Homosexual Behavior in Males by Avoidance Learning," *Behavior Research and Therapy* 11 (1973): 214.

154. Farrall Instrument Company advertisement, "Aversion Therapy," *Advocate* Records. See also McGuire and Vallance, "Aversion Therapy by Electric Shock," 151; Rachman, "Aversion Therapy," 293.

155. "Farrall Instruments: Spectrum of Behavior Modification Instruments," box 2, folder 9, Barbara Gittings and Kay Tobin Lahusen Papers, John J. Wilcox, Jr., LGBT Archives, William Way LGBT Community Center, Philadelphia, PA.

156. See Lee Birk, William Huddleston, Elizabeth Miller, and Bertram Cohler, "Avoidance Conditioning for Homosexuality," *Archives of General Psychiatry* 25:4 (October 1971): 315.

157. Feldman, "Aversion Therapy for Sexual Deviations," 74.

158. Ivan Toby Rutner, "A Double-Barrel Approach to Modification of Homosexual Behavior," *Psychological Reports* 26:2 (1970): 358; S. Rachman, "Sexual Disorders and Behavior Therapy," *American Journal of Psychiatry* 118:3 (September 1961): 235.

159. David H. Barlow, Harold Leitenberg, and W. Stewart Agras, "The Experimental Control of Sexual Deviation through Manipulation of the Noxious Scene in Covert Sensitization," *Journal of Abnormal Psychology* 74:5 (1969): 598.

160. J. G. Thorpe, E. Schmidt, and D. Castell, "A Comparison of Positive and Negative (Aversive) Conditioning in the Treatment of Homosexuality," *Behaviour Research and Therapy* 1 (October 1963): 361.

161. Feldman, "Aversion Therapy for Sexual Deviations," 77.

162. Barlow, Leitenberg, and Agras, "Experimental Control of Sexual Deviation," 598.

163. Edward J. Callahan and Harold Leitenberg, "Aversion Therapy for Sexual Deviation: Contingent Shock and Covert Desensitization," *Journal of Abnormal Psychology* 81:1 (1973): 62.

164. Michael M. Miller, "Hypnotic-Aversion Treatment of Homosexuality," *Journal of the National Medical Association* 55:5 (1963): 412.

165. David H. Barlow, "Increasing Heterosexual Responsiveness in the Treatment of Sexual Deviation: A Review of the Clinical and Experimental Evidence," *Behavior Therapy* 4 (1973): 656.

166. *Dallas Morning News*, "Team Says Homosexuals Can Be Heterosexual," February 2, 1973, 11.

167. *Dallas Morning News*, "Team Says Homosexuals Can Be Heterosexual."

168. Barlow, "Increasing Heterosexual Responsiveness," 659.

169. Jennifer Lambe shows that insulin and electroshock treatments were used for their punitive rather than putatively curative effects in Cuba as well. See Jennifer L. Lambe, *Madhouse: Psychiatry and Politics in Cuban History* (Chapel Hill: University of North Carolina Press, 2017), 164. See also Bernard Weiner, "The Clockwork Cure," *Nation*, April 3, 1972, 433–36.

170. Rob Cole, notes, "Atascadero—II," box 1, folder 51, *Advocate* Records.

171. Manuscript, no author, no title, n.d., box 15, folder 5, Tommi Avicolli Mecca Collection, John J. Wilcox, Jr., LGBT Archives, William Way LGBT Community Center, Philadelphia, PA.

172. Don Jackson, "California Runs an Atascadero 'Dachau' for Queers," clipping, box 1, folder 51, *Advocate* Records.

173. "Scaring the Devil Out," *Medical World News* 11:42 (October 9, 1970): 29. The author of this article notes that in 1969, the practice was witnessed and exposed by a visiting Harvard law student and was discontinued.

174. Nick DiSpoldo, "The Edison Medicine," *Berkeley Barb* (January 10–16, 1975), clipping, "Aversion Therapy" file, *Advocate* Records. See also "Suffocation 'Therapy' Halted, State Institutions Say," *Advocate* 4:23 (January 6–19, 1971): 10. Alondra Nelson discusses the mobilization of the Black Panther Party against psychosurgery performed on Black radicals incarcerated at Vacaville in *Body and Soul: The Black Panther Party and the Fight against Medical Discrimination* (Minneapolis: University of Minnesota Press, 2011), 167–69.

175. *Dallas Morning News*, "Team Says Homosexuals Can Be Heterosexual."

176. *Los Angeles Times*, "Behavior Modification: Fascism or the Future?," May 17, 1973, C5.

177. Judd Marmor to Roy Menninger, February 11, 1971, box 20, folder 6, Judd Marmor Papers, Charles E. Young Research Library, University of California, Los Angeles, CA. See also Lawrence Hatterer, *Changing Homosexuality in the Male: Treatment for Men Troubled by Homosexuality* (New York: McGraw-Hill, 1970), 64.

178. Irving Bieber, "Clinical Aspects of Male Homosexuality," in *Sexual Inversion: The Multiple Roots of Homosexuality*, ed. Judd Marmor (New York: Basic Books, 1965), 266.

179. Wilbur, "Clinical Aspects of Female Homosexuality," 279.

180. Hatterer, *Changing Homosexuality*, 58.

181. Hatterer, *Changing Homosexuality*, 58.

182. Lawrence Hatterer, "A Psychiatrist Offers Hope: Homosexuality can be Conquered," *Philadelphia Inquirer Magazine*, clipping, box 9, folder 4, Barbara Gittings and Kay Tobin Lahusen Gay History Papers and Photographs, Manuscripts and Archives Division, New York Public Library.

183. Hatterer, *Changing Homosexuality*, 65.

CHAPTER THREE

1. Edmund White, *My Lives* (New York: Ecco, 2006); White, *City Boy: My Life in New York during the 1960s and '70s* (New York: Bloomsbury, 2009), 17.

2. John D'Emilio doubts that acceptance of the medical model of homosexuality "extended even to the whole middle class" (D'Emilio, "The Stuff of History: First-Person Accounts of Gay Male Lives," *Journal of the History of Sexuality* 3:2 [1992]: 314–19).

3. Karpman, memorandum, box 9, Benjamin Karpman Papers, Jean-Nickolaus Tretter Collection in Gay, Lesbian, Bisexual, and Transgender Studies, University of Minnesota, Minneapolis, MN (hereafter cited as Karpman Papers). See also Nathan G. Hale Jr., *The Rise and Crisis of Psychoanalysis in the United States: Freud and the Americans* (New York: Oxford University Press, 1995), 75.

4. Patricia Highsmith, November 30, 1948, in *Patricia Highsmith, Her Diaries and Notebooks, 1941–1995*, ed. Anna von Planta (New York: Norton, 2021), 435.

5. Paul Moor, "The View from Irving Bieber's Couch: 'Heads I Win, Tails You Lose,'" *Journal of Gay & Lesbian Psychotherapy* 5:3–4 (2001): 30.

6. Martin Duberman, *Cures: A Gay Man's Odyssey* (New York: Dutton, 1991), 44.

7. Martin Duberman, *Cures: A Gay Man's Odyssey*, 10th anniversary edition (New York: Basic Books, 2002), 306.

8. Barbara Taylor, *The Last Asylum: A Memoir of Madness in Our Times* (Chicago: University of Chicago Press, 2015), 137. 4.

9. Quoted in Elizabeth Ann Danto, *Freud's Free Clinics: Psychoanalysis and Social Justice, 1918–1938* (New York: Columbia University Press, 2005), 14.

10. Newton Arvin, "The Past Recaptured," unpub. ms., box 436, 82, David E. Lilienthal Papers, Seeley G. Mudd Library, Princeton University, Princeton, NJ (hereafter cited as Lilienthal Papers); Arvin to David Lilienthal, July 17, 1920, box 47, Lilienthal Papers.

11. Patricia Highsmith, June 25, 1943, in *Patricia Highsmith*, 238.

12. Eli Zaretsky, *Secrets of the Soul: A Social and Cultural History of Psychoanalysis* (New York: Knopf, 2004), 5. Deborah Cohen argues that many middle-class British gay men embraced psychoanalytic explanations of homosexuality, writing that "for those who had been oppressed or rejected by their families, the idea that homosexuality could be traced to aberrant child-rearing had obvious appeal" (Deborah Cohen, *Family Secrets: Shame and Privacy in Modern Britain* [New York: Oxford University Press, 2013], 174).

13. Duberman, *Cures* (New York: Dutton, 1991), 33.

14. Eli Zaretsky, *Political Freud: A History* (New York: Columbia University Press, 2015), 5.

15. Dan Wakefield, *New York in the Fifties* (Boston: Houghton Mifflin, 1992), 208.

16. Donald Webster Cory (pseudonym of Edward Sagarin), *The Homosexual in America: A Subjective Approach* (1951; reprint, New York: Castle Books, 1960), 153, 59.

17. KP27, responses to questionnaire, 5, Karpman Papers.

18. Jennifer Terry, *An American Obsession: Science, Medicine, and Homosexuality in Modern Society* (Chicago: University of Chicago Press, 1999), 15.

19. See Samuel B. Hadden, "Attitudes toward and Approaches to the Problem of Homosexuality," paper delivered at the meeting of the Pennsylvania Psychiatric Society, Philadelphia, PA, October 26, 1965, 2, box 2, folder 24, Samuel Bernard Hadden Papers, University Archives and Records Center, University of Pennsylvania, Philadelphia, PA (hereafter cited as Hadden Papers); Ernest Bien, "Why Do Homosexuals Undergo Treatment?" *Medical Review of Reviews* 40:1 (January 1934): 5.

20. May E. Romm, "Sexuality and Homosexuality in Women," in *Sexual Inversion: The Multiple Roots of Homosexuality*, ed. Judd Marmor (New York: Basic Books, 1965), 282. See also William V. Silverberg, introduction, in Richard C. Robertiello, *Voyage from Lesbos: The Psychoanalysis of a Female Homosexual* (New York: Citadel, 1959), 11; Cornelia B. Wilbur, "Clinical Aspects of Female Homosexuality," in *Sexual Inversion: The Multiple Roots of Homosexuality*, ed. Judd Marmor (New York: Basic Books, 1965), 279.

21. Hadden, "Trends in Treatment of Homosexuality and Sexual Deviants, October 10, 1955, unpublished ms., box 2, folder 23, Hadden Papers.

22. Sigmund Freud, "The Psychogenesis of a Case of Female Homosexuality," *International Journal of Psycho-Analysis* 1:2 (January 1920): 127, 126.

23. Freud, "Psychogenesis of a Case of Female Homosexuality," 128.

24. Charles G. Hitchcock, "Psychiatric Attitudes toward Homosexuality," unpub. ms., 1972, box 5 folder 3, Evelyn C. Hooker Papers, Department of Special Collections, Charles E. Young Research Library, University of California, Los Angeles (hereafter cited as Hooker Papers).

25. Romm, "Sexuality and Homosexuality in Women," 282.

26. Paul J. Poinsard, M.D., to John S., September 9, 1954, box 143, folder 10, Barbara Gittings and Kay Tobin Lahusen Gay History Papers and Photographs, Manuscripts and Archives Division, New York Public Library, New York, NY (hereafter cited as Gittings and Lahusen NYPL).

27. John S. Gittings to Dr. Poinsard, August 26, 1954, box 143, folder 10, Gittings and Lahusen NYPL; Poinsard to Gittings, September 9, 1954, box 143, folder 10, Gittings and Lahusen NYPL.

28. See Elizabeth Lunbeck, *The Psychiatric Persuasion: Knowledge, Gender, and Power in Modern America* (Princeton: Princeton University Press, 1994), 82.

29. Albert Merland, "Lunacy Procedure under the Law," box 9, Records of Saint Elizabeths Hospital, National Archives and Records Administration, RG 418, Wash-

ington, DC (hereafter cited as Saint Elizabeths Records); U.S. Congress, House, H.R. 6598, 80th Cong., 2nd sess., May 18, 1948, box 8, Saint Elizabeths Administrative Files, Saint Elizabeths Records.

30. See Grob, *Mental Illness and American Society, 1875–1940* (Princeton: Princeton University Press, 1983), 9; Richard T. Fox, *So Far Disordered in Mind: Insanity in California, 1870–1930* (Berkeley: University of California Press, 1978); Lunbeck, *Psychiatric Persuasion*, 82.

31. KP9, Notes taken by Dr. Griffin, case history, May 5, 1933, Karpman Papers.

32. KP9, Karpman Papers.

33. Samuel Hadden, "Treatment of Homosexuality by Individual and Group Psychotherapy," *American Journal of Psychiatry* 114 (1958): 811.

34. Quoted in Benjamin Karpman, "From the Emotional and Dream Life of a Transvestite, II," *Archives of Criminal Psychodynamics* 5:1 (Winter 1962): 67.

35. Morton M. Hunt, *Mental Hospital: A Vivid Insight into the World of the Mentally Disturbed* (New York: Pyramid, 1962), 49.

36. Margaret Deirdre O'Hartigan, "The GID Controversy: Transsexuals Need the Gender Identity Disorder Diagnosis," *Transgender Tapestry*, no. 79 (Summer 1997): 30.

37. Nahman H. Greenberg, Alan K. Rosenwald, and Paul E. Nielson, "A Study in Transsexualism," *Psychiatric Quarterly* 34:2 (June 1960): 203–35.

38. See Joanne Meyerowitz, *How Sex Changed: A History of Transsexuality in the United States* (Cambridge, MA: Harvard University Press, 2002), 224–25. Beans Velocci argues that the requirement that prospective gender transition patients undergo a psychiatric evaluation served to provide legal cover to surgeons anxious about being sued, in "Standards of Care: Uncertainty and Risk in Harry Benjamin's Transsexual Classifications," *TSQ: Transgender Studies Quarterly* 8:4 (November 2021): 466–67.

39. Jules Gill-Peterson, "A Trans History of Conversion Therapy," *Sad Brown Girl* (blog), April 22, 2021, https://sadbrowngirl.substack.com/p/a-trans-history-of-conversion-therapy.

40. "Socarides Attacks Transsexuals," *Gay News* 1:27 (August 10, 1970).

41. Nancy Hunt, *Mirror Image: The Odyssey of a Male-to-Female Transsexual* (New York: Holt, Rinehart and Winston, 1978), 18, 25.

42. Manfred S. Guttmacher, "The Homosexual in Court," *American Journal of Psychiatry* 112:8 (February 1956): 592.

43. See Anna Lvovsky, *Vice Patrol: Cops, Courts, and the Struggle over Gay Life before Stonewall* (Chicago: University of Chicago Press, 2021).

44. See Risa Goluboff, *Vagrant Nation: Police Power, Constitutional Change, and the Making of the 1960s* (New York: Oxford University Press, 2016), 47, 164–65; William Eskridge, *Dishonorable Passions: Sodomy Laws in America, 1861–2003* (New York: Viking, 2008), 86–88.

45. See George Chauncey, "The Forgotten History of Gay Entrapment," *Atlantic*, June 25, 2019, https://www.theatlantic.com/ideas/archive/2019/06/before-stonewall-biggest-threat-was-entrapment/590536/.

46. Goluboff, *Vagrant Nation*, 50.

47. See Clare Sears, *Arresting Dress: Cross-Dressing, Law, and Fascination in Nineteenth-Century San Francisco* (Durham: Duke University Press, 2014); Kate Redburn, "Before Equal Protection: The Fall of Cross-Dressing Bans and the Transgender Legal Movement, 1963–86," *Law & History Review* (2023): 1–45; William N. Eskridge, Jr., *Gaylaw: Challenging the Apartheid of the Closet* (Cambridge, MA: Harvard University Press, 1999): 17–137.

48. Interview of Miss Major Griffin-Gracy by Abram J. Lewis, December 16, 2017, New York City Trans Oral History Project, https://nyctransoralhistory.org/interview/miss-major/.

49. Guttmacher, "Homosexual in Court," 595.

50. Guttmacher, "Homosexual in Court," 596.

51. Lvovsky reads this judicial discretion as having a softening impact on the criminal legal system and disempowering police, arguing that the "medicalization of homosexuality . . . often had a surprisingly liberal effect" in *Vice Patrol*, 121. See also Michael Willrich, *City of Courts: Socializing Justice in Progressive Era Chicago* (Cambridge: Cambridge University Press, 2003); Cornelius F. Collins, "N.Y. Court Requests Psychiatric Service Clinic for Criminals Supplemental Memorandum," *Journal of Criminal Law and Criminology* 19:3 (November 1928): 337–43. On judicial discretion in lower courts, see Malcolm M. Feeley, *The Process is the Punishment: The Handling of Cases in a Lower Criminal Court* (New York: Russell Sage Foundation, 1992).

52. Samuel Hadden, "Attitudes toward and Approaches to the Problem of Homosexuality," 2, paper delivered to the meeting of the Pennsylvania Psychiatric Society, Philadelphia, PA, October 26, 1956, box 2, folder 24, Hadden Papers.

53. Samuel Hadden, "A Way Out for Homosexuals," *Harpers* 234:1402 (March 1967): 114.

54. Samuel E. Hadden, "Trends in Treatment of Homosexuality and Sexual Deviants," October 10, 1955, box 2, folder 23, Hadden Papers.

55. KP37, keywords, Karpman Papers.

56. KP38, Karpman Papers.

57. "DOB Questionnaire Reveals Some Comparisons between Male and Female Homosexuals," *Ladder* 4 (September 1960): 11.

58. See John D'Emilio, *Sexual Politics, Sexual Communities: The Making of a Homosexual Minority in the United States, 1940–1970* (Chicago: University of Chicago Press, 1983), 157.

59. Daughters of Bilitis, "What to Do in Case of Arrest," *Ladder* 1:2 (November 1956): 6.

60. Alexander B. Smith and Alexander Bassin, "Group Therapy with Homosexuals," *Journal of Social Therapy* 5:3 (1959): 229.

61. L. Covi, "A Group Psychotherapy Approach to the Treatment of Neurotic Symptoms in Male and Female Patients of Homosexual Preference," *Psychotherapy and Psychosomatics* 20:3–4 (1972): 176–80.

62. The Miller Law went on to prohibit such invitations "upon any avenue, street, road, highway, open space, alley, public square, enclosure, public building or other public place, store, shop, or reservation at any public gathering or assembly in the District of Columbia, to accompany, go with, or follow him or her to his or her residence, or to any other home or building, enclosure, or other place," for prostitution "or any other immoral or lewd purpose" (U.S. Congress, Senate, *Providing for the Treatment of Sexual Psychopaths in the District of Columbia*, S. Rep. No. 1377, 80th Cong., 2nd sess., May 21, 1948, 9).

63. U.S. Congress, House, Committee on the District of Columbia, *Criminal Sexual Psychopaths*, 80th Cong., 2nd sess., 1948, 114. When Representative Miller introduced the bill to Congress, on the other hand, he observed that "the present laws of the District of Columbia do not seem adequate to handle sex crimes against children" (Arthur Miller, speaking on H.R. 6071, April 26, 1948, 80th Cong., 2nd sess., *Congressional Record* 80, pt. 4, 4886).

64. Blanche Baker, draft of speech, no title, 1959, *Advocate* Records, ONE. William Eskridge determines that "half of the first hundred sexual psychopaths adjudicated in New Jersey were convicted of adult sodomy, fellatio, and 'lewdness,' New Jersey's code word for homosexual overtures," and almost a quarter of Indiana's committed psychopaths were in jail for sodomy or "unnatural" sex with consenting adults (William N. Eskridge, *Dishonorable Passions: Sodomy Laws in America, 1861–2003* [New York: Viking, 2008], 95).

65. KP30, "My Life History," 29–30, Karpman Papers.

66. See Simon Cole, "From the Sexual Psychopath Statute to 'Megan's Law': Psychiatric Knowledge in the Diagnosis, Treatment, and Adjudication of Sex Criminals in New Jersey, 1949–1999," *History of Medicine and Allied Sciences* 55:3 (2000): 308; Stephen Robertson, "Separating the Men from the Boys: Masculinity, Psychosexual Development, and Sex Crime in the United States, 1930s–1960s," *Journal of the History of Medicine* 56 (January 2001): 3–35.

67. Stephen Robertson, *Crimes against Children: Sexual Violence and Legal Culture in New York City, 1880–1960* (Chapel Hill: University of North Carolina Press, 2005).

68. Alfred B. Vuocolo found that 12 percent of people convicted as sex offenders under New Jersey's Sex Offender Act in its first year, from July 1, 1959, to June 30, 1960, were nonwhite; this was around twice their percentage in population in the state (Alfred B. Vuocolo, *The Repetitive Sex Offender: An Analysis of the Administration of the New Jersey Sex Offender Program from 1949 to 1965* [Roselle, NJ: Quality Printing, 1969], 66).

69. KP72, Karpman Papers.

70. Leonard M. Rothstein, M.D., to James W. McAllister, Esq., April 29, 1969, box 13, folder 4, Frank Kameny Papers, Library of Congress, Washington, DC (hereafter cited as Kameny Papers).

71. Arthur Alston to Frank Kameny, January 7, 1971, box 13, folder 4, Kameny Papers.

72. Kameny to Alston, January 9, 1971, box 13, folder 4, Kameny Papers.

73. Albert Ellis, *Homosexuality: Its Causes and Cure* (New York: Lyle Stewart, 1965), 74.

74. Ellis, *Homosexuality*, 79.

75. "LOPLO," transcription of session with patient, May 14, 1958, box 57, folder 69, Albert Ellis Papers, Rare Book and Manuscript Collection, Columbia University, New York, NY (hereafter cited as Ellis Papers).

76. Ellis, *Homosexuality*, 191.

77. "LOPLO," May 16, 1958.

78. Ellis, *Homosexuality*, 208.

79. KP14, Karpman Papers.

80. KP14, Karpman Papers.

81. "My First Year in Rational Therapy," May 15, 1968, box 129, folder 11, Ellis Papers.

82. Earl Johnson to Albert Ellis, January 26, 1966, box 123, folder 15, Ellis Papers.

83. Charles W. Socarides, *The Overt Homosexual* (New York: Grune & Stratton, 1968), 105.

84. KP40, re memorandum, 10, box 8, Karpman Papers.

85. Letter to Albert Ellis, September 7, 1966, box 125, folder 10, Ellis Papers.

86. Ann Aldrich (pseudonym of Marijane Meaker), *We Walk Alone* (1955; reprint, New York: Feminist Press, 2006), 127–28.

87. William H. Masters and Virginia E. Johnson, *Homosexuality in Perspective* (Boston: Little Brown, 1979), 364.

88. Albert Abarbanel-Brandt, "Homosexuals in Hypnotherapy," *Journal of Sex Research* 2:2 (July 1966): 130–31.

89. KP56, questions and answers, 121, Karpman Papers.

90. KP80, session no. 19, February 2, 1951, Karpman Papers.

91. Betty Berzon, "Homosexuality Then and Now: A Gay Perspective," unpublished ms, n.d., box 4, folder 58, Betty Berzon Papers, ONE National Gay and Lesbian Archives, Los Angeles, CA.

92. Hadden, "Homosexuality: An Experientially Determined and Treatable Condition," unpublished book ms., 1981, box 2, folder 41, Hadden Papers.

93. KP50, "Terror, Frustration, Revulsion," September 15, 1945.

94. For 'G and G,'" 1975, in "Psychiatrists and Psychologists," ONE Archive Subject Files, ONE Archives, USC Libraries, Los Angeles, CA.

95. David H. Barlow, Harold Leitenberg, and W. Stewart Agras, "The Experimental Control of Sexual Deviation through Manipulation of the Noxious Scene in Covert Sensitization," *Journal of Abnormal Psychology* 74:5 (1969): 598.

96. Albert J. Sbordone, "An Interview with Charles Silverstein," *Journal of Gay & Lesbian Psychotherapy* 7:4 (2003): 52.

97. Duberman, *Cures* (1991), 92.

98. Duberman, *Cures* (1991), 20, 31.

99. KP27, responses to questionnaire, Karpman Papers.

100. KP50, "Persecution, Security," September 5, 1945, Karpman Papers.

101. KP82, case history, box 15, 6, Karpman Papers.

102. White, *My Lives*, 29.

103. John Money to Martin Duberman, June 6, 1991, in *Cures* correspondence, Martin Duberman Papers, Manuscripts and Archives Division, New York Public Library, New York, NY.

104. Didier Eribon, *Insult and the Making of the Gay Self* (Durham: Duke University Press, 2004), 16.

105. Erving Goffman, *Stigma: Notes on the Management of Spoiled Identity* (New York: Prentice-Hall, 1963), 19.

106. Gary Alinder, "Psychiatry: Crime against Nature," June 15, 1970, Newspaper and Periodical Clippings, Digital Transgender Archive, https://www
.digitaltransgenderarchive.net/catalog?utf8=%E2%9C%93&search_field=all_fields&q
=psychiatry.

107. KP 31, Karpman Papers.

108. Barbara Gittings, "Gays in Library Land," 1990, box 1, folder 6, Barbara Gittings and Kay Tobin Lahusen Papers, ONE National Gay and Lesbian Archives, USC Libraries, University of Southern California, Los Angeles, CA.

109. Betty Berzon, *Surviving Madness: The Betty Berzon Story* (Midway, FL: Spinsters Ink, 2011), 9.

110. Charles Silverstein, *For the Ferryman: A Personal History* (New York: Chelsea Station Editions, 2011), 78.

111. Ronald Gold, "Stop It, You're Making Me Sick," box 100, folder 6, 6, Gittings and Lahusen NYPL.

112. Cei Bell, "The Radicalqueens Trans-formation," in *Smash the Church, Smash the State!: The Early Years of Gay Liberation*, ed. Tommi Avocolli Mecca (San Francisco: City Lights Books, 2009), 118.

113. Samuel Delany, "The Possibility of Possibilities," in *In the Life: A Black Gay Anthology*, ed. Joseph Beam (Boston: Alyson Publications, 1986), 194–95.

114. Bergler, *One Thousand Homosexuals*, vii.

115. Albert Ellis, "Are Homosexuals Necessarily Neurotic?" *ONE* 3:7 (April 1955): 12; Ellis to Randy Wicker, New York City League for Sexual Freedom, February 18, 1965, box 123, folder 9, Ellis Papers. See also Albert Ellis, "The Use of Psychotherapy with Homosexuals," *Mattachine Review* 2:1 (February 1956): 14–16; Albert Ellis, "How Homosexuals Can Combat Anti-Homosexualism," *ONE* 5 (1957): 7–9; Albert Ellis, "On the Cure of Homosexuality," *Mattachine Review* 6 (November–December 1955): 6–9.

116. Gilberto Davis to Albert Ellis, September 12, 1969, box 132, folder 13, Ellis Papers.

117. Quoted in Rebecca L. Davis, "My Homosexuality Is Getting Worse Every Day':

Norman Vincent Peale and the Liberal Protestant Response to Same-Sex Desires in Mid-Twentieth Century America," in *American Christianities: A History of Dominance and Diversity*, ed. Catherine A. Brekus and W. Clark Gilpin (Chapel Hill: University of North Carolina Press, 2011), 347, 351. On *Look*'s readership, see *Time* magazine, "Shake-up at *Look*," January 11, 1954, https://content.time.com/time/subscriber/article/0,33009,819349,00.html.

118. Davis, "My Homosexuality Is Getting Worse," 357.

119. Davis, "My Homosexuality Is Getting Worse," 360.

120. Thaddeus Russell, "The Color of Discipline: Civil Rights and Black Sexuality," *American Quarterly* 60:1 (March 2008): 101–28.

121. Martin Luther King Jr., "Advice for Living," *The Papers of Martin Luther King, Jr., Volume 4, Symbol of the Movement, January 1957—December 1958*, ed. Clayborne Carson, Susan Carson, Adrienne Clay, Virginia Shadron, and Kieran Taylor (Berkeley: University of California Press, 2000), 348. See also Michael G. Long, *Martin Luther King Jr., Homosexuality, and the Early Gay Rights Movement: Keeping the Dream Straight?* (New York: Palgrave Macmillan, 2012), 39–53.

122. *Hartford Courant*, "Ann Lander's Advice," March 14, 1961, 32. See Patrick M. Johnson and Kwame A. Holmes, "Gaydar, Marriage, and Rip-Roaring Homosexuals: Discourses about Homosexuality in Dear Abby and Ann Landers Advice Columns, 1967–1982," *Journal of Homosexuality* 66:3 (January 2019): 389–406.

123. *Minneapolis Morning Tribune*, "Ann Talks about That 'Unspeakable Topic,'" January 22, 1964, 9.

124. Ann Landers, "Love," *Washington Post*, January 9, 1973, box 123, folder 11, Kameny Papers.

125. Dear Abby, *Atlanta Constitution*, October 29, 1969, 3B.

126. Dear Abby, *Minneapolis Star*, July 9, 1967, 47.

127. *Hartford Courant*, "Men Whistle at My Boyfriend," November 11, 1965, 49.

128. Ann Landers, *Hartford Courant*, August 20, 1972, 18A.

129. Ann Landers, *Aberdeen Daily News*, July 20, 1970.

130. Ann Landers, *Austin Statesman*, March 11, 1967, A8.

131. Ann Landers, *Detroit Free Press*, September 8, 1968, 61.

132. Dear Abby, *Courier-Journal & Times* (Louisville, KY), February 1, 1970, G15.

133. Dear Abby, *Courier-Journal & Times*, February 1, 1970.

134. Dear Abby, *Atlanta Constitution*, May 29, 1972, 2B

135. Dear Abby, *Courier Journal & Times* (Louisville, KY), April 12, 1970, G1.

136. *Life* magazine, "Homosexuality in America," June 26, 1964, 66–74, 76–80.

137. Ernest Havemann, "Scientists Search for the Answers to a Touchy and Puzzling Question: Why?" *Life* magazine, June 26, 1964, 77.

138. *Time* magazine, "Homosexuals Can Be Cured," February 12, 1965, 44–45.

139. *Time* magazine, "The Homosexual in America," January 21, 1966, 40–41.

140. See Leisa Meyer, "'Strange Love': Searching for Sexual Subjectivities in Black Print Popular Culture during the 1950s," *Feminist Studies* 38:3 (Fall 2012): 625–57.

141. "Is There Hope for Homosexuals?" *Jet* 2:15 (August 7, 1952): 26.

142. See Allan Bérubé, *Coming Out under Fire: The History of Gay Men and Women in World War Two* (New York: Free Press, 1990), 8–33; Naoko Wake, "The Military, Psychiatry, and 'Unfit' Soldiers, 1939–1942," *Journal of the History of Medicine and Allied Sciences* 62:4 (October 2007): 461–94.

143. Kenneth Lewes, Elizabeth Young-Bruehl, Ralph Roughton, Maggie Mageee, and Diana C. Miller, "Homosexuality and Psychoanalysis I: Historical Perspectives," *Journal of Gay & Lesbian Mental Health* 12:4 (2008): 303.

## CHAPTER FOUR

1. Erving Goffman, *Asylums: Essays on the Social Situation of Mental Patients and Other Inmates* (New York: Anchor Press, 1961), 12.

2. Goffman, *Asylums*, 14.

3. Michel Foucault, *Psychiatric Power: Lectures at the Collège de France, 1973–1974*, trans. Graham Burchell (New York: Picador, 2006), 33. About psychiatric power, Foucault writes that "of course, the doctor's power is not the only power exercised, for . . . power is never something that someone possesses, any more than it is something that emanates from someone. Power does not belong to anyone or even to a group; there is only power because there is dispersion, relays, networks, reciprocal supports, differences of potential, discrepancies, etcetera. It is in this system of differences which have to be analyzed, that power can start to function" (Foucault, *Psychiatric Power*, 4). Jennifer Terry offers a brilliant analysis of how people exploited those opportunities in "Theorizing Deviant Historiography," *differences* 3:2 (1991): 55–74.

4. Benjamin Karpman, *Case Studies in the Psychopathology of Crime*, vol. 3 (Washington, DC: Medical Science Press, 1948).

5. Newton Arvin to David Lilienthal, January 21, 1920, box 47, David E. Lilienthal Papers, Seeley G. Mudd Manuscript Library, Princeton University, Princeton, NJ.

6. Newton Arvin, diary, March 9, 1940, box 43, folder 8, Newton Arvin Papers, Smith College Library, Mortimer Rare Book Collection, Northampton, MA.

7. KP27, responses to questions, February 7, 1942, Benjamin Karpman Papers, Jean-Nickolaus Tretter Collection in Gay, Lesbian, Bisexual, and Transgender Studies, University of Minnesota, Minneapolis, MN (hereafter cited as Karpman Papers).

8. Nikolas Golosow and Elliott L. Weitzman, "Psychosexual and Ego Regression in the Male Transsexual," *Journal of Nervous and Mental Disease* 149:4 (1969): 333.

9. Robert Bogdan, ed., *On Being Different: The Autobiography of Jane Fry* (New York: Wiley and Sons, 1974), 123.

10. Alan Helms, *Young Man from the Provinces: A Gay Life before Stonewall* (1995; reprint, Minneapolis: University of Minnesota Press, 2003), 76.

11. Karl Bryant, "The Politics of Pathology and the Making of Gender Identity Disorder" (PhD dissertation, University of California, Santa Barbara, 2007), 10. See Jules Gill-Peterson, "A Trans History of Conversion Therapy," *Sad Brown Girl* (blog),

April 22, 2021, https://sadbrowngirl.substack.com/p/a-trans-history-of-conversion-therapy.

12. Donald Webster Cory (pseudonym of Edward Sagarin), *The Homosexual in America: A Subjective Approach* (1951; reprint, New York: Castle Books, 1960), 67, 72.

13. Ann Aldrich, *We Walk Alone* (1955; reprint, New York: Feminist Press, 2006), 24.

14. Edmund White, *My Lives: An Autobiography* (New York: Harper Collins, 2006), 23.

15. Mart Crowley, *The Boys in the Band*, Samuel French Acting Edition (1968; reprint, New York: Concord Theatricals, 2018), 27, 106.

16. See, for example, KP35, Karpman Papers.

17. KP25, case file notes, March 5, 1949, Karpman Papers.

18. Letter to Albert Ellis, September 7, 1966, box 125, folder 10, Ellis Papers.

19. KP59, "Special Attention!," Karpman Papers.

20. JKP34, "The Hurdle," September 13, 1954, Karpman Papers.

21. KP34, therapy session notes, June 26, 1956, Karpman Papers.

22. KP34, "The Hurdle," September 13, 1954, Karpman Papers.

23. Karpman, Yearly Report, July 1, 1954–June 30, 1955, Annual Reports of Subordinate Units, box 11, Records of Saint Elizabeths Hospital, National Archives and Records Administration, RG 418, Washington, DC (hereafter cited as Saint Elizabeths Records).

24. KP83, questions and answers, May 25, 1942, box 16, Karpman Papers.

25. KP83, questions and answers, May 25, 1942, box 16, Karpman Papers.

26. KP35, "The Life of Walter Horne, Second Installment," Karpman Papers.

27. KP56, June 5, 1937, Karpman Papers.

28. KP40, "Impotence in the Male," Karpman Papers.

29. KP40, 51, Karpman Papers.

30. KP40, Karpman Papers.

31. KP18, Karpman Papers.

32. KP25, "Comments on Survey No. 2," Karpman Papers.

33. KP45, case history, Karpman Papers.

34. Martin Duberman, *Cures: A Gay Man's Odyssey* (New York: Dutton, 1991), 58.

35. Paul Moor, "The View from Irving Bieber's Couch: 'Heads I Win, Tails You Lose,'" *Journal of Gay & Lesbian Psychotherapy* 5:3–4 (2001): 27, 33.

36. KP74, "In Regard to My Being Normal and Falling in Love with a Man," March 11, 1945, Karpman Papers.

37. KP45, case history, 110, Karpman Papers.

38. KP45, case history, Karpman Papers.

39. KP9, psychoautobiography, Karpman Papers.

40. KP9, journals, Karpman Papers.

41. Hyman S. Barahal, "Female Transvestism and Homosexuality," *Psychiatric Quarterly* 27:1–4 (January 1953): 392, 400, 393.

42. Bogdan, *On Being Different*, 20.

43. Bogdan, *On Being Different*, 215.

44. Christine Jorgensen, *A Personal Autobiography* (New York: Paul S. Ericksson, 1967), 101.

45. KP26, autobiography, 20, Karpman Papers.

46. KP27, responses to questionnaire, Karpman Papers.

47. KP27, responses to questions, January 1942, Karpman Papers.

48. KP92, "Questions and Answers," Karpman Papers.

49. Box 2, Karpman Papers.

50. Joshua Muyiwa, "The Collage Is Queer: Three Artists' Approaches," Serendipity Arts, accessed November 15, 2022, https://serendipityarts.org/the-collage-is-queer%3A-three-artists%2C-three-approaches. See also Anna Poletti, "Periperformative Life Narrative: Queer Collages," *GLQ: A Journal of Lesbian and Gay Studies* 22:3 (June 2016): 359–76; Freya Gowrley, "Collage as Queer Protest," *Art Quarterly* (Spring 2021): 48; Robert Dewhurst, "Gay Sunshine, Pornopoetic Collage, and Queer Archive," in *Porn Archives*, ed. Tim Dean, Steven Ruszczycky, and David Squires (Durham: Duke University Press, 2014): 213–33; Zachary Small, "The Quintessentially Queer Art of Collage," November 28, 2016, Hyperallergic, https://hyperallergic.com/341239/the-quintessentially-queer-art-of-collage/.

51. Karpman explains this method in "'Blitz' Psychotherapy," *Medical Annals of the District of Columbia* 11:8 (August 1942): 291–96, box 136, folder 2009, Richard Wright Papers, Beinecke Library, Yale University, New Haven, CT.

52. KP56, Karpman Papers.

53. KP30, November 9, 1943, Karpman Papers.

54. KP30, memorandum, November 9, 1943, Karpman Papers.

55. KP13, "A Personal Note for Better Understanding with Dr. Karpman," November 18, 1950, Karpman Papers.

56. KP37 to Karpman, July 30, 1942, Karpman Papers.

57. KP35, diary #2, Karpman Papers.

58. KP35, diary, April 22, Karpman Papers.

59. KP100, Karpman Papers.

60. Karpman, *The Sexual Offender and His Offenses: Etiology, Pathology, Psychodynamics and Treatment* (New York: Julian Press, 1954), xii. Karpman described his questionnaire method in *Case Studies in the Psychopathology of Crime*, vol. 1 (Washington, DC: Mimeoform Press, 1933), cases 1–5. "The patient is asked to write his own history (which is usually very brief and inadequate) and on the basis of the material obtained, questions are made out, the answers to which are then incorporated in the original and

serve as the basis of another questionnaire; the process being continued until the history is satisfactorily completed" (vii). See also Karpman, "'Blitz' Psychotherapy," 292.

61. KP34, therapy session notes, October 25, 1955, Karpman Papers.

62. KP55, "Comments on Freud, Vol. II," Karpman Papers.

63. KP56, responses to questions, Karpman Papers.

64. KP37, Karpman Papers.

65. See Jennifer Terry, *An American Obsession: Science, Medicine, and Homosexuality in Modern Society* (Chicago: University of Chicago Press, 1999); Henry L. Minton, *Departing from Deviance: A History of Homosexual Rights and Emancipatory Science in America* (Chicago: University of Chicago Press, 2002).

66. KP35, diary #2, Karpman Papers.

67. KP35, "Comments on Sex Variation," Karpman Papers.

68. KP35, "Comments on Sex Variation," 75.

69. KP35, "Comments on Sex Variation."

70. Karpman, "The Problem of Homosexuality," review of George Henry, *Sex Variants*, *American Journal of Psychiatry* 100:3 (1943): 429–33.

71. KP27, Karpman memorandum, November 10, 1941, Karpman Papers. Harris was one of the cases that Karpman wrote about in *The Alcoholic Woman: Case Studies in the Psychodynamics of Alcoholism* (Washington, DC: Linacre Press, 1953).

72. KP92, "Homeric Expressions," February 14, 1950, Karpman Papers.

73. Testimony of Benjamin Karpman, 1943, box 6, Karpman Papers.

74. Karpman, "The Evolution of a Psychiatrist," *Quarterly Review of Psychiatry and Neurology* 1 (1946): 412.

75. Karpman, *Case Studies in the Psychopathology of Crime*, 3:xxvii. Nathan G. Hale Jr. identifies an "eclecticism" among American psychoanalysts generally in this period, who drew on Adler and Jung as well as Freud (Hale, *The Rise and Crisis of Psychoanalysis in the United States: Freud and the Americans, 1917–1985* [New York: Oxford University Press, 1995], 27).

76. Karpman, "A Yardstick for Measuring Psychopathy," *Federal Probation* 10 (1946): 29. See also Karpman's testimony in U.S. Congress, House, Committee on the District of Columbia, *Criminal Sexual Psychopaths*, 115.

77. Karpman, *Sexual Offender and His Offenses*, 612, 417.

78. KP45, case history, Karpman Papers.

79. Benjamin Karpman, "Homosexuality," Karpman Papers.

80. Karpman, *Sexual Offender and His Offenses*, 469. See David K. Johnson, *The Lavender Scare: The Cold War Persecution of Gays and Lesbians in the Federal Government* (Chicago: University of Chicago Press, 2004); Genny Beemyn, *A Queer Capital: A History of Gay Life in Washington, D.C.* (New York: Routledge, 2015).

81. KP45, case history, 36, Karpman Papers. Karpman was not alone among psy-

chiatrists in criticizing the Cold War persecution of homosexuals as security threats. See Johnson, *Lavender Scare*, 143.

82. Karpman, "Considerations Bearing on the Problems of Sexual Offenses," *Journal of Criminal Law & Criminology* 43 (May 1952): 26.

83. Benjamin Karpman, "Memorandum," Karpman Papers.

84. Karpman, *Sexual Offender and His Offenses*, 468.

85. Karpman, *Sexual Offender and His Offenses*, 466.

86. U.S. Congress, House, Committee on the District of Columbia, *Criminal Sexual Psychopaths*, 112.

87. Benjamin Karpman, "Yardstick for Measuring Psychopathy," 29.

88. Karpman, memorandum, 2, box 9, Karpman Papers.

89. Benjamin Karpman to Richard Wright, April 21, 1943, Richard Wright Papers, box 100, fol. 1416, Beinecke Library, Yale University; Karpman to Wright, July 1, 1943, box 100, fol. 1416, Wright Papers. On the relationship between Karpman and Wright, see Eli Zaretsky, *Political Freud: A History* (New York: Columbia University Press, 2015), 55–59; Jay Garcia, *Psychology Comes to Harlem: Rethinking the Race Question in Twentieth-Century America* (Baltimore: Johns Hopkins University Press, 2012), 71.

90. Benjamin Karpman, "Psychosexual Inventory," KP 9.

91. Karpman, "Considerations Bearing on the Problems of Sexual Offenses," 24. This would be a political strategy that gay activists like Donald Webster Cory (pseudonym of Edward Sagarin) would also use in his influential 1951 book, *The Homosexual Minority in America*, to argue for rights and understanding for homosexuals. On the importance of race to arguments about gay rights, see Kevin J. Mumford, "The Trouble with Gay Rights: Race and the Politics of Sexual Orientation in Philadelphia, 1969–1982," *Journal of American History* 98:1 (June 2011): 49–72.

92. KP36, psychogenic survey, Karpman Papers.

93. KP83, questions and answers, 1942, Karpman Papers.

94. KP42, "Miscellaneous," June 5, 1955, Karpman Papers.

95. KP25, comments on survey no. 2, Karpman Papers.

96. KP35, diary #2, Karpman Papers

97. KP35, "Flop Houses," Karpman Papers.

98. KP26, autobiography, Karpman Papers.

99. KP59, responses to questions, Karpman Papers.

100. KP48, "New Ideas," October 16, 1953, Karpman Papers. Saint Elizabeths was racially segregated until 1954. On the life of Black patients and the racial regime at Saint Elizabeths in these years, see Martin Summers, *Madness in the City of Magnificent Intentions: A History of Race and Mental Illness in the Nation's Capital* (Oxford University Press, 2019); Gambino, "'These Strangers within Our Gates': Race, Psychiatry, and Mental Illness among Black Americans at St. Elizabeths Hospital in Washington, D.C., 1900–1940," *History of Psychiatry* 19:4 (2008): 387–408.

101. KP48, case file, autobiography, 112–13, Karpman Papers.

102. See, for example, Seymour Parker and Robert J. Kleiner, *Mental Illness in the Urban Negro Community* (New York: Free Press, 1966).

103. KP48, autobiography, Karpman Papers. On the tradition of Black creative literary expression that critiqued structures of confinement and incarceration, see Jess Waggoner, "Race, Gender, and Sanism: Remapping Mad Feminist Genealogies," *Signs: Journal of Women in Culture and Society* 47:4 (Summer 2022): 885–904. Pell antici-pated arguments later made by psychiatrists and activists that mental illness was caus-ally linked to racism. Martin Summers's study of African American patients at Saint Elizabeths suggests that Pell's experience may have been unusual. While Summers finds that some Black patients underwent intensive psychotherapy, "they were hardly the typical patients to receive this particular type of intervention" (Summers, *Madness in the City of Magnificent Intentions*, 5). On the relationship of African Americans to psy-chiatry in this period, see Jonathan M. Metzl, *The Protest Psychosis: How Schizophrenia Became a Black Disease* (Boston: Beacon, 2009); Charles Prudhomme and David F. Musto, "Historical Perspectives on Mental Health and Racism in the United States," in Charles V. Willie, Bernard M. Kramer, and Bertram S. Brown, eds., *Racism and Mental Health* (Pittsburgh: University of Pittsburgh Press, 1973), 25–57; Jay Garcia, *Psychol-ogy Comes to Harlem: Rethinking the Race Question in Twentieth-Century America* (Baltimore: Johns Hopkins University Press, 2012); Catherine A. Stewart, "'Crazy for This Democracy': Postwar Psychoanalysis, African American Blues, and the Lafargue Clinic," *American Quarterly* 65:2 (June 2013): 371–95; Mab Segrest, *Administrations of Lunacy: Racism and the Haunting of American Psychiatry at the Milledgeville Asylum* (New York: New Press, 2020); Gabriel N. Mendes, *Under the Strain of Color: Harlem's Lafargue Clinic and the Promise of an Antiracist Psychiatry* (Ithaca, NY: Cornell Univer-sity Press, 2015).

104. Matthew Gambino finds that Saint Elizabeths and psychiatrists affiliated with the hospital were key in developing a psychiatry of race and that physicians at Saint Elizabeths "devoted a substantial amount of time and energy to the question of black mental illness. Indeed, the institution rapidly became a center for research in what became known as 'comparative psychiatry'" (Matthew Gambino, "Mental Health and Ideals of Citizenship: Patient Care at St. Elizabeths Hospital in Washington, D.C., 1903–1962" [PhD dissertation, University of Illinois, 2010], 58–59). Carl Jung visited Saint Elizabeths in 1912 to analyze the dreams and statements of fifteen Black patients there. In 1914, Saint Elizabeths psychiatrist Mary O'Malley found a higher incidence of "insanity" in Black patients than in whites. In 1916, Saint Elizabeths psychiatrist John E. Lind delivered a paper before the Washington Psychoanalytic Society describing Black patients as possessed of an "inferior psychological nature" (Martin Summers, "'Suit-able Care of the African When Afflicted with Insanity': Race, Madness, and Social Or-der in Comparative Perspective," *Bulletin of the History of Medicine*, 84:1 [Spring 2010]: 50). See also Gambino, "'These Strangers within Our Gates'"; Metzl, *Protest Psychosis*; Prudhomme and Musto, "Historical Perspectives on Mental Health and Racism"; Sum-mers, *Madness in the City of Magnificent Intentions*.

105. Walter Bromberg and Girard H. Franklin, "Treatment of Sexual Deviates with Group Psychodrama," *Group Psychotherapy* 4 (1952): 289, 278.

106. Bromberg and Franklin, "Treatment of Sexual Deviates," 277.

107. Bromberg and Franklin, "Treatment of Sexual Deviates," 276.

108. Bromberg and Franklin, "Treatment of Sexual Deviates," 286.

109. See Chauncey, *Gay New York: Gender, Urban Culture, and the Making of the Gay World, 1890–1940* (New York: Basic Books, 1994); Nan Alamilla Boyd, *Wide-Open Town: A History of Queer San Francisco to 1965* (Berkeley: University of California Press, 2003); Marc Stein, *City of Sisterly and Brotherly Loves: Lesbian and Gay Philadelphia, 1945–1972* (Chicago: University of Chicago Press, 2000).

110. KP37, Sexual History, Karpman Papers.

111. KP50, dream: "Eroticism Fear Hate," October 20, 1945, Karpman Papers.

112. KP50, dream: "Anger, Frustration," September 13, 1946, Karpman Papers.

113. KP31, responses to questions, 56, Karpman Papers.

114. KP 31 file, responses to questions, 30, Karpman Papers.

115. KP59, responses to questions, Karpman Papers.

116. Raymond Robertson to Albert Ellis, March 15, 1966, box 123, folder 11, Ellis Papers.

117. JP92, diary, February 7, 1950, Karpman Papers.

118. KP92, diary, February 7, 1950, Karpman Papers; KP92, diary, December 27, 1949, Karpman Papers.

119. KP92, diary, January 31, 1950, Karpman Papers.

120. KP92, diary, April 13, 1950, Karpman Papers.

121. KP27, "Marjorie," Karpman Papers.

122. "Whitey," in Nancy Adair and Casey Adair, *Word Is Out: Stories of Some of Our Lives* (San Francisco: New Glide Publications, 1978), 7.

123. Gustavus Stadler, *Woody Guthrie: An Intimate Life* (Boston: Beacon Press, 2020), 159.

124. See Lisa Duggan, *Sapphic Slashers: Sex, Violence, and American Modernity* (Durham: Duke University Press, 2001), 89–119.

125. See Emily Skidmore, *True Sex: The Lives of Trans Men at the Turn of the Twentieth Century* (New York: NYU Press, 2017), 29–30.

126. P. M. Wise, "Case of Sexual Perversion," *Alienist and Neurologist* 4:1 (January 1883): 88. See also Skidmore, *True Sex*, 27–37; Bambi Lobdell, *"A Strange Sort of Being": The Transgender Life of Lucy Ann/Joseph Israel Lobdell, 1829–1912* (Jefferson, NC: McFarland & Company, 2012); James G. Kiernan, "Psychological Aspects of the Sexual Appetite," *Alienist and Neurologist* 12 (April 1891): 202–3; Carolyn Dinshaw, "Born Too Soon, Born Too Late: The Female Hunter of Long Eddy, *circa* 1855," in David A. Powell, ed., *21st Century Gay Culture* (Newcastle, UK: Cambridge Scholars Publishing, 2008), 1–12.

127. Magora Kennedy, interview, in *Cured*, directed by Patrick Sammon and Benjamin Singer (2020).

128. Author's interview with Miriam Wolfson, July 27, 2015, New York, NY.

129. Jason Victor Serinus, "From the Closets of New Haven to the Collectives of New York GLF," in *Smash the Church, Smash the State! The Early Years of Gay Liberation*, ed. Tommi Avocolli Mecca (San Francisco: City Lights Books, 2009), 58.

130. Gary Atkins, *Gay Seattle: Stories of Exile and Belonging* (Seattle: University of Washington Press, 2013), 34.

131. Evelyn Hooker, "Reflections of a 40-Year Exploration: A Scientific View on Homosexuality," *American Psychologist* 48:4 (April 1993): 451.

132. Michael Warner develops the concept of queer counterpublics in *Publics and Counterpublics* (New York: Zone Books, 2002).

133. Betty Berzon, *Surviving Madness: The Betty Berzon Story* (Midway, FL: Spinsters Ink, 2011), 76.

134. Mark Rees, *Dear Sir or Madam: The Autobiography of a Female-to-Male Transsexual* (London: Cassell, 1996), 37.

135. KP3, case file, Karpman Papers.

136. KP35, Karpman Papers.

137. Sara Ahmed, *Strange Encounters: Embodied Others in Post-Coloniality* (London: Routledge, 2000), 8.

CHAPTER FIVE

1. Meeting of the Executive Committee, January 27, 1964, Committee on Public Health of the New York Academy of Medicine, Minutes, 1964, New York Academy of Medicine Collection, New York, New York.

2. "Homosexuality: A Report by the Committee on Public Health," *Bulletin of the New York Academy of Medicine* 40:7 (July 1964): 578.

3. *Wall Street Journal*, "Homosexuality Is an Illness and Is Curable in Some Cases, Major Doctors' Group Says," May 19, 1964.

4. "Homosexuality: A Report by the Committee on Public Health."

5. *New York Times*, "Homosexuals Proud of Deviancy," May 19, 1964, 1.

6. Evelyn Hooker, "Reflections of a 40-Year Exploration: A Scientific View on Homosexuality," *American Psychologist* 48:4 (April 1993): 450.

7. Laud Humphreys, "An Interview with Evelyn Hooker," *Alternative Lifestyles* 1:2 (May 1978): 199–200; Dorr W. Legg, ed., *Homophile Studies in Theory and Practice* (Los Angeles: ONE Institute Press and GLB Publishers, 1994), 166–67.

8. See Jim Kepner, "A Memory of Dr. Evelyn Hooker," *ONE/IGLA Bulletin*, no. 3 (1997): 10–11; Andrew M. Boxer and Joseph M. Carrier, "Evelyn Hooker: A Life Remembered," *Journal of Homosexuality* 36:1 (1998): 6–7; "Evelyn Hooker," *American Psychologist* 47 (1992): 499–501; Henry L. Minton, *Departing from Deviance: A History of Homosexual Rights and Emancipatory Science in America* (Chicago: University of Chicago Press, 2002), 222.

9. "Dr. Hooker Sees Nixon as Obstacle to Gay Reform," *Advocate*, no. 54 (March 3–16, 1971): 1.

10. Humphreys, "An Interview with Evelyn Hooker," 195, box 1, folder 5, Hooker Papers.

11. Evelyn Hooker, "The Psychologist: Dr. Evelyn Hooker," in *Making History: The Struggle for Gay and Lesbian Equal Rights, 1945–1990: An Oral History*, ed. Eric Marcus (New York: HarperCollins, 1992), 18.

12. Humphreys, "An Interview with Evelyn Hooker."

13. Evelyn Hooker, "An Empirical Study of Some Relations between Sexual Patterns and Gender Identity in Male Homosexuals," in *Sex Research: New Developments*, ed. John Money (New York: Holt, Rinehart and Winston, 1965), 27.

14. Hooker, "Male Homosexuality in the Rorschach," *Journal of Projective Techniques* 22 (1958): 33.

15. Psychiatrist William Wheeler wrote that the Rorschach test "could be of practical value to Army psychiatrists who may be confronted . . . with soldiers accused of homosexuality which they deny" (William Marshall Wheeler, "An Analysis of Rorschach Indices of Male Homosexuality," *Rorschach Research Exchange and Journal of Projective Techniques* 13:2 [1949], 100). See also Carl J. Nitsche, J. Franklin Robinson, and Edward T. Parsons, "Homosexuality and the Rorschach," *Journal of Consulting Psychology* 20:3 (1956): 196; Floyd O. Due and M. Erik Wright, "The Use of Content Analysis in Rorschach Interpretation: 1. Differential Characteristics of Male Homosexuals," *Rorschach Research Exchange* 9 (December 4, 1945): 169–77; Martin S. Bergmann, "Homosexuality on the Rorschach Test," *Bulletin of the Menninger Clinic* 9:3 (May 1945): 78–84; Peter Hegarty, "Homosexual Signs and Heterosexual Silences: Rorschach Research on Male Homosexuality from 1921 to 1969," *Journal of the History of Sexuality* 12:3 (2003): 409.

16. Due and Wright, "The Use of Content Analysis in Rorschach Interpretation," 170. In 1949, psychologist William Wheeler reinforced the alleged usefulness of the Rorschach test for detecting homosexuality, compiling a list of twenty indices of homosexuality that became known as "Wheeler signs" (Wheeler, "An Analysis of Rorschach Indices of Male Homosexuality"). See also Marvin R. Goldfried, "On the Diagnosis of Homosexuality from the Rorschach," *Journal of Consulting Psychology* 30:4 (1966): 338–49.

17. Hooker, "The Psychologist: Dr. Evelyn Hooker," 24.

18. Hooker, "The Adjustment of the Male Overt Homosexual," *Journal of Projective Techniques* 21:1 (March 1957): 18.

19. Hooker, "Adjustment of the Male Overt Homosexual," 21.

20. Hooker, "Adjustment of the Male Overt Homosexual," 30.

21. Humphreys, "An Interview with Evelyn Hooker," box 1, folder 5, Hooker Papers.

22. Hooker, "Adjustment of the Male Overt Homosexual"; Arthur C. Carr, *The Prediction of Overt Behavior through the Use of Projective Techniques* (Springfield, IL: Charles C. Thomas, 1960), 3.

23. Hooker, "The Homosexual Community," 40.

24. See for example, Evelyn Hooker, "Male Homosexuality," in *Taboo Topics*, ed. N. L. Farberow (New York: Atherton, 1963): 44–55; Evelyn Hooker, "The Homosexual

Community," *Proceedings of the XIV International Congress of Applied Psychology*, vol. 2, *Personality Research*, ed. G. Nielson (Oxford, UK: Munksgaard, 1962), 40–59; Evelyn Hooker, "A Preliminary Analysis of Group Behavior," *Journal of Psychology* 42 (1956): 217–25; Evelyn Hooker, "Male Homosexuals and Their 'Worlds,'" in *Sexual Inversion: The Multiple Roots of Homosexuality*, ed. Judd Marmor (New York: Basic Books, 1965), 83–107.

25. Legg, *Homophile Studies*, 1.

26. Lyn Pedersen (pseudonym of Jim Kepner), "Who's Got the Microscope?" *ONE* 3:5 (February 1955): 19.

27. D.S., "Mental Health and Homosexuality," ONE 7:2 (1959): 16.

28. Albert Ellis, *Reason and Emotion in Psychotherapy* (New York: Lyle Stuart, 1962), 251. See also Albert Ellis, "New Hope for Homosexuals," in *The Third Sex*, ed. Isadore Rubin (New York: New Book Co., 1961), 54.

29. Albert Ellis, "Are Homosexuals Necessarily Neurotic?" *ONE* 3:7 (April 1955): 8–12; Albert Ellis, *Homosexuality: Its Causes and Cure* (New York: Lyle Stewart, 1965), 109; Ellis, introduction, in Donald Webster Cory (pseudonym of Edward Sagarin), *The Lesbian in America* (New York: Citadel Press, 1964), 18.

30. Ellis, "Are Homosexuals Necessarily Neurotic?," 12.

31. Responses to Ellis, "Are Homosexuals Necessarily Neurotic?" *ONE* 3:6 (June 1955): 8–12.

32. Ronald Anderson, "Neurosis and the Homosexuals," *ONE* 3:9 (September 1955): 5.

33. Albert Ellis, "How Homosexuals Can Combat Anti-Homosexualism," *ONE* 5 (1957): 8.

34. See Ellis, *Homosexuality: Its Causes and Cure*, 82; Ellis, "Homosexuality: The Right to be Wrong," *Journal of Sex Research* 4:2 (May 1968): 99; Ellis, introduction to *The Lesbian in America*, 12.

35. Randy Wicker to Albert Ellis, February 16, 1965, box 123, folder 9, Albert Ellis Papers, Rare Book and Manuscript Library, Columbia University, New York, NY (hereafter cited as Ellis Papers).

36. Albert Ellis to Randy Wicker, February 18, 1965, box 123, folder 9, Ellis Papers.

37. See Marcia M. Gallo, *Different Daughters: A History of the Daughters of Bilitis and the Rise of the Lesbian Rights Movement* (New York: Carroll & Graf Publishers, 2006), 1.

38. Florence Conrad (pseudonym for Florence Jaffy), "Bergler on the Air," *Ladder* 6:1 (1961): 14.

39. Florence Conrad (pseudonym for Florence Jaffy), "Homosexuality," *Ladder* 6:8 (1962): 18.

40. Daughters of Bilitis, "Statement of Purpose," 1955, ONE National Gay and Lesbian Archives.

41. See Gallo, *Different Daughters*, 11

42. Kay Tobin to Foster Gunnison, December 9, 1969, box 5, folder 1, Frank

Kameny Papers, Library of Congress, Washington, DC (hereafter cited as Kameny Papers).

43. Conrad, "New Research on Lesbians Begins This Fall," *Ladder* 7:9 (1962): 4.

44. Ralph H. Gundlach, "Why Is a Lesbian?" *Ladder* 7:12 (1963): 5.

45. F.I.B., "Readers Respond," *Ladder* 8:2 (1963): 23.

46. L.E.R., "The Psychiatrist as Social Tranquilizer," *Ladder* 8:12 (1964): 14.

47. Karpman statement, ms., n.d., box 44, folder 4, Kameny Papers.

48. Frank Kameny, lecture to New York Mattachine Society, July 1964, quoted in John D'Emilio, *Sexual Politics, Sexual Communities: The Making of a Homosexual Minority in the United States, 1940–1970* (Chicago: University of Chicago Press, 1983), 163. On Kameny and the Mattachine Society of Washington, DC, see David K. Johnson, *Lavender Scare: The Cold War Persecution of Gays and Lesbians in the Federal Government* (Chicago: University of Chicago Press, 2004), 179–208; D'Emilio, *Sexual Politics, Sexual Communities*, 154–62; Minton, *Departing from Deviance*, 242–44.

49. Franklin E. Kameny, "Does Research into Homosexuality Matter?," *Ladder* 9:8 (1965): 17.

50. Kameny, "Does Research into Homosexuality Matter?," 14.

51. "Policy of the Mattachine Society of Washington," adopted March 4, 1965, Mattachine Society of Washington file, Institute for Sex Research, Kinsey Institute.

52. Kameny, "Does Research into Homosexuality Matter?," 20.

53. Kameny, "Does Research into Homosexuality Matter?," 15.

54. Kameny, "Does Research into Homosexuality Matter?," 16.

55. Florence Conrad, "Research Is Here to Stay," *Ladder* 9:10 (1965): 17–18.

56. Barbara Gittings to Frank Kameny, February 21, 1965, box 6, folder 11, Barbara Gittings and Kay Tobin Lahusen Gay History Papers and Photographs, Manuscripts and Archives Division, New York Public Library, New York, New York (hereafter cited as Gittings and Lahusen NYPL).

57. Barbara Gittings, Editorial, *Ladder* 8:11 (1964): 4.

58. Dick Leitsch to Frank Kameny, June 14, 1968, box 6, folder 11, Kameny Papers.

59. See Gary Alinder, "Psychiatry: Crime against Nature," *Great Speckled Bird* 3:24 (June 15, 1970): 6–7.

60. See Alondra Nelson, *Body and Soul: The Black Panther Party and the Fight against Medical Discrimination* (Minneapolis: University of Minnesota Press, 2011).

61. See Abram J. Lewis, "'We Are Certain of Our Own Insanity': Antipsychiatry and the Gay Liberation Movement, 1968–1980," *Journal of the History of Sexuality* 25:1 (January 2016): 83–113.

62. Ronald D. Lee, "Mental Health and Gay Liberation," April 1972, unpub. ms., box 104, folder 9, Gittings and Lahusen NYPL.

63. Author's interview with William Bennett, Cambridge, MA, September 26, 2015.

64. Duberman, "How Different?," introduction to *Issues in Lesbian and Gay Life:*

*Psychiatry, Psychology, and Homosexuality*, ed. Ellen Herman (New York: Chelsea House, 1995), 11.

65. Edmund White, *City Boy: My Life in New York during the 1960s and '70s* (New York: Bloomsbury, 2009), 54.

66. Edmund White, *My Lives: An Autobiography* (New York: Harper Collins, 2006), 24.

67. Duberman, "How Different?," 11.

68. American Psychiatric Association, *Diagnostic and Statistical Manual of Mental Disorders* (Washington, DC: American Psychiatric Association, 1952), 38–39.

69. *Diagnostic and Statistical Manual of Mental Disorders*, 2nd ed. (American Psychiatric Association, 1968), 44.

70. Gary Alinder, "Gay Liberation Meets the Shrinks," *Come Out!* 1:4 (June–July 1970): 23.

71. Alinder, "Gay Liberation Meets the Shrinks," 23.

72. "1970 Annual Meeting Preliminary Program," *American Journal of Psychiatry* 126:9 (March 1970): 1345–88.

73. Alinder, "Gay Liberation Meets the Shrinks," 23. Gay activists were not the first to take on the APA. In 1969, the annual meeting of the APA in Miami was also the occasion for protests from the organization's Black Caucus, Women's Caucus, and newly formed Radical Caucus. See Lucas Richert, *Break on Through: Racial Psychiatry and the American Counterculture* (Cambridge, MA: MIT Press, 2019).

74. "Gay Raiders Seize Stage at D.C. Psychiatrist Meet," *Advocate* 60 (May 26–June 8, 1971): 3.

75. "Gay Raiders Seize Stage at D.C. Psychiatrist Meet," 3.

76. "Lifestyles of the Non-Patient Homosexual," transcript of panel discussion, American Psychiatric Association Annual Meeting, Washington, DC, May 6, 1971, box 13, folder 1, Lilli Vincenz Papers, Library of Congress, Washington, DC.

77. "Speech for the American Psychiatric Association," May 3, 1971, box 52, folder 6, Gittings and Lahusen NYPL.

78. John Fryer, speech presented at the American Psychiatric Association's Annual Meeting, May 2, 1972, John Fryer Papers, Historical Society of Pennsylvania, Philadelphia, PA.

79. Silverstein, "Even Psychiatry Can Profit from Its Past Mistakes," *Journal of Homosexuality* 2:2 (Winter 1976–77): 155.

80. Charles Silverstein, "Are You Saying Homosexuality Is Normal?" *Journal of Gay and Lesbian Mental Health* 12:3 (2008): 279; Silverstein, "Even Psychiatry Can Profit from Its Past Mistakes," *Journal of Homosexuality* 2:2 (Winter 1976–77): 153-58; see also George Weinberg, *Society and the Healthy Homosexual (New York: St. Martin's Press, 1972)*; Marcel T. Saghir, Eli Robins, Bonnie Walbran, and Kathye A. Gentry, "Homosexuality. III. Psychiatric Disorders and Disabilities in the Female Homosexual," *American Journal of Psychiatry* 127:8 (February 1970): 1079-86.

81. Charles Silverstein, "Statement to the Nomenclature Committee of the American Psychiatric Association," box 3, folder 7, Eromin Center Records, Special Collections Research Center, Temple University, Philadelphia, PA (hereafter cited as Eromin Records).

82. Richard O. Hire, "An Interview with Robert Jean Campbell III," *Journal of Gay and Lesbian Psychotherapy* 6:3 (2002): 84.

83. A diverse set of critiques of psychiatry, lodged by ex-patients, psychiatric dissidents, and academics, is often collected together under the rubric of "antipsychiatry." On antipsychiatry, see Michael Staub, *Madness Is Civilization: When the Diagnosis Was Social, 1948–1980* (Chicago: University of Chicago Press, 2011); Thomas Szasz, *The Myth of Mental Illness* (New York: Hoeber-Harper, 1960); R. D. Laing, *The Divided Self: An Existential Study of Sanity and Madness* (London: Tavistock, 1960); T. J. Scheff, *Being Mentally Ill: A Sociological Theory* (New York: Aldine, 1966); David Cooper, *Psychiatry and Anti-Psychiatry* (London: Tavistock, 1967).

84. Staub, *Madness Is Civilization*, 142.

85. See Staub, *Madness Is Civilization*.

86. Vernon Rosario, "An Interview with Judd Marmor, MD," in *American Psychiatry and Homosexuality: An Oral History*, ed. Jack Drescher and Joseph P. Merlino (New York: Harrington Park Press, 2007), 84.

87. Eric Marcus, "The Good Doctor: Judd Marmor," in *Making History: The Struggle for Gay and Lesbian Equal Rights, 1945–1990: An Oral History* (New York: HarperCollins, 1992), 250.

88. Marcus, "The Good Doctor," 251.

89. Judd Marmor, ed., *Sexual Inversion: The Multiple Roots of Homosexuality* (New York: Basic Books, 1965).

90. Marcus, "The Good Doctor," 252.

91. Judd Marmor, paper delivered at the annual meeting of the America Psychiatric Association, May 9, 1973, Eromin Center, box 1, folder 7, Eromin Records.

92. See Hannah Decker, *The Making of DSM-III: A Diagnostic Manual's Conquest of American Psychiatry* (New York: Oxford University Press, 2013); Mitchell Wilson, "*DSM-III* and the Transformation of American Psychiatry," *American Journal of Psychiatry* 150:3 (March 1993): 399–410; Herb Kutchins and Stuart Kirk, *Making Us Crazy: DSM: The Psychiatric Bible and the Creation of Mental Disorders* (New York: Free Press, 1997), 68–70.

93. Jack Drescher, "An Interview with Robert L. Spitzer, M.D.," *Journal of Gay & Lesbian Psychotherapy* 7:3 (2003): 100.

94. Robert Spitzer, "Homosexuality and Mental Disorder: A Reformulation of the Issues," 7, box 3, David Kessler Papers, GLBT Historical Society, San Francisco, CA (hereafter cited as Kessler Papers).

95. Spitzer, "Homosexuality and Mental Disorder," On psychiatrists' efforts to eliminate psychoanalytic influences from the *DSM*, see Kutchins and Kirk, *Making Us Crazy*, 65; Elisabeth Roudinesco, *Why Psychoanalysis?*, trans. Rachel Bowlby (New

York: Columbia University Press, 2001), 35; Wilson, "*DSM-III* and the Transformation of American Psychiatry"; Dagmar Herzog, *Cold War Freud: Psychoanalysis in an Age of Catastrophes* (Cambridge: Cambridge University Press, 2017), 72–74.

96. Robert J. Stoller, "Criteria for Psychiatric Diagnosis," *American Journal of Psychiatry* 130:11 (November 1973): 1207.

97. Philip Kennicott, "At Smithsonian, Gay Rights Is out of the Closet, into the Attic," *Washington Post*, September 8, 2007.

98. Quoted in Eric Marcus, *Making History*, 225.

99. Robert L. Spitzer, "A Proposal about Homosexuality and the APA Nomenclature: Homosexuality as an Irregular Form of Sexual Behavior and Sexual Orientation Disturbance as a Psychiatric Disorder," *American Journal of Psychiatry* 130:11 (November 1973): 1214.

100. Change in *DSM-II*, 6th Printing, approved by APA Board of Trustees, Dec. 15, 1973, 44, box 164, folder 39, National Gay and Lesbian Task Force Records, Rare Books and Manuscripts, Cornell University, Ithaca, NY (hereafter cited as NGLTF Records).

101. Robert Spitzer, "The Diagnostic Status of Homosexuality in DSM-III: A Reformulation of the Issues," *American Journal of Psychiatry* 138:2 (1981): 210.

102. Drescher, "An Interview with Robert L. Spitzer, M.D.," 103.

103. Spitzer, "The Diagnostic Status of Homosexuality in DSM-III," 213.

104. Spitzer, "Homosexuality and Mental Disorder."

105. Richard Green to Rick Friedman, December 1, 1976, box 3, Kessler Papers. See Decker, *The Making of DSM-III*, 210.

106. Judd Marmor to Richard Pillard, March 15, 1977, American Psychiatric Association Melvin Sabshin Library and Archives, DSM Collection, Washington, D.C.

107. Ronald Bayer and Robert L. Spitzer, "Edited Correspondence on the Status of Homosexuality in DSM-III," *Journal of the History of the Behavioral Sciences* 18:1 (1982): 34.

108. Judd Marmor to Robert Spitzer, April 15, 1977, box 3, Kessler Papers.

109. Judd Marmor to Robert Spitzer, September 9, 1977, box 21, folder 2, Judd Marmor Papers, Department of Special Collections, Charles E. Young Research Library, University of California, Los Angeles, CA (hereafter cited as Marmor Papers ONE).

110. Robert Spitzer to Richard Pillard, May 10, 1977, in Bayer and Spitzer, "Edited Correspondence on the Status of Homosexuality," 39.

111. Harold I. Lief, "Sexual Survey No. 4: Current Thinking of Homosexuality," *Medical Aspects of Human Sexuality* 11 (1977): 110, quoted in Kenneth Lewes, *The Psychoanalytic Theory of Male Homosexuality* (New York: Simon and Schuster), 223.

112. Memo, Franklin Kameny to "Those Who Contributed to My May 1973 Trip to Honolulu to Attend the Meeting of the American Psychiatric Association," December 15, 1973, ONE Archive Subject Files: "Psychiatry and Gays."

113. *Gay, Lesbian, and Bisexual Caucus of the American Psychiatric Association Newsletter* 3:2 (June 1978): 3, in "American Psychiatric Association, Gay Caucus Members," NGLTF Records, Cornell University, Ithaca, NY.

114. Gittings to Charles Brydon and Lucia Valeska, Co-Executive Directors, National Gay Task Force, March 24, 1980, box 164, folder 40, NGLTF Records.

115. Robert Cabaj, "Strike While the Iron Is Hot: Science, Social Forces, and Ego-Dystonic Homosexuality," *Journal of Gay and Lesbian Mental Health* 13:2 (2009): 89.

116. Barbara Gittings to Charles Brydon and Lucia Valeska, National Gay Task Force, March 24, 1980, box 164, folder 40, NGLTF Records. While Kameny was publicly cavalier about the inclusion of ego-dystonic homosexuality in the *DSM-III*, in private correspondence with Spitzer he pushed him to reconsider his support of the new category, urging him to remember that "the issue is Dyshomophilia *NOT—NOT—NOT Homosexuality*." Dyshomophila, Kameny emphasized "is as much a product of the past misdeeds and crimes of psychiatry itself as it is of anything else, and don't ever forget it!!!" (Kameny to Spitzer, April 18, 1977, in Bayer and Spitzer, "Edited Correspondence on the Status of Homosexuality in DSM-III," 38, 39).

117. Donald Webster Cory (pseudonym of Edward Sagarin), "Can Homosexuality Be Cured?" *Sexology* 18 (October 1951): 153–54.

118. "Psychotherapy vs. Public Opinion," *Ladder* 1 (1957): 9.

119. Carol Hales, "Accept the Challenge!" *Ladder* 1:7 (1957): 12.

120. "DOB Questionnaire Reveals Some Facts about Lesbians," *Ladder* 3:12 (1959): 9; "Coming in June: A Lesbian Questionnaire," *Ladder* 2:8 (1958): 9. See also Gallo, *Different Daughters*, 47–55.

121. "DOB Questionnaire Reveals Some Facts," 5, 6, 18.

122. See, for example, Minton, *Departing from Deviance*, 220.

123. Hooker, "The Psychologist: Dr. Evelyn Hooker," 22.

124. Evelyn Hooker, "Male Homosexuals and Their 'Worlds,'" in *Sexual Inversion: The Multiple Roots of Homosexuality*, ed. Judd Marmor (New York: Basic Books, 1965), 92; Hooker, foreword, in David H. Rosen, ed., *Lesbianism: A Study of Female Homosexuality* (Springfield, MA: Charles C. Thomas, 1973), viii.

125. "Dr. Hooker Sees Nixon as Obstacle to Gay Reform," *Advocate* 54 (March 3–16, 1971): 1.

126. Task Force on Homosexuality, meeting notes, 56, box 1, folder 3, Marmor Papers ONE.

127. "Final Report of the Task Force on Homosexuality," October 10, 1969, *ONE Institute Quarterly: Homophile Studies* 8 (1970): 6, 5–6, box 4, folder 3, Hooker Papers.

128. John M. Livingood, ed., *National Institute of Mental Health Task Force on Homosexuality: Final Report and Background Papers* (Rockville, MD: U.S. Department of Health, Education, and Welfare, 1972), 2.

129. Livingood, *National Institute of Mental Health Task Force on Homosexuality*, 5.

130. Hooker talk transcription, February 9, 1971, "Psychiatry," ONE Archive Subject Files.

131. Barbara Gittings, Remarks to APA at "Lifestyles of Non-Patient Homosexuals" panel, May 6, 1971, in Kameny Papers.

132. Deborah B. Gould, *Moving Politics: Emotion and ACT UP's Fight against AIDS* (Chicago: University of Chicago Press, 2009), 28.

133. Lewis, "'We Are Certain of Our Own Insanity,'" 92.

134. Sara Ahmed, *The Promise of Happiness* (Durham: Duke University Press, 2011), 91, 11, 112. See also Daniel Horowitz, *Happier? The History of a Cultural Movement That Aspired to Transform America* (New York: Oxford University Press, 2018); Elizabeth D. Samet, *Looking for the Good War: American Amnesia and the Violent Pursuit of Happiness* (New York: McMillan, 2021).

135. Franklin Kameny, "Emphasis on Research Has Had Its Day," *Ladder* 10:1 (1965): 13.

136. Kameny, "Does Research into Homosexuality Matter?" *Ladder* 9:8 (1965): 16–17.

137. Kameney also objected to gay activists who wanted to integrate an antiwar position into their politics, writing that "it has no logical or other relationship to us whatever, and involvement in it, in any slightest way can only do us—and the entire movement— . . . very lasting harm. . . . As for homosexuality and Vietnam, 'The separation must be complete!!!!'" Kameny to Don Slater, April 3, 1966, box 6, folder 13, Gittings and Lahusen NYPL.

138. Jonathan M. Metzl, "Why against Health?," in *Against Health: How Health Became the New Morality*, ed. Jonathan M. Metzl and Anna Kirkland (New York: NYU Press, 2010), 5.

139. In particular, the 1952 Immigration and Nationality Act barred individuals "afflicted with psychopathic personality" and the 1967 Supreme Court decision *Boutilier v. Immigration and Naturalization Service* concluded that the language of that law was intended to exclude homosexuals, even in the face of opposition from psychiatrists. See Margot Canaday, *The Straight State: Sexuality and Citizenship in Twentieth-Century America* (Princeton: Princeton University Press, 2009): 241–49; Marc Stein, "Boutilier and the U.S. Supreme Court's Sexual Revolution," *Law and History Review* 23:3 (Fall 2005): 491–536; Siobhan B. Somerville, "Queer Loving," *GLQ: A Journal of Lesbian and Gay Studies* 11:3 (2005): 335–70. On the use of psychiatric assessments in custody hearings, see Daniel Rivers, *Radical Relations: Lesbian Mothers, Gay Fathers, and Their Children in the United States since World War II* (Chapel Hill: University of North Carolina Press, 2013): 67–72, 92–95.

140. Emily Thuma, *All Our Trials: Prisons, Policing, and the Feminist Fight to End Violence* (Champaign: University of Illinois Press, 2019), 67. At the center of the protest against those developments, Thuma shows, were radical feminists, prison rights activists, and disability activists.

141. See Joanne Meyerowitz, *How Sex Changed: A History of Transsexuality in the United States* (Cambridge, MA: Harvard University Press, 2002); Jennifer Terry, *An American Obsession: Science, Medicine, and Homosexuality in Modern Society* (Chicago: University of Chicago Press, 1999); Jules Gill-Peterson, *Histories of the Transgender Child* (Minneapolis: University of Minnesota Press, 2019), 13; David Valentine, *Imagining Transgender: An Ethnography of a Category* (Durham: Duke University Press, 2007).

142. Jay Prosser writes that "the reading of sexual inversion as about homosexuality

is profoundly ironic," given its primary focus on gender ( Jay Prosser, "Transsexuals and the Transsexologists: Inversion and the Emergence of Transsexual Subjectivity," in *Sexology in Culture: Labelling Bodies and Desires*, ed. Lucy Bland and Laura Doan [Cambridge: Polity Press, 1998], 117–18. See also Gill-Peterson, *Histories of the Transgender Child*, 13–16.

143. Meyerowitz, *How Sex Changed*, 177.

144. Craig Loftin, "Unacceptable Mannerisms: Gender Anxieties, Homosexual Activism, and Swish in the United States, 1945–1965," *Journal of Social History* 40:3 (Spring 2007): 579.

145. Blanche Baker, "Toward Understanding," *ONE* 7 (1959): 26.

146. Donald Webster Cory (pseudonym of Edward Sagarin), *The Homosexual in America: A Subjective Approach* (1951; reprint, New York: Castle Books, 1960), 92.

147. Cory, *Homosexual in America*, 37.

148. Gallo, *Different Daughters*, 7.

149. Tracy Baim, *Barbara Gittings: Gay Pioneer* (Chicago: Prairie Avenue Productions, 2015), 51.

150. Finn Enke calls for a more complicated understanding of the trans politics of 1970s feminism and recognition of a history of transfeminism, one attuned to the presence of trans feminists and the support of trans women by some lesbian feminists, in "Collective Memory and the Transfeminist 1970s: Toward a Less Plausible History," *TSQ: Transgender Studies Quarterly* 5:1 (2018): 9–29.

151. Kameny to Leitsch, June 19, 1968, box 6, folder 11, Kameny Papers.

152. Ron Gold, "Stop It, You're Making Me Sick," paper delivered at the APA convention, May 9, 1973, Honolulu, Hawaii.

153. Kameny to Spitzer, April 18, 1977, box 3, Kessler Papers.

154. Farrall Instruments brochure, box 9, folder 153, Paul Lowinger Papers, University of Pennsylvania, Kislak Center for Special Collections, Rare Books and Manuscripts, Philadelphia, PA. See 125th Annual Meeting of the American Psychiatric Association, May 1–5, 1972, Dallas, Texas, program, box 122, folder 8, Kameny Papers.

155. Farrall Instruments advertisements, box 53, folder 9, Gittings and Lahusen NYPL.

156. "Visually Keyed Shocker," box 53, folder 9, Gittings and Lahusen NYPL.

157. "Visually Keyed Shocker," Gittings and Lahusen NYPL.

158. Harry Benjamin, *The Transsexual Phenomenon: A Scientific Report on Transsexualism and Sex Conversion in the Human Male and Female* (New York: Julian Press, 1966).

159. Dallas Denny, "The Politics of Diagnosis and a Diagnosis of Politics," *Chrysalis* 1:3 (1993): 11. See Meyerowitz, *How Sex Changed*; Sandy Stone, "The Empire Strikes Back: A Posttransexual Manifesto," in *The Transgender Studies Reader Remix*, ed. Susan Stryker and Dylan McCarthy Blackston (New York: Routledge, 2022), 15–30; Gill-Peterson, *Histories of the Transgender Child*.

160. See Meyerowitz, *How Sex Changed*, 141, 159–62.

161. Beans Velocci, "Standards of Care: Uncertainty and Risk in Harry Benjamin's Transsexual Classifications," *TSQ: Transgender Studies Quarterly* 8:4 (November 2021): 462–80.

162. See Judith Butler, "Introduction: Acting in Concert," in *Undoing Gender* (New York: Routledge, 2004), 1–16.

163. Joost Meerloo, "Change of Sex and Collaboration with the Psychosis," *American Journal of Psychiatry* 124 (1976): 263; Charles Socarides, "A Psychoanalytic Study of the Desire for Sexual Transformation ('transsexualism'): The Plaster-of-Paris Man," *International Journal of Psycho-Analysis* 51 (1970): 346; B. Stinson, "A Study of Twelve Applicants for Transsexual Surgery," *Ohio State Medical Journal* 68 (1972): 246; Vanik Volkan and Tajammul Bhatti, "Dreams of Transsexuals Awaiting Surgery," *Comprehensive Psychiatry* 14 (1973): 278.

164. Angelo Tornabene to Lou Sullivan, September 25, 1970, Lou Sullivan Collection, GLBT Historical Society, San Francisco, CA, https://www.digitaltransgenderarchive.net/files/p5547r43n.

165. American Psychiatric Association, *Diagnostic and Statistical Manual*, 3rd ed. (*DSM-III*) (Washington, DC: APA, 1980), 261. See Valentine, *Imagining Transgender*, 55; Judith Butler, *Undoing Gender*, 5; Eve Kosofsky Sedgwick, "How to Bring Your Kids Up Gay: The War on Effeminate Boys," *Social Text* 29 (1991): 18–27.

166. *DSM-III*, 261–62.

167. *DSM-III*, 280, 282.

168. *DSM-III*, 282.

169. See James O. Stallings, "How a Man Becomes a Woman," *She*, May 1978, Newspaper and Periodical Clippings, Transgender Archives, University of Victoria, Victoria, BC, Canada, https://www.digitaltransgenderarchive.net/files/p2676v65f.

170. Erickson Educational Foundation, *Counseling the Transsexual: Five Conversations with Professionals in Transsexual Therapy* (Baton Rouge, LA: Printed by the author, 1973), Transgender Archives, University of Victoria, https://archive.org/details/counselingtranse0000noau/mode/2up.

171. Harry Gershman, "The Effect of Group Therapy on Compulsive Homosexuality in Men and Women," *American Journal of Psychoanalysis* 35:4 (January 1975): 305.

172. Richard Green, *The "Sissy Boy Syndrome" and the Development of Homosexuality* (New Haven: Yale University Press, 1987).

173. See Green, *"Sissy Boy Syndrome"*; Marcel Saghir and Eli Robins, *Male and Female Homosexuality* (Baltimore: Williams and Wilkins, 1973); Alan Bell, M. S. Weinberg, and S. K. Hammersmith, *Sexual Preference: Its Development in Men and Women* (Bloomington: Indiana University Press, 1981).

174. Eve Kosofsky Sedgwick, "How to Bring Your Kids Up Gay," *Social Text*, no. 29 (1991): 20, 21. Karl Edward Bryant points to limitations of this critique, in "The Politics of Pathology and the Making of Gender Identity Disorder" (PhD dissertation, University of California, Santa Barbara, 2007). See also Jack Drescher, "Transsexualism, Gender Identity Disorder, and the DSM," *Journal of Gay and Lesbian Mental Health*

14:2 (April 2010): 109–22; Kenneth J. Zucker and Robert L. Spitzer, "Was the Gender Identity Disorder of Childhood Diagnosis Introduced into DSM-III as a Backdoor Maneuver to Replace Homosexuality? A Historical Note," *Journal of Sex and Marital Therapy* 31 (2005): 31–42.

175. John Money to Robert Spitzer, August 8, 1977, American Psychiatric Association Melvin Sabshin, M.D. Library and Archives, *DSM* Collection, Washington, DC.

176. See, for example, John Money and Anke A. Ehrhardt, *Man & Woman, Boy & Girl: Differentiation and Dimorphism of Gender Identity from Conception to Maturity* (Baltimore: Johns Hopkins University Press, 1972); Robert Stoller, *Sex and Gender: On the Development of Masculinity and Femininity* (New York: Science House, 1968); Richard Green and John Money, *Transsexualism and Sex Reassignment* (Baltimore: Johns Hopkins University Press, 1969); Richard Green, *Sexuality Identity Conflict in Children and Adults* (New York: Basic Books, 1974); Robert J. Stoller, *Sex and Gender: The Transsexual Experiment* (London: Hogarth Press, 1968).

177. Sarah Seton, "Transsexual Theatre," *Twenty Minutes*, May 1991, 3. See also Mary C. Burke, "Resisting Pathology: GID and the Contested Terrain of Diagnosis in the Transgender Rights Movement," *Sociology of Diagnosis* 12 (2011): 183–210.

178. Riki Ann Wilchins, "The GID Controversy: Gender Identity Disorder Diagnosis Harms Transsexuals," *Transgender Tapestry* 79 (1997): 44-45; Deirdre O'Hartigan, "The GID Controversy: Transsexuals Need the Gender Identity Disorder Diagnosis," *Transgender Tapestry* 79 (1997): 30–45.

179. O'Hartigan, "The GID Controversy: Transsexuals Need the Gender Identity Disorder Diagnosis," *Transgender Tapestry*, 45.

180. O'Hartigan, "The GID Controversy: Transsexuals Need the Gender Identity Disorder Diagnosis."

181. Wilchins, "The GID Controversy: Gender Identity Diagnosis Harms Transsexuals," *Transgender Tapestry* 44. See also Melanie Erin Spritz, "Psychiatric Labels: Still Hard to Shake," *Transgender Treatment Bulletin* 1:2 (February 1998): 6–7. Cameron Awkward-Rich argues that the claim by trans people that "we are not mentally ill" is a "habit of trans thought" that undergirds the formation of trans studies and claims to trans rights (Cameron Awkward-Rich, *The Terrible We: Thinking with Trans Maladjustment* [Durham: Duke University Press, 2022], 3).

182. Florence Ashley, "The Misuse of Gender Dysphoria: Toward Greater Conceptual Clarity in Transgender Health," *Association for Psychological Science* 16:6 (2021): 1159.

183. Wilchins, "The GID Controversy: Gender Identity Diagnosis Harms Transsexuals," 31. Cameron Awkward-Rich argues that "the disavowal of *sick*" was a foundational claim on which academic trans studies was based (*The Terrible We*, 3). Karl Bryant makes a powerful and persuasive argument that GIDC works to produce gender-conforming homosexuals by targeting "certain kinds of pre-homosexual children: gender nonconforming pre-homosexual children" (Bryant, "The Politics of Pathology and the Making of Gender Identity Disorder," 249). See also Mary C. Burke, "Resisting Pathology: GID and the Contested Terrain of Diagnosis in the Transgender Rights Movement," *Sociology of Diagnosis* 12 (2011): 183–210; "GID and the Transgender Movement: A Joint Statement by the International Conference on Transgender

Law and Employment Policy (ICTLEP) and the National Center for Lesbian Rights (NCLR)," Fifth International Conference on Transgender Law and Employment Policy, July 1996, Appendix A.

184. American Psychiatric Association, *Diagnostic and Statistical Manual of Mental Disorders*, 5th ed. (*DSM-V*) (Washington, DC: APA, 2013), 451.

## EPILOGUE

1. American Psychiatric Association, "Position Statement on Homosexuality and Civil Rights," *American Journal of Psychiatry* 131:4 (1974): 497.

2. Louis Landerson, Discussion of "Behavioral Therapy—Bag of Tricks or Point of View? Treatment for Homosexuality," *Psychotherapy: Theory, Research, and Practice* 9:3 (Fall 1972): 286.

3. Mary Ann Jones and Martha A. Gabriel, "Utilization of Psychotherapy by Gay Men, Lesbians, and Bisexuals," *American Journal of Orthopsychiatry* 64:2 (April 1999): 210. Alan P. Bell and Martin S. Weinberg's 1978 study of men and women in the San Francisco Bay area found that 56 percent of the gay men (compared to 27 percent of the heterosexual male control group) and 66 percent of the lesbians (compared to 41 percent of the heterosexual female control group) reported having consulted with a psychotherapist at some time in their lives (Alan P. Bell and George Weinberg, *Homosexualities: A Study of Diversity among Men and Women* [New York: Simon & Schuster, 1978]). See also Kris S. Morgan and M. J. Eliason, "Caucasian Lesbians' Use of Psychotherapy: A Matter of Attitude," *Psychology of Women Quarterly* 16 (1992): 127–30.

4. Judith Bradford, Caitlin Ryan, and Esther D. Rothblum, "National Lesbian Health Care Survey: Implications for Mental Health Care," *Journal of Consulting and Clinical Psychology* 62:2 (April 1994): 234. The survey also showed that over half the sample of lesbians surveyed had had thoughts about suicide, and 18 percent had attempted suicide.

5. Walt Odets, *Out of the Shadows: Reimagining Gay Men's Lives* (New York: Farrar, Straus and Giroux, 2019), xiv.

6. Dorr W. Legg, ed., *Homophile Studies in Theory and Practice* (Los Angeles: ONE Institute Press and GLB Publishers, 1994), 172.

7. See Katie Batza, *Before AIDS: Gay Health Politics in the 1970s* (Philadelphia: University of Pennsylvania Press, 2018); Alondra Nelson, *Body and Soul: The Black Panther Party and the Fight against Medical Discrimination* (Minneapolis: University of Minnesota Press, 2013); Joseph P. Shapiro, *No Pity: People with Disabilities Forging a New Civil Rights Movement* (New York: Times Books, 1993).

8. Paul E. Lynch, "An Interview with Richard C. Pillard, MD," *Journal of Gay & Lesbian Psychotherapy* 7:4 (2003): 66.

9. Author's interview with Charles Silverstein, July 28, 2015, New York, NY.

10. "Homosexual Counseling Center Opens," press release, October 1, 1971, box 5, folder 3, Gittings and Lahusen NYPL.

11. *Gay House Newsletter*, No. 1, May 9, 1971, box 12, folder 19, Gittings and Lahusen NYPL.

12. Cindy Hanson and John Preston, "Editor's Note," *Gay People and Mental Health* 1:1 (October 1972), 1.

13. "For 'G and G,'" 1975, in ONE Archive Subject Files, "Psychiatrists and Psychologists," ONE National Gay and Lesbian Archives, USC Libraries, University of Southern California, Los Angeles, CA.

14. R.H.J., "Peer Counseling," *Gay People and Mental Health* 4:3 (May–June 1975): 1.

15. Charna Klein, *Counseling Our Own: The Lesbian/Gay Subculture Meets the Mental Health System* (Seattle: Consultant Service Northwest, 1986), 11.

16. Ronald D. Lee, "Mental Health and Gay Liberation," unpub. ms., April 1972, box 104, folder 9, Gittings and Lahusen NYPL.

17. See Batza, *Before AIDS*, 25–26, 77–78.

18. Alan K. Malyon, "Some Suggested Guidelines for Psychotherapy with Gay Men," June 1979, unpublished ms, "Society for the Psychological Study of Lesbian and Gay Issues" records, box 8, folder 35, Human Sexuality Collection, Cornell University Rare and Manuscript Collections, Ithaca, NY.

19. Gay Activists Alliance, *20 Questions about Homosexuality: A Political Primer*, pamphlet, Gittings and Tobin collection, box 2, Gerber / Hart Library and Archives, Chicago, IL.

20. Judd Marmor, "Notes on Some Psychodynamic Aspects of Homosexuality," in *National Institute of Mental Health Task Force on Homosexuality: Final Report and Background Papers*, ed. John Livingood (Rockville, MD: U.S. Department of Health, Education, and Welfare, 1972), 55.

21. "On Our Own: Gay Men in Consciousness-Raising Groups," 1972, 51, in John R. Yoakem Papers, box 22, folder 26, Jean-Nickolaus Tretter Collection in Gay, Lesbian, Bisexual, and Transgender Studies, University of Minnesota, Minneapolis, MN.

22. Eromin Center, Inc., brochure, box 1, folder 72, Harry Langhorne Papers, Division of Rare and Manuscript Collections, Cornell University Library, Ithaca, NY. Eromin was not alone in dedicating itself to "sexual minorities" in this period. The Seattle Counseling Services for Sexual Minorities was founded in 1969 and the Center for Counseling Sexual Minorities opened in 1972 in Pittsburgh.

23. Arlene Lieb, "Sexually Different—Mentally Sound," reprinted from the *Drummer*, November 6, 1973, Eromin Center, box 1, folder 19, Eromin Center Records, Special Collections Research Center, Temple University, Philadelphia, PA (hereafter cited as Eromin Records); "About Eromin Center, Inc.," n.d., box 4, folder 12, Eromin Records.

24. Intake questionnaire form, n.d., box 2, folder 6, Eromin Records.

25. "The Philosophy of the Counseling Staff of the Eromin Center, Inc.," n.d., box 2, folder 6, Eromin Records.

26. "Eromin Center Clinical Philosophy," 1978, box 2, folder 9, Eromin Records.

27. "Mental Health: Walking the Straight and Narrow," 1974, box 4, folder 5, Eromin Records.

28. See Stephen Vider, *The Queerness of Home: Gender, Sexuality, and the Politics*

*of Domesticity after World War II* (Chicago: University of Chicago Press, 2021), 171–78; David S. Byers, Stephen Vider, and Amelia Smith, "Clinical Activism in Community-Based Practice: The Case of LGBT Affirmative Care at the Eromin Center, Philadelphia, 1973–1984," *American Psychologist* 74:8 (November 2019): 868–81. On the U.S. gay community's engagement with the Mariel boatlift more broadly, see Julio Capó Jr., "Queering Mariel: Mediating Cold War Foreign Policy and U.S. Citizenship among Cuba's Homosexual Exile Community, 1978–1994," *Journal of American Ethnic History* 29:4 (Summer 2010): 78–106.

29. Report of the Ad Hoc Committee on Board Structure and Composition, October 18, 1979, box 1, folder 19, Eromin Records.

30. Katie Batza makes the important point that gay and lesbian health services that were formed in the 1970s provided a crucial infrastructure before the AIDS crisis in the early 1980s in *Before AIDS*. The devastating irony of gayness being remedicalized and repathologized so soon after homosexuality was deleted from the *Diagnostic and Statistical Manual of Mental Disorders*, this time through a virus purportedly linked to gay sexual behavior rather than as an attribution of mental disorder, was felt painfully by gay men and lesbians. See Lance Wahlert, "The Painful Reunion: The Remedicalization of Homosexuality and the Rise of the Queer," *Bioethical Inquiry* 9 (2012): 261–75; Peter Conrad and Alison Angell, "Homosexuality and Remedicalization," *Society* 41:5 (July 2004): 32–39.

31. John Money to Martin Duberman, June 6, 1991, in Duberman Papers, bound volume for *Cures*, NYPL.

32. C. Bard Cole, "Pulling Down the Ivory Tower: An Interview with Martin Bauml Duberman, New York Native, 419, April 29, 1991, in bound volume for *Cures*, Duberman Papers, NYPL.

33. Ray Olson, review of Martin Duberman's *Cures*, *Booklist*, March 15, 1991, in bound volume for, Duberman Papers, NYPL.

34. Steve Wileman to Martin Duberman, May 18, 1991, in bound volume for *Cures*, Duberman Papers.

35. Jasper Lynch to Martin Duberman, July 24, 1991, in bound volume for *Cures*, Duberman Papers.

36. "A Patient Stronger Than the 'Cure': A *New York Newsday* Interview with Martin Duberman," *New York Newsday*, April 8, 1991, in bound volume for *Cures*, Duberman Papers.

37. *Time* magazine, "Sick Again?," February 29, 1978, clipping, box 164, folder 40, Association of Gay and Lesbian Psychologists Records, Division of Rare and Manuscript Collections, Cornell University. See also Harold I. Lief, "Sexual Survey No. 4: Current Thinking of Homosexuality," *Medical Aspects of Human Sexuality* 11:110 (1977), quoted in Kenneth Lewes, *The Psychoanalytic Theory of Male Homosexuality* (New York: Simon and Schuster, 1988), 223.

38. Tom Waidzunas makes this important point in *The Straight Line: How the Fringe Science of Ex-Gay Therapy Reoriented Sexuality* (Minneapolis: University of Minnesota Press, 2015). See also Tanya Erzen, *Straight to Jesus: Sexual and Christian Conversions in the Ex-Gay Movement* (Berkeley: University of California Press, 2006).

39. Waidzunas, *Straight Line*, 11. Waidzunas urges us to take seriously the ex-gay movement's engagement with scientific institutions and its effect on scientific knowledge.

40. Jack Drescher, "An Interview with Robert L. Spitzer, M.D.," *Journal of Gay & Lesbian Psychotherapy* 7:3 (2003): 104; Robert L. Spitzer, "Can Some Gay Men and Lesbians Change Their Sexual Orientation? 200 Participants Reporting a Change from Homosexual to Heterosexual Orientation," *Archives of Sexual Behavior* 32:5 (October 2003): 403.

41. Spitzer, "Can Some Gay Men and Lesbians Change Their Sexual Orientation?," 412.

42. Jack Drescher, "The Spitzer Study and the Culture Wars," *Archives of Sexual Behavior* 32:5 (October 2003): 431. See also Sean Lund and Cathy Renna, "An Analysis of the Media Response to the Spitzer Study," in *Ex-Gay Research: Analyzing the Spitzer Study and Its Relation to Science, Religion, Politics, and Culture*, ed. Jack Drescher and Kenneth J. Zucker (New York: Harrington Park Press, 2006), 277–90; Wayne Besen, "*Political* Science," in Drescher and Zucker, *Ex-Gay Research*, 291–307.

43. Gabriel Arana, "My So-Called Ex Gay Life," *American Prospect*, April 11, 2012, 50–57.

44. Spitzer, "Can Some Gay Men and Lesbians Change Their Sexual Orientation?"

45. Lawrence Hartmann, "Too Flawed: Don't Publish," *Archives of Sexual Behavior* 32:5 (October 2003): 436.

46. John Bancroft, "Can Sexual Orientation Change? A Long-Running Saga," *Archives of Sexual Behavior* 32:5 (October 2003): 421.

47. Milton L. Wainberg, Donald Bux, Alex Carballo-Dieguez, Gary W. Dowsett Terry Dugan, Marshall Forstein, Karl Goodkin, Joyce Hunter, Thomas Irwin, Paulo Mattos, Karen McKinnon, Ann O'Leary, Jeffrey Parsons, and Edward Stein, "Science and the Nuremberg Code: A Question of Ethics and Harm," *Archives of Sexual Behavior* 32:5 (October 2003): 457.

48. Mark Potok, "Quacks: 'Conversion Therapists,' the Anti-LGBT Right, and the Demonization of Homosexuality," Special Report, Southern Poverty Law Center, May 25, 2016, 11.

49. Arana, "My So-Called Ex-Gay Life,"; Robert L. Spitzer, "Spitzer Reassesses His 2003 Study of Reparative Therapy of Homosexuality," *Archives of Sexual Behavior* 41 (2012): 757.

50. Joseph Nicolosi, *Reparative Therapy of Male Homosexuality* (Northvale, NJ: Jason Aronson, 1991).

51. Alliance for Therapeutic Choice and Scientific Integrity, accessed October 27, 2022, https://www.therapeuticchoice.com/.

52. Alliance for Therapeutic Choice and Scientific Integrity, "Transgender," accessed January 11, 2023, https://www.therapeuticchoice.com/transgender.

53. See Jules Gill-Peterson, "A Trans History of Conversion Therapy," *Sad Brown Girl* (blog), April 22, 2021, https://sadbrowngirl.substack.com/p/a-trans-history-of-conversion-therapy.

54. The 2016 platform of the Republican Party opposed the banning of conversion therapy in thinly coded language by supporting the right of parents "to determine the proper medical treatment and therapy for their minor children" (https://www .presidency.ucsb.edu/documents/2016-republican-party-platform). The Texas Republican Party platform of 2022 abandoned coded language in asserting that "homosexuality is an abnormal lifestyle choice," opposing "all efforts to validate transgender identity," and declaring that "therapists, psychologists, and counselors licensed with the State of Texas shall not be forbidden or penalized by any licensing board for practicing Reintegration Therapy or other counseling methods when counseling clients of any age with gender dysphoria or unwanted same-sex attraction" (Texas Republican Party, "Report of the Permanent 2022 Platform & Resolutions Committee," 2022, 21, https:// texasgop.org/wp-content/uploads/2022/06/6-Permanent-Platform-Committee -FINAL-REPORT-6-16-2022.pdf/).

55. On the relationship of psychiatric and carceral power, see Emily Thuma, "Against the 'Prison/Psychiatric State': Anti-Violence Feminisms and the Politics of Confinement," *Feminist Formations* 26:2 (Summer 2014): 26–51.

56. Martin Duberman, *Cures: A Gay Man's Odyssey*, Tenth Anniversary Edition (New York: Basic Books, 2002), 309.

# Index

Abarbanel-Brandt, Albert, 84
active analysis, 23
activism. *See* declassification; gay rights
   movement; homophile movement;
   Mattachine Society; resistance
adaptation, 23, 94, 106
adjustment therapy, 23, 50–54. *See also*
   curing
advice columns, 88–91
"Advice for Living" (King Jr.), 89
Ahmed, Sara, 8, 116, 140–41
AIDS. *See* HIV/AIDS
Alcoholics Anonymous, 44–45
Aldrich, Ann, 84, 96
Alinder, Gary, 87, 128
Alston, Arthur, 81
American Civil Liberties Union (ACLU),
   109
*American Journal of Psychiatry*, 106
American Psychiatric Association
   (APA), 1–2, 7, 29–30, 35–36, 118,
   128–39, 144, 147, 150–51, 154–57,
   212n73. See also *Diagnostic and
   Statistical Manual of Mental Disorders
   (DSM)*; "golden age"
American Psychoanalytic Association, 24
American Psychological Association,
   121
Amin, Kadji, 10
analogies, 9–10, 110, 126
anti-cross-dressing laws, 77
antipsychiatry, 127, 131–32, 213n83
apomorphine, 62
Arana, Gabriel, 158
*Archives of Sexual Behavior*, 158

"Are Homosexuals Necessarily Neurotic?"
   (ONE), 122–23
art. *See* erotic art
Arvin, Newton, 71–72, 95
Ashley, Florence, 148
Association for the Advancement of
   Behavior Therapy, 130
*Asylums* (Goffman), 94
Atascadero, 68
Atkins, Gary, 115
Auden, W. H., 119
Austria, 23–24
aversive conditioning, 2, 14, 54, 61–68,
   129, 141, 144
Awkward-Rich, Cameron, 7, 219n181,
   219n183

Bachardy, Don, 119
Baker, Blanche, 80, 142–43, 151
Barahal, Hyman, 100
Barlow, David, 66
Batza, Katie, 222n30
Bayer, Ronald, 2
Beach, Frank, 130
Bell, Alan P., 220n3
Bell, Cei, 87
Benjamin, Harry, 28, 145
Bennett, William, 127
Bergler, Edmund, 1, 26–27, 29, 43, 46–47,
   50, 87–88, 123, 137
Berlant, Lauren, 6
Bérubé, Allan, 33
Berzon, Betty, 48, 85, 87, 116
Bieber, Irving, 1, 26–27, 29, 32, 38, 41, 44,
   46, 50, 68, 71, 99, 123, 133

Bien, Ernest, 41
bisexuality, 20–21, 23, 25, 31, 42, 48, 107.
    *See also* constitutional bisexuality
Black Caucus (American Psychiatric
    Association), 212n73
Black Panther Party, 127, 151, 192n174
Blair, Ralph, 152
Bloch, Iwan, 20
Bogdan, Robert, 100
Boutilier, Clive Michael, 182n101
Bowman, Karl, 34
*Boys in the Band, The* (Crowley),
    96–97
Bromberg, Walter, 112
Bryant, Karl, 95–96
Bussee, Michael, 158

Cabaj, Robert, 136
Cabeen, Charles, 33
Campbell, Robert Jean, 130
Canaday, Margot, 3, 182n100
carceral archipelago, 4
carceral spaces, 4–6, 13–14, 34–36, 55–56,
    67–68, 81–82, 112–16, 141–42. *See also*
    Saint Elizabeths Hospital
case files, 5–7, 75, 80. *See also* encounter;
    gay history; Karpman, Benjamin;
    LGBT history
*Case Studies in the Psychopathology of
    Crime* (Karpman), 203n60
Cauldwell, David O., 28
change. *See* adaptation
Chauncey, George, 3, 10, 113
Chenier, El, 182n91
citizenship, 3, 32, 36, 125
*Claiming Disability* (Linton), 9
Clare, Eli, 10
class. *See* social class
classification, 19–20, 142, 145–48
Cohen, Deborah, 193n12
Coleman, James, 33
colonialism, 8
Commission on Mental Health, 74–75
Committee of the American Bar Associa-
    tion, 35
communism, 12, 19, 32
community, 22–23, 43–44, 112–16
Conrad, Florence, 123

constitution, 41–45, 48–49. *See also*
    organic
constitutional bisexuality, 20, 25, 98.
    *See also* bisexuality
contrary sexual inversion. *See* inversion
conversion therapy, 76, 82–85, 96, 157–59,
    224n54. *See also* sexual conversion
Cooper, Gary, 158
Cory, Donald Webster, 45, 72, 96, 122,
    137, 143, 186n58, 205n91
counseling centers, 151–53
court clinics, 76–79
Covi, Lino, 79
*Criminal Intimacy* (Kunzel), 4
criminalization. *See* carceral spaces;
    court clinics; expertise; power; sexual
    psychopath laws
critical health studies, 9, 11, 125, 136–42
cross-gender identification, 17, 28, 38,
    41–43, 63, 68, 87, 100, 142
Crowley, Mart, 96–97
Cuban migrants, 154, 192n169
cultural hostility. *See* discrimination;
    exclusion; homophobia; insult; stigma
*Cures* (Duberman), 2, 154–55, 159
curing: and eradication, 10–11, 30, 63;
    and failure, 50, 62, 64, 69, 101, 108,
    131; and judgment, 39–41, 66, 85, 91;
    the language of, 66, 89, 91–92, 94,
    97–98, 105; in literature, 87–88; and
    motivation, 68–69, 83–86; opposition
    to, 22–23, 44–46; and psychiatry, 1–2,
    18–19, 23–25, 46, 94–95, 109; rates, 26,
    68, 90, 92, 122; and sex, 100–101. *See
    also* adjustment therapy; aversive con-
    ditioning; electroconvulsive shock;
    lobotomy; optimism; pathological
    (homosexuality as); pessimism; sexual
    conversion

Daughters of Bilitis (DOB), 79, 123–27,
    137–38, 143
Davis, Rebecca, 89
Dear Abby, 89–90
declassification, 1, 7–8, 11–12, 74, 89, 118,
    128, 133–35, 143–44, 147, 154–56
Delany, Samuel, 87–88
D'Emilio, John, 3, 193n2

Department of Homeland Security, 4
depression, 55, 57–58, 85, 101, 153
de-propagandizing, 40–41, 43, 46
Deutsch, Danica, 28
*Diagnostic and Statistical Manual of Mental Disorders* (*DSM*), 7, 11–12, 29–30, 33, 36, 118, 128–36, 143–44, 150, 154–56, 222n30. *See also* American Psychiatric Association; *DSM-II*; *DSM-III*
Dinerstein, Russell, 55
disability studies, 9–11, 141, 151
discrimination, 2, 7, 46, 52, 108–11, 118, 122, 125, 129–30, 150–51. *See also* employment; homophobia; military
Doan, Laura, 16
"Does Research into Homosexuality Matter?" (*Ladder*), 125–26
Drager, Emmet Harsin, 16
dream analysis, 39, 107
Dr. H. Anonymous, 129–30
*DSM-II*, 128, 132, 134
*DSM-III*, 133–35, 144–48, 215n116
Duberman, Martin, 2, 71–72, 85, 99, 127–28, 154–55, 159
due process, 35
dyshomophilia, 215n116

*Ebony*, 89
effeminacy, 56, 68, 87, 96, 142–43, 147
ego-dystonic homosexuality, 135–37, 140–41, 144, 147, 215n116
Elbe, Lili, 42
electroconvulsive shock, 2, 14, 54–56, 64–65, 67–68, 75, 95, 141, 192n169
Elliott, Beth, 143
Ellis, Albert, 23, 28, 40–41, 46–47, 82–84, 88, 97, 113, 122–23, 186n58
Ellis, Havelock, 20, 22, 41, 87
emetics, 64, 66
employment, 32, 53, 79, 86, 108, 125, 137–38, 150
encounter, 8, 12–13, 71, 93–98, 103–6, 110–14, 141, 150. *See also* case files
endocrinology, 25, 28, 42
Enke, Finn, 217n150
Eribon, Didier, 86
Eromin Center, 153–54

erotic art, 101, *102–3*
Eskridge, William, 197n64
ethics, 17, 108
etiology. *See* constitution; masochism; neuroses; organic; pathological (homosexuality as); trauma
Europe, 19, 24–25
exclusion, 6, 11, 15, 32, 36, 52, 84, 140–41, 150–51, 182n101. *See also* homophobia; stigma
ex-gay movement, 157–58
Exodus International, 158
expertise, 12–13, 19, 31–32, 36–37, 76, 91, 105–9, 128–31

Farrall Instruments, 65, 144
fear (of heterosexuality), 67, 96
Feldman, M. P., 62, 65
femininity, 14, 20–21, 25, 42, 63–64, 105, 138, 158
feminism, 131, 143, 151, 216n140, 217n150. *See also* women
fetishism, 28, 62, 64, 68, 122
Ford, Clellen S., 130
Foucault, Michel, 3–4, 6, 13, 94–95, 201n3
free association, 39
Freeman, Walter, 57–59
Freud, Sigmund: on external compulsion, 73; followers of, 23–25; influence of, 71–72, 87, 107, 204n75; and pessimism, 2, 25; and psychoanalysis, 2, 39; rejection of, 128; theories of, 20–22, 28, 31, 98, 104–5; works of, 73
Freund, Kurt, 62, 64
From, Sam, 119
Fry, Jane, 43, 95, 100
Fryer, John, 129–30

Gambino, Matthew, 206n104
Gay, Lesbian, and Bisexual Caucus (American Psychiatric Association), 136
"Gay, Proud, and Healthy," 139
Gay Activists Alliance (GAA), 129, 153
gay-affirmative mental health services, 152–54
*Gay American History* (Katz), 2
gay cruising, 76, 83, 113, 125

gay history, 1–9, 11, 16, 27, 73, 124–27, 144, 150–53. *See also* case files; LGBT history; normal homosexuals
Gay House, 152
gay identity, 47–48, 117–18, 140
"Gay Is Good," 139
Gay Liberation Front (GLF), 129
*Gay New York* (Chauncey), 3
gay rights movement, 3, 44, 46, 110, 129, 132, 139, 150–51, 186n58
gender-affirming care, 42–43, 75–76, 86, 145, 148–49, 158–59, 195n38. *See also* trans life
gender deficit, 158
gender dysphoria, 145, 149, 158
gender identification, 100, 146–47
Gender Identity Disorder (GID), 11–12, 145–49
Gender Identity Disorder of Childhood, 146, 149, 219n183
gender role, 147
*General Introduction to Psychoanalysis, A* (Freud), 105
General Services Administration, 4
George W. Henry Foundation, 52–54
Gerber, Henry, 32
Germany, 23–24
Gill-Peterson, Jules, 3, 76, 142, 184n16
Ginsberg, Allen, 51
Gittings, Barbara, 2, 74, 87, 124–27, 129, 132, 136, 138–40, 143–44
glamor, 43–44, 49, 92
Glueck, Bernard, 55
Goffman, Erving, 86, 94, 141
Gold, Ron, 87, 133, 143
"golden age," 12, 19, 107
Goldfarb, Warren, 47–48
Goldman, Emma, 71
Goluboff, Risa, 77
Goodman, Bernice, 152
Gould, Deborah, 140
Great Britain, 19, 23–24, 193n12
Green, Richard, 95–96, 133, 135, 146–47
Griffin-Gracy, Miss Major, 77
Gross, Alfred A., 52–54, 188n97
group therapy, 43–44, 47, 78–79, 85
Gundlach, Ralph, 124
Guttmacher, Manfred, 35, 76–78

Hadden, Samuel, 36, 43–44, 47, 73, 78, 91
Hale, Nathan G., Jr., 204n75
Hall, Radclyffe, 74
Hamburger, Christian, 42
Hanson, Cindy, 152
happiness, 140–41, 151
Harper, Robert, 43
Hartmann, Lawrence, 158
Hatterer, Lawrence, 68–69
Havemann, Ernest, 91
Hay, Harry, 45
health. *See* critical health studies
Helms, Alan, 95
Henry, George W., 18, 52–54, 105–6, 188n97
hereditary degeneration, 20, 25
Herman, Ellen, 31
Herzog, Dagmar, 29, 31
Highsmith, Patricia, 71–72
Hirschfeld, Magnus, 20, 22–23, 41, 87
HIV/AIDS, 151, 154, 222n30
Homophile Community Health Center, 151–52
homophile movement, 110, 119, 121–22, 125–27, 136–38, 151. *See also* Mattachine Society; ONE
*Homophile Studies*, 138
homophobia, 19, 28–31, 43–44. *See also* discrimination
Homosexual Counseling Center, 152
*Homosexual in America, The* (Cory), 45, 96, 122
"Homosexual in America, The" (*Time*), 92
*Homosexuality: A Psychoanalytic Study of Male Homosexuals* (Bieber), 26–27, 38
*Homosexuality: Disease or Way of Life* (Bergler), 26, 88
*Homosexuality: Its Causes and Cure* (Ellis), 88
"Homosexuality in America" (*Life*), 91
*Homosexual Minority in America, The* (Cory), 205n91
"Homosexuals Proud of Deviancy" (*New York Times*), 117
Hooker, Evelyn, 115, 118–21, 130–31, 137–38
Horney, Karen, 40

"How to Bring Your Kids Up Gay" (Sedgwick), 147
human constitution, 20
Hunt, Nancy, 76
hypnosis, 23

identification. *See* terminology
Identity House, 152
immigration, 32, 36, 141
Immigration and Nationality Act, 216n139
indoctrination, 47
injustice collecting, 46, 90
insanity, 115, 119
Institute of Sexual Science, 22–23
insulin, 2, 54–55, 192n169
insult, 86
intersex embodiment, 20, 42, 184n16
inversion, 20, 22–23, 25, 105, 142
involuntary psychiatric commitment, 74–82, 86, 115
Isay, Richard, 40
Isherwood, Christopher, 115, 119
"Is There Hope for Homosexuals?" (*Jet*), 92

Jaffy, Florence, 123–24, 126
*Jet*, 92
Jewish people, 30, 119
Johnson, Thomas, 78–79
Johnson, Virginia, 31, 84
Jones, Basil, 64
Jones, Ernest, 24, 30
Jorgensen, Christine, 42–43, 100
Joseph, Gilbert, 8
Jung, Carl, 87, 204n75

Kameny, Frank, 81–82, 125–29, 132, 134, 136, 139–41, 143–44, 148, 215n116, 216n137
Kantorovich, N. V., 61
Karpman, Benjamin: and adjustment therapy, 51–52; background on, 4–5, 107; on homosexuality, 13, 98, 106–9, 181n81; methods of, 103–4, 107, 113; patients of, 5–7, 41–43, 47–52, 59, 79, 83–85, 97–101, 104–5, 110–11; on psychiatrists, 15; and race, 109–10; on sexual psychopathy, 33; on

transvestism, 28, 41, 49–50. *See also* case files; Saint Elizabeths Hospital
Katz, Jonathan Ned, 2, 50–51
Kaufman, Benjamin, 156
Kennedy, Magora, 115
Kennedy, Rosemary, 57
Kepner, Jim, 32
Kiernan, James G., 23–24
King, Martin Luther, Jr., 89
Kinsey, Alfred, 31, 45–46
Klein, Charna, 152
Klopfer, Bruno, 119–20
Krafft-Ebing, Richard von, 20, 23

*Ladder* (Daughters of Bilitis), 123–27
Lahusen, Kay, 124
Lambe, Jennifer, 192n169
Landers, Ann, 89–91
Landerson, Louis, 150
language. *See* terminology
law. *See* anti-cross-dressing laws; court clinics; due process; gay cruising; race; sex offenders; sexual psychopath laws; social class; vagrancy laws; *and specific laws*
learning theory, 15, 60–68
Lee, Ronald, 127, 153
Legg, Dorr, 151
Leitsch, Dick, 127, 143
lesbian history: and counseling centers, 151–53; and disability history, 9; and erotic art, 101–3; and gender conformity, 143; and healthiness, 125–26, 137; and literature, 27–28, 96; and nightlife, 113; and psychiatry, 11, 73–74, 123–24, 150–51; and resistance, 99; and terminology, 16; and trans people, 143–44. *See also* Daughters of Bilitis; women
Lewes, Kenneth, 2, 30, 36–37, 93
Lewis, Abram J., 140
LGBT history, 3–8, 16, 154. *See also* case files; gay history
Liebman, Samuel, 56
*Life*, 91
"Lifestyles of Non-Patient Homosexuals," 129, 138
Linton, Simi, 9

Lobdell, Joseph Israel, 115
lobotomy, 2, 14, 49, 54, 56–60, 101, 141
Loftin, Craig, 142
loneliness, 22, 44, 89, 113
*Look*, 88
Love, Heather, 10
Love in Action, 158
Lunbeck, Elizabeth, 12

MacKinnon, George, 35, 80
Make-a-Picture-Story Test (MAPS), 120
*Man into Woman* (Elbe), 42
Marcus, Sharon, 171n25
Marmor, Judd, 68, 131–33, 135, 153
Martin, Emily, 9
masculinity, 14, 20–21, 25, 63–64, 68, 105, 119, 138, 158
masochism, 26, 46, 100, 140
Masters, William, 31, 84
*Mattachine Review*, 88
Mattachine Society, 45, 79, 81, 109, 119, 122–25, 127
Max, Louis, 61
McCarran-Walter Act, 36
McRuer, Robert, 10–11
Meaker, Marijane, 84, 96
Mendocino State Hospital, 112
mental disorder (homosexuality as a). *See* carceral spaces; curing; declassifica-tion; homophobia; Hooker, Evelyn; normal homosexuals; pathological (homosexuality as); psychoanalysis; Saint Elizabeths Hospital; sexual psychopath laws
"Mental Health and Homosexuality" (Midwinter Institute), 122
metrazol, 54–55
Meyerowitz, Joanne, 142
Midwinter Institute, 122–23
military, 5, 32–33, 47–48, 92, 120, 125
Miller, Arthur, 34, 197n63
Miller, Michael, 66–67
Miller Law, 34–35, 80, 108, 110, 197n62. *See also* sexual psychopath laws
Minnesota. *See* University of Minnesota
Minton, Henry, 188n97
Mitchell, Alice, 115
Mollow, Anna, 10

momism, 27
Money, John, 86, 147, 154
Moniz, Egas, 56–57
morality, 2, 18, 80, 130, 141
Morgan, Robin, 143
*My Lives* (White), 70

National Association for Research and Therapy of Homosexuality (NARTH), 156, 158
National Institute of Mental Health (NIMH), 118, 131, 138
National Mental Health Act, 31
national security, 12–13, 19, 30, 32
*Native Son* (Wright), 110
Nelson, Alondra, 192n174
neuroses, 21, 28, 40–43, 46–51, 88, 98–99, 104–5, 122–23, 142–43, 153. *See also* trauma
New York Academy of Medicine, 29, 117, 126
New York Psychoanalytic Institute, 131
New York Psychoanalytic Society, 24–25
*New York Times*, 117
Nicolosi, Joseph, 156, 158
Nielson, Kim, 9
nightlife, 113, 119
Nixon, Richard, 138
normal homosexuals, 118–21, 131, 137–38, 147. *See also* gay history
normal pervert, 108
normativity: and activism, 15, 84, 140; and curing, 68; and disability studies, 10–11; and Kinsey, 45–46; and law, 34; psychiatrists as arbiters of, 13, 19–22, 31, 76; and psychiatry, 2
Nugent, Walter, 67

Odets, Walt, 151
O'Hartigan, Margaret Deirdre, 75, 148
Oliven, John, 16
ONE, 88, 119, 121–23, 151
optimism, 18–19, 22–26, 36–38, 60, 69, 88–91, 94, 107–8, 117, 124. *See also* pessimism
organic, 2, 20, 22, 28, 41–43, 45, 47, 60, 132. *See also* constitution

Overholser, Winfred, 32–33, 35, 55, 57, 108

Ovesey, Lionel, 26, 48

Owensby, Newdigate, 55

Paganini, Albert, 59

pathological (homosexuality as): and counseling centers, 154; effects of, 154–55; and gender identification, 147; and hierarchies, 14, 80; and the military, 32–33; opposition to, 6–8, 32, 48–49, 118, 124–39, 156–58, 174n52; and power, 10, 96; and scholarship, 1; and sexual criminality, 77; theory, 21, 26–29, 123, 135–37; and treatment, 38–39, 44–47. *See also* curing

Pavlov, Ivan, 60–61

Payne Whitney Psychiatric Center, 95

Peale, Norman Vincent, 88–89

pedophilia, 138, 197n63

"Pervert Elimination Campaign," 108

pessimism, 2, 18, 22, 25, 41, 60. *See also* optimism

Pilgrim State Hospital, 59, 75, 100

Pillard, Richard, 135, 151–52

Platero, Lucas, 16

plethysmograph, 67, 144

Poinsard, Paul J., 74

politics. *See* gay rights movement

power: and case files, 6–7, 12; and expertise, 12–13, 19, 31–32, 36–37, 76, 106, 108–9, 128–31; and gatekeeping, 76, 145; and pathology, 2, 10, 38; and privilege, 70; and psychiatric encounters, 94–98, 127, 150, 201n3; and regulatory structures, 3, 7, 15, 76–82, 92–93, 97–98, 108–9

Preston, John, 152

prevention, 138

Prince, Virginia, 16

prison. *See* carceral spaces

projective psychological tests, 120–21

propaganda. *See* de-propagandizing

psychiatric encounter. *See* encounter

psychiatric hospitals, 114–16. *See also* specific hospitals

psychiatry. *See* adaptation; American Psychiatric Association; court clinics;

curing; encounter; expertise; "golden age"; involuntary psychiatric commitment; pathological (homosexuality as); power; psychoanalysis; reading "Psychiatry: Friend or Foe to Homosexuals—a Dialogue," 129

psychic interiority, 2, 72, 95

psychoanalysis: background on, 6–7, 13; and external compulsion, 73–83; fees, 71; and Jewish practitioners, 30–31; and mass culture, 86–87; and neutrality, 39–40; and prestige, 31–36, 70–72; and privilege, 70–71; and refugees, 24, 26; and resistance, 98–100; and scholarship, 30; and sex, 98–99; theories of, 21–29, 38, 40–41, 98. *See also* homophobia; *and specific psychoanalysts*

"Psychogenesis of a Case of Female Homosexuality, The" (Freud), 73

psychopathia transexualis, 28

psychopathic personality, 182nn100–101

psychotherapeutic groups. *See* group therapy

psychotherapy. *See* curing

Quakers, 52

queer studies, 9–10, 16

race: and civil rights, 127–28; and criminalization, 14, 36, 77–82; and immigration, 36; and Karpman, 109–10; and male effeminacy, 142; and mental illness, 111–12, 206nn103–4; and popular magazines, 89, 92; and psychoanalysis, 5, 27, 70–71; and queer, 174n55; and scholarship, 9; and segregation, 205n100; and shock treatments, 56, 60. *See also* analogies; carceral spaces

Rachman, Stanley, 64–65

Radical Caucus (American Psychiatric Association), 212n73

Rado, Sandor, 25–26

Rational-Emotive Behavior Therapy, 40

Raz, Mical, 60

reading, 87–92, 114, 171n25

Rees, Mark, 116

Rekers, George, 158
religion, 10, 18, 45, 49, 89, 110, 130, 156–58
repression, 21, 39, 56, 71, 97
Republican Party, 159, 224n54
resistance, 95–96, 98–100, 103, 105–6, 110, 112, 124
Robertson, Stephen, 81
Romm, May E., 73–74
Rorschach inkblot test, 120–21, 209nn15–16
Rowland, Chuck, 151
Russell, Thaddeus, 89

Sagarin, Edward, 45, 48, 72, 96, 122, 126, 137, 143, 186n58, 205n91
Saint Elizabeths Hospital, 4–6, 24, 57, 74–75, 80, 94–97, 100–106, 110–16, 206nn103–4. *See also* carceral spaces; Karpman, Benjamin
Sakel, Manfred, 54
Schilder, Paul, 55
schizophrenia, 55, 57–58, 120, 145
Schrenck-Notzing, Albert von, 22
Sedgwick, Eve Kosofsky, 16, 19, 147
Selective Service Act, 32, 92
self-knowledge, 87–88, 97–98, 104–5, 114, 117, 140
Serber, Michael, 63
Serinus, Jason, 115
Seton, Sarah, 148
sexism, 111–12
Sex Offender Act, 197n68
sex offenders, 33–35, 40, 59, 77–82, 97, 112, 197n68
sexology, 3, 12–13, 19–25, 41, 45, 115, 142, 158
*Sexual Behavior in Human Males* (Kinsey), 45
sexual conversion, 2, 13, 26, 37, 68, 131. *See also* conversion therapy; curing
*Sexual Inversion* (Marmor), 131–32
*Sexual Offender and His Offenses, The* (Karpman), 108
"Sexual Orientation Disturbance," 134–35
Sexual Psychopath Act (California), 112
sexual psychopath laws, 5, 13, 33–35, 76, 79–82, 141, 182n91, 182n94. *See also* Miller Law

*Sex Variants* (Henry), 18, 105–6
shame, 95, 111, 116
shame aversion therapy, 63
shell shock, 32
Sheppard and Enoch Pratt hospital, 32
"Should Homosexuality Be in the APA Nomenclature?," 133
Silverstein, Charles, 47, 51, 85, 87, 130, 152
Skinner, B. F., 60–61
Socarides, Charles, 1, 26, 29, 50, 76, 83, 133, 156
social class, 77–79, 142, 193n2
somatic theory, 20–21, 29, 54–60, 132
Somerville, Siobhan, 174n55
Spitzer, Robert, 130, 132–35, 144, 156–58
Stadler, Gustavus, 114
Stekel, Wilhelm, 23, 87, 107
Steward, Samuel, 50
stigma, 10–11, 30, 52, 82–86, 90, 98, 105, 116, 118, 141–42, 148, 151, 154–56. *See also* exclusion
Stoller, Robert, 47, 133, 147
Stonewall Rebellion, 128
Sullivan, Harry Stack, 12, 32
Sullivan, Lou, 145
sympathy, 23–24, 32, 51–53, 89–92, 155
Szasz, Thomas, 127

taxonomy. *See* classification
Taylor, Barbara, 71
terminology, 15–17, 106–7, 135–36, 142, 145–46, 149
Terry, Jennifer, 6, 72, 142
testosterone injections, 62, 67
Thematic Apperception Test (TAT), 120
therapeutic psychodrama, 112
third sex, 20
Thompson, George N., 55
Thorpe, J. G., 66
Thuma, Emily, 142, 216n140
*Time*, 91–92
Tocqueville, Alexis de, 18
Tontonoz, Matthew, 31
transfeminism, 217n150
*Transgender Tapestry*, 148
trans life: and hostility, 143–48; and intersex discourses, 184n16; and mental illness, 219n181; and power,

7, 76, 149–50; and psychoanalysis, 41–43; and reactions to GID, 147–49; and scholarship, 3; and shock therapy, 56, 62–63; and terminology, 16, 28, 41, 145–46, 149. See also *DSM-III*; gender-affirming care

transsexuality, 28, 100, 142–46, 148

*Transsexual Phenomenon, The* (Benjamin), 145

trans studies, 7, 9–10, 16. *See also* LGBT history

*Transvestia* (Prince), 16

transvestism, 28–29, 41–42, 49, 56, 62, 63, 68, 90, 97, 100, 142–43

trauma, 25, 28, 47, 60, 66, 86–87, 90, 100, 127. *See also* neuroses

Tretter, Jean-Nickolaus, 3–4

UCLA (University of California at Los Angeles), 118–19

Ulrichs, Karl Heinrich, 20

University of Minnesota, 3–4, 75

U.S. Supreme Court, 125, 182n101, 216n139

Vacaville, 68

vagrancy laws, 76–77, 115

Van Buren, Abigail, 89–91

Velocci, Beans, 195n38

Vuocolo, Alfred B., 197n68

Wahlert, Lance, 174n52

Wake, Naoko, 186n68

Wakefield, Dan, 72

Walt Whitman Guidance Center, 151

Washington Psychoanalytic Society, 24

Watts, James, 57–59

Weinberg, George, 130

Weinberg, Martin S., 220n3

*Well of Loneliness* (Hall), 74

West Coast Lesbian Conference, 143

*We Walk Alone* (Aldrich), 96

Wheeler, William, 209nn15–16

White, Edmund, 70–71, 85–86, 96, 128

White, William Alanson, 4, 33

Whitman, Walt, 22

"Why Is a Lesbian?" (*Ladder*), 124

Wicker, Randy, 123

Wilbur, Cornelia, 27–28, 68

Wilchins, Riki Ann, 148–49

Willard Insane Asylum, 115

Wise, P. M., 115

Wolfson, Miriam, 115

Wolpe, Joseph, 61, 67

women, 27, 118–21, 128, 131, 151. *See also* lesbian history

Women's Caucus (American Psychiatric Association), 212n73

Wright, Richard, 110

Wylie, Philip, 27

Zaretsky, Eli, 24, 72

Zlotlow, Moses, 59

www.ingramcontent.com/pod-product-compliance
Lightning Source LLC
Chambersburg PA
CBHW030211280125
20961CB00010B/477